RESTENOSIS AFTER INTERVENTION WITH NEW
MECHANICAL DEVICES

Developments in Cardiovascular Medicine

VOLUME 131

RESTENOSIS
after Intervention with New Mechanical Devices

edited by

PATRICK W. SERRUYS
Professor of Interventional Cardiology,
Cardiac Catheterization Laboratory, Thorax Center,
Erasmus University, Rotterdam,
The Netherlands

BRADLEY H. STRAUSS
Cardiac Catheterization Laboratory, Thorax Center,
Erasmus University, Rotterdam,
The Netherlands

and

SPENCER B. KING III
Director, Andreas Gruentzig Cardiovascular Center
Emory University, Atlanta, Georgia, U.S.A.

With a foreword by
ERIC J. TOPOL

Kluwer Academic Publishers
Dordrecht / Boston / London

Library of Congress Cataloging-in-Publication Data

Restenosis after intervention with new mechanical devices / edited by
  Patrick W. Serruys, Bradley H. Strauss, and Spencer B. King III ;
  with a foreword by Erik J. Topol.
        p.   cm. -- (Developments in cardiovascular medicine ; v. 131)
  Includes index.
  ISBN 0-7923-1555-3 (hb : alk. paper)
        1. Coronary artery stenosis. 2. Transluminal angioplasty-
  -Complications and sequelae. 3. Endarterectomy--Complications and
  sequelae. 4. Laser angioplasty--Complications and sequelae.
  I. Serruys, P. W. II. Strauss, Bradley H., 1957-   . III. King,
  Spencer B., 1937-   . IV. Series.
        [DNLM: 1. Angiography--methods. 2. Angioplasty, Laser--methods.
  3. Angioplasty, Transluminal, Percutaneous Coronary--methods.
  4. Coronary Disease--diagnosis. 5. Coronary Disease--therapy.
  6. Recurrence. 7. Ultrasonography--methods.   W1 DE997VME v. 131 /
  WG 300 R436]
  RC685.C58R47 1992
  DNLM/DLC
  for Library of Congress   91-35390

ISBN 0-7923-1555-3

Published by Kluwer Academic Publishers,
P.O. Box 17, 3300 AA Dordrecht, The Netherlands.

Kluwer Academic Publishers incorporates the publishing programmes of
D. Reidel, Martinus Nijhoff, Dr W. Junk and MTP Press.

Sold and distributed in the U.S.A. and Canada
by Kluwer Academic Publishers,
101 Philip Drive, Norwell, MA 02061, U.S.A.

In all other countries, sold and distributed
by Kluwer Academic Publishers Group,
P.O. Box 322, 3300 AH Dordrecht, The Netherlands.

Printed on acid-free paper

Foreword

Many investigators in the field of interventional cardiology have passed through at least two distinct phases in the new era of evaluating percutaneous transcatheter technologies to treat coronary artery disease. The first phase was sheer excitement. Who would have thought that by the end of the 1980's we could physically remove atherosclerotic plaque or laser ablate it? Who would have conceived of placing permanent prostheses inside such relatively small, tortuous and diseased coronary arteries? With these completely different mechanistic approaches and radically altered goals, a strong hope was that debulking the plaque or buttressing the arterial wall we would markedly limit the chances for subsequent restenosis. Although preliminary data from multiple observational studies of the new device technologies suggest that this is not the case so far, it remains quite possible that properly directed or applied use of any of the alternative technologies will ultimately have a place in reducing the likelihood for recurrence. The true evaluation of the promise will only be known after careful, prospective, randomized controlled trials are complete.

The second phase that we are entering is one of some relative disillusionment. That is, with respect to the early high, pervasive restenosis rates with new technologies, some investigators have voiced a sense of hopelessness. This is particularly unfortunate because it may reflect premature assessment and unrealistic demands of a novel front of technologies.

We have already learned a considerable amount about the underlying process of restenosis directly from the new technologies. Although easily overlooked, it is quite important to underscore some of these pivotal findings. For example, prior to directional atherectomy, we had to rely on necropsy specimen tissue to analyze the histologic process of restenosis. Already it is clear from literally thousands of specimens from live, symptomatic patients what is found in the culprit atherosclerotic or restenotic lesion and adjacent vessel wall. Sophisticated analysis of atherectomy-derived tissue specimens have involved use of *in situ* hybridization and cell culture techniques. This has revealed several important markers that "light up" with specific messenger RNA probes including platelet derived growth factor, tissue factor, plasminogen activator inhibitor, and fibroblast growth factor. The role of platelets and the hemostatic system has long been emphasized in the process of vessel wall repair. However, cell culture from atherectomy specimens suggest that white cells, and in particular macrophages and monocytes, may have a critical role.

Beyond these scientific advances from "live" atherectomy specimens, we have taken home many lessons from the stents with respect to restenosis. Precise quantitative coronary angiography of stented patients with 6 month follow-up has revealed a near ubiquitous presence of re-narrowed target vessel lumens. Only a few years ago, we had no concept that intimal hyperplasia could occur inside the stent. Furthermore, the theory that "hyperexpansion" of the vessel lumen with a stent may compensate for some degree of underlying hyperplasia or recoil deserves careful study.

These are only a few examples of vital lessons occurring as an outgrowth of the new device era. In this monograph, Drs. Serruys, Strauss and King have orchestrated a comprehensive assessment of restenosis from the perspective of new technologies. In the first sections, a critical chapter addresses the issues of angiography in restenosis research, which is a remarkably controversial topic. As clinical trials are designed to date, some of the most frequently asked questions are: (1) What should be the angiographic endpoint?; (2) Is an angiographic endpoint meaningful?; (3) Can or should continuous measurements of absolute minimal diameter be used? The section following angiographic assessment that precedes the actual technique discourse is devoted to intravascular imaging. This is especially appropriate and important. Just as we have garnished vital insights from working in the coronary arteries with new tools, so are we gaining critical perspective from "looking" inside the artery rather than simply relying on angiographic shadows. For example, with on-line two-dimensional intravascular echocardiography, the actual extent of vessel recoil can be observed and quantitated. Three-dimensional reconstructed panarterial imaging will undoubtedly play a key role in the future, with its unique capacity to delineate all three layers of the coronary artery. The longstanding debate of what really constitutes restenosis: regrowth, recoil, or "pseudorestenosis" simply due to inadequate primary dilatation will likely be fully resolved by intravascular imaging.

In the subsequent sections of this beautifully integrated text, fully developed discussions of the various new technologies including stenting, atherectomy, rotational angioplasty, and lasers are provided. Of particular note, great care has been taken to provide a full menu, with inclusion of all of the more widely tested techniques and lucid summaries provided by internationally revered investigators. Whenever possible or appropriate, the editors have included chapters from both sides of the Atlantic which is particularly valuable given the diverse experience to date.

As a whole, this monograph is exceptionally worthwhile owing to its complete, up-to-date, balanced, and visionary elements. There is no question that the new coronary device era has ushered in some excitement, and some despair. This book serves a pivotal purpose by weaving so many new concepts together, establishing the groundwork for further development of mechanical approaches to limit restenosis. I heartily recommend this text to all interventional cardiologists interested in practical and research aspects of restenosis. It certainly appears that we are all "junior" students in a very complex field and educational efforts such as the accompanying text can help us take a giant step beyond elementary school.

Eric J. Topol
Cleveland, August 1991

Contents

Foreword *by* Eric J. Topol   v

List of contributors   xiii

PART ONE: ASSESSMENT OF STENOSIS/RESTENOSIS –
            PRESENT AND FUTURE

Introduction *by* J. Richard Spears   3

1. Methodologic aspects of quantitative coronary angiography
   (QCA) in interventional cardiology   11
   by Bradley H. Strauss, Marie-Angèle M. Morel, Eline J.
   Montauban van Swijndregt, Walter R. M. Hermans, Victor
   A. W. Umans, Benno J. W. M. Rensing, Peter de Jaegere,
   Pim J. de Feyter and Patrick W. Serruys

PART TWO: INTRAVASCULAR IMAGING

Introduction *by* Klaas Bom, C. T. Lancée, Wilma J. Gussenhoven
and Jos R. T. C. Roelandt   53
Historical aspects of intravascular imaging

2. Potential of intravascular ultrasound imaging in the evaluation
   of morphology, elastic properties and vasomotor function of
   coronary arteries   63
   by Natesa G. Pandian, Tsui-Lieh Hsu and Andrew Weintraub

3. Intravascular ultrasound imaging following mechanical coronary
   interventions: theoretic advantages and initial clinical experience   73
   by Steven E. Nissen and John C. Gurley

4. Ultrasound guidance for catheter-based plaque removal and
   ablation techniques: potentional impact on restenosis   97

by Paul G. Yock, Peter J. Fitzgerald, Krishnankutty Sudhir, Victor K. Hargrave and Thomas A. Ports

5. Intravascular ultrasound: potential for optimizing mechanical solutions to restenosis   111
by Jeffrey M. Isner, Kenneth Rosenfield, Douglas W. Losordo and Ann Pieczek

6. Evaluation of restenosis following new coronary interventions   149
by Richard E. Kuntz and Donald S. Baim

PART THREE: STENTS RESTENOSIS AND NEW TECHNIQUES

Introduction *by* Ulrich Sigwart
Stenting for restenosis?   163

7. The Wallstent experience: 1986–1990   167
by Patrick W. Serruys and Bradley H. Strauss

8. Restenosis after Palmaz-Schatz stent implantation   191
by David L. Fischman, Michael P. Savage, Stephen G. Ellis, Richard A. Schatz, Martin B. Leon, Donald Baim and Sheldon Goldberg

9. Restenosis after Gianturco-Roubin stent. Placement for acute closure   207
by James A. Hearn, Spencer B. King III, John S. Douglas and Gary S. Roubin

10. Immediate and long-term morphologic changes in stenosis geometry after Wiktor™ stent implantation in native coronary arteries for recurrent stenosis following balloon angioplasty. Report on the first fifty consecutive patients   215
by Peter De Jaegere, Patrick W. Serruys, Wim van der Giessen and Pim de Feyter

PART FOUR: ATHERECTOMY

Introduction *by* John B. Simpson   237

11. Restenosis: directional coronary atherectomy   241
by Tomoaki Hinohara, John B. Simpson, Gregory C. Robertson and Matthew R. Selmon

12. Transluminal extraction endarterectomy   259
by Roger S. Gammon, Michael H. Sketch Jr. and Richard S. Stack

PART FIVE: ROTATIONAL ABLATION

Introduction *by* David Auth   275
Angioplasty with high speed rotary ablation

13. Percutaneous transluminal coronary rotary ablation with
    Rotablator: European experience   289
    by Michel E. Bertrand, Jean M. Lablanche, Fabrice Leroy,
    Christophe Bauters, Peter De Jaegere, Patrick W. Serruys,
    Jurgen Meyer, Ulrich Dietz and Raimund Erbel

14. Percutaneous coronary rotational atherectomy: the William
    Beaumont Hospital experience   297
    by Mark S. Freed, Khusrow Niazi and William W. O'Neill

15. Percutaneous transluminal coronary rotational ablation: serial
    follow-up by quantitative angiography   313
    by Kirk L. Peterson, Isabel Rivera, Martin McDaniel, John
    Long, Allan Bond, Mikki Bhargava and the clinical
    investigators of the multicenter trial of the Rotablator

PART SIX: LASERS

Introduction *by* Warren Grundfest, Frank Litvack, James Margolis,
James Laudenslager and Tsvi Goldenberg   331

16. Improved luminal dimensions and local pharmacological therapy
    with laser balloon angioplasty for potential mitigation of
    angioplasty restenosis   347
    by J. Richard Spears

17. Laser balloon angioplasty: European experience   359
    by H. W. Thijs Plokker and E. Gijs Mast

18. Coronary laser angioplasty   373
    by Timothy A. Sanborn

19. Restenosis following laser angioplasty   385
    by J. Michael Koch, Stephan Friedl, James M. Seeger,
    Gérald Barbeau and George S. Abela

20. Sapphire-probe laser angioplasty – European experience   415
    by Johannes Lammer

21. Excimer laser assisted angioplasty of peripheral vessels   427
    by Giancarlo Biamino, P. Skarabis, H. Böttcher, G. Kampmann,
    C. Ragg, U. Flesch and H. Witt

22. Clinical results of percutaneous coronary excimer laser
    angioplasty trials   475

by Warren S. Grundfest, Frank Litvack, James Margolis,
James Laudenslager and Tsvi Goldenberg

23. Direct laser ablation of coronary arterosclerotic plaque in
humans – the German experience   485
by Andreas Baumbach, Karl K. Haase and Karl R. Karsch

24. Summary   497
by Spencer B. King III

List of Contributors

George S. Abela
  Institute for Prevention of CV Disease, New England Deaconess Hospital,
  Kennedy Bldg., 5th floor, 1 Autumn Street, Boston, MA 02215, U.S.A.
  Co-authors: J. Michael Koch, Stephan Friedl, James M. Seeger and Gérald
  Barbeau

David C. Auth
  Heart Technology Inc., 2515 140th Avenue NE, Bellevue, WA 98005,
  U.S.A.

Michel E. Bertrand
  Division of Cardiology B, University of Lille, Hospital Cardiologique,
  Boulevard du Professeur Leclerc, F-59037 Lille, France
  Co-authors: Jean M. Lablanche, Fabrice Leroy, Christophe Bauters, Peter
  De Jaegere, Patrick W. Serruys, Jurgen Meyer, Ulrich Dietz and Raimund
  Erbel

Giancarlo Biamino
  Institute of Radiology, University Clinic, Rudolf Virchow/Wedding, Free
  University of Berlin, DW-1000 Berlin 45, Germany
  Co-authors: P. Skarabis, H. Böttcher, G. Kampmann, C. Ragg, U. Flesch
  and H. Witt

Klaas Bom
  Thoraxcentre, Erasmus University, P.O. Box 1738, 3000 DR Rotterdam,
  The Netherlands
  Co-authors: C. T. Lancée, Wilma J. Gussenhoven and Jos R. T. C.
  Roelandt

Peter De Jaegere
Thoraxcentre, Erasmus University, P.O. Box 1738, 3000 DR Rotterdam, The Netherlands
Co-authors: Patrick W. Serruys, Wim van der Giessen and Pim de Feyter

Mark S. Freed
Cardiology Division, William Beaumont Hospital, 3601 West 13 Mile Road, Royal Oak, MI 48073–6769, U.S.A.
Co-authors: Khusrow Niazi and William W. O'Neill

Roger S. Gammon, M.D.
Senior Interventional Cardiovascular Fellow, Duke University Medical Center, Durham, NC 27710, U.S.A.

Sheldon Goldberg
Director, Division of Cardiology, Thomas Jefferson University, Medical College, 403 College, 1025 Walnut Street, Philadelphia, PA 19107–5083, U.S.A.
Co-authors: David L. Fischman. Michael P. Savage, Stephen G. Ellis, Richard A. Schatz, Martin B. Leon and Donald Baim

Warren S. Grundfest
Laser Research and Technology Development, Cedars-Sinai Medical Center, 8700 Beverly Boulevard, Los Angeles, CA 90048–1869, U.S.A.
Co-authors: Frank Litvack, James Laudenslager and Tsvi Goldenberg

Tomoaki Hinohara
Cardiovascular Medicine, Coronary Interventions & Cardiac Arrhythmias, 770 Welch Road, Suite 100, Palo Alto, CA 94304, U.S.A.
Co-authors: John B. Simpson, Gregory C. Robertson and Mattew R. Selmon

Jeffrey M. Isner
St. Elizabeth's Hospital of Boston, 736 Cambridge Street, Boston, MA 02135, U.S.A.
Co-authors: Kenneth Rosenfield, Douglas W. Losordo and Ann Pieczek

Karl R. Karsch
Department of Internal Medicine III, Eberhard-Karls-University, Medical University Clinic, Otfried-Müller-Strasse 10, DW-7400 Tübingen 1, Germany
Co-authors: Andreas Baumbach and Karl K. Haase

Spencer B. King III
Andreas Gruentzig Cardiovascular Center, Emory University Hospital, Suite F606, 1364 Clifton Rd, NE, Atlanta, GA 30322, U.S.A.
Co-authors: James A. Hearn, John S. Douglas and Gary S. Roubin

Richard E. Kuntz
Beth Israel Hospital, Cardiovascular Division, 330 Brookline Avenue, Boston, MA 02215, U.S.A.
Co-author: Donald S. Baim

Johannes Lammer
Department of Radiology, Karl-Franzens-University Graz, Auenbrugger-platz 9, A-8036 Graz, Austria

Steven E. Nissen
Division of Cardiology, University of Kentucky Medical Center, Lexington VA Hospital, 800 Rose Street, Lexington, KY 40536, U.S.A.
Co-author: John C. Gurley

Natesa G. Pandian
Non-invasive Cardiac Laboratory, Tufts-New England Medical Center, 750 Washington Street, Box 32, Boston, MA 02111, U.S.A.
Co-authors: Tsui-Lieh Hsu and Andrew Weintraub

Kirk L. Peterson
Core Angiography Laboratory, Sharp Memorial Hospital/UCSD, 225 W. Dickinson Street, San Diego, CA 92103, U.S.A.
Co-authors: Isabel Rivera, Martin McDaniel, John Long, Allan Bond, Mikki Bhargava and the clinical investigators of the multi-center trial of the Rotablator

H. W. Thijs Plokker
Department of Cardiology, St. Antonius Hospital, Koekoekslaan 1, 3435 CM Nieuwegein, The Netherlands
Co-author: E. Gijs Mast

Timothy A. Sanborn
Division of Cardiology, Box 1030, Mount Sinai Medical Center, 1 Gustave L. Levy Place, New York, NY 10029, U.S.A.

Patrick W. Serruys
Thoraxcenter, Erasmus University, P.O. Box 1738, 3000 DR Rotterdam, The Netherlands
Co-author: Bradley H. Strauss

Ulrich Sigwart
Department of Invasive Cardiology, The Royal Brompton and National Heart Hospital, 22 Upper Wimpole Street, London, W1M 7TA, U.K.

John B. Simpson
Cardiovascular Medicine, Coronary Interventions & Cardiac Arrythmias, 770 Welch Road, Suite 100, Palo Alto, CA 94304, U.S.A.

Michael H. Sketch Jr., M.D.
Assistant Professor of Medicine, Cardiology Division, Duke University Medical Center, Durham, NC 27710, U.S.A.

J. Richard Spears
Cardiac Laser Laboratory, Louis M. Elliman Research Building, Wayne State University School of Medicine, 421 E. Canfield Road, Detroit, MI 48201, U.S.A.

Richard S. Stack
Interventional Cardiovascular Program, Duke University Medical Center, Box 3111, Durham, NC 27710, U.S.A.
Co-authors: Roger S. Gammon and Michael H. Sketch Jr.

Bradley Strauss
Presently at: St. Michael's Hospital Division of Cardiology, 30 Bond Street, Toronto, Ontario, Canada M5B 1W8. Erasmus University, Thoraxcenter, P.O. Box 1738, 3000 DR Rotterdam, The Netherlands.
Co-authors: Marie-Angèle M. Morel, Eline J. Montauban van Swijndregt, Walter R. M. Hermans, Victor A. W. Umans, Benno J. W. M. Rensing, Peter P. de Jaegere, Pim J. de Feyter and Patrick W. Serruys

Eric J. Topol
Chairman, Department of Cardiology, The Cleveland Clinic Foundation, One Clinic Center, 9500 Euclid Avenue, Cleveland, OH 44195, U.S.A.

Paul G. Yock
Division of Cardiology, University of California, 505 Parnassus Avenue, M1186, San Francisco, CA 94143–0124, U.S.A.
Co-authors: Peter J. Fitzgerald, Krishnankutty Sudhir, Victor K. Hargrave and Thomas A. Ports

PART ONE

Assessment of Stenosis/Restenosis – Present and Future

Introduction

J. RICHARD SPEARS

Defining the Restenosis Problem

Followlng percutaneous transluminal coronary angioplasty, most patients demonstrate at least some lesion progression over a six month period [1, 2]. When the issue of restenosis is raised clinically, however, lesion progression which is deemed unacceptable is the more relevant problem. It is difficult to provide a definition of unacceptable restenosis, and any such attempt to do so may result in a somewhat misleading binary assignment of patients into two groups – those who meet and those who do not meet a criterion specified by the definition – despite the fact that the long-term results lie on a continuum. Ideally, when comparing different treatment strategies for prevention of restenosis, all data in a frequency histogram of long-term angiographic luminal results should be used, e.g., the population means of either the minimum diameter or percent stenosis can be compared, obviating the need to use any criterion of restenosis. On the other hand, it is more convenient in some studies to use a binary assignment based on a simple criterion and compare the incidence of restenosis between groups. In addition, the latter approach may be more applicable to the management of individual patients, e.g., when the referring physician wishes to know the angiographic restenosis status of his patient.

How restenosis is examined is important not only for facilitating comparisons of treatment strategies, but also for setting practical, clinical goals. A commonly used criterion, when a binary assignment is employed, is a diameter stenosis >50% (Table 1). In general, a greater cutoff value is required before a "critical" stenosis is attained, so that this value allows for slight underestimation of lesion severity and/or mild further progression before a blunted hyperemic flow response would be expected to occur. The use of a criterion of less than a 20% improvement in percent stenosis at the time of follow-up, compared to the pre-PTCA value, also has clinical relevance, but requires the analysis of two films, thereby increasing the variability of the measurement compared to the analysis of the follow-up film alone.

P.W. Serruys, B.H. Strauss and S.B. King III (eds), *Restenosis after Intervention with New Mechanical Devices*, 3–9.
© 1992 *Kluwer Academic Publishers. Printed in the Netherlands.*

4   J.R. Spears

Table 1. Common definitions for binary assignment of restenosis.

	Advantages	Disadvantages
>50% DS	Independent of vessel size. Allows underestimation &/or mild progression before "critical" stenosis reached. Permits visual/caliper measurements. Could be more important than absolute values in terms of prognosis of lesion progression.	Depends on variable definition of reference segment. Analysis of 2 segments to obtain % DS increases variability compared to use of Dmin.
Dmin	Independent of reference segment. Less variability compared to % DS since only 1 segment is analyzed. May be the most important parameter governing epicardial coronary resistance.	Different values required for vessels of differing size. Requires computer image processing for accurate measurement. Particularly for Dmin <1 mm, values may differ between image processing labs.
>50% loss of % DS gain	Provides rough estimate of new plaque growth.	Often may not be as clinically relevant as % DS. Requires analysis of 2 films, which is combersome and increases variability of measurement.
Dloss ≥.72 mm	Provides statistical estimate of new plaque growth based on computer analysis of films.	Often may not be clinically as relevant as % DS. Requires computer image processing of 2 films. Criterion (≥.72 mm) may vary between labs.
Densitometric area	Measurements are potentially rotationally invariant for nonaxisymmetric lumina.	Potentially subject to multiple sources of error: heterogeneity of contrast medium mixing; overlapping branches; nonlinear H & D curve; orientation of vessel axis may differ between reference and stenotic segments.

D = diameter.
S = stenosis.
H & D = Hurter-Driffield (film characteristic curve).

Although absolute values of stenotic diameter have utility when adjacent reference segments are narrowed, this advantage may be offset by the fact that % stenosis measurements are more independent of vessel size and thus allow pooling of data from vessels of differing size. In addition, percent stenosis values could have greater prognostic utility than the simple use of the minimum absolute luminal diameter, since flow patterns, such as turbulence and separated flow immediately distal to a stenosis, have been implicated in the localization of atherosclerotic lesions [3]. However, the definition of the reference segment, used in the calculation of percent stenosis, varies between angiographers. While the largest proximal luminal diameter is used by some groups, the larger of either of the proximal and distal segments has been used in our studies of laser balloon angioplasty, and a mean of the proximal and distal reference segments is used by others. Obviously, approaches which tend to reduce the size of the reference segment will reduce the apparent severity of percent stenosis.

The minimum absolute diameter is the most important geometric factor governing flow [4], and its measurement is independent of a reference segment measurement. Although a scaling device, such as the shaft of a guide catheter, needs to be analyzed to obtain absolute dimensions, the inter-observer variability in such measurements is likely to be considerably less than that associated with reference segment measurements. Moreover, if care is taken to reproduce the same radiographic conditions (angle, skew, table and image intensifier height) between serial angiographic studies, a single magnification factor can be applied to all images of the same luminal segment over time, thereby potentially further reducing variability in comparison to percent stenosis measurements which require two measurements for each value. Absolute diameter measurement of the reference segment can also be performed in the same manner, which may be helpful, unlike percent stenosis measurements, in assessing the effect of an intervention on this location. A potential drawback in the use of absolute diameter measurements, however, is that different criteria of restenosis may need to be applied for vessels of differing size.

From the above discussion, it is apparent that measurements of both absolute luminal dimensions and percent stenosis have utility, and they probably both should be employed in rigorous comparisons of the long-term efficacy of various treatment modalities.

Another important type of definition of restenosis is the magnitude of the chronic loss of the acute gain in luminal dimensions, as an estimate of the degree of lesion progression [5]. Use of this type of definition should provide some insight as to the relative magnitude of lesion progression between different treatment strategies, but it requires the analysis of two films, so that the variability of the measurement will be greater than that associated with measurements of the follow-up film alone. As used by the image processing center at the Thoraxcenter in Rotterdam, the loss of 0.72 mm over time, representing two standard deviations of mean absolute diameter measurements between angiographic studies [6], also may not be applicable to other image processing systems, which may differ in the variability of such measurements [7]. There are two additional potential constraints in the use of this type of definition. Firstly, some patients having a marked acute improvement in luminal dimensions may be categorized as having restenosis by this definition without having a clinically significant stenosis at follow-up while others with a clinically important stenosis could be categorized as not having restenosis. Secondly, a larger acute luminal result may inherently be at greater risk for restenosis, since the velocity of blood flow at the luminal surface will be lower than that associated with a smaller luminal result; a relatively low blood flow velocity at the potentially thrombogenic luminal surface of the mechanically injured arterial wall may potentiate the growth of thrombus (and other components of an atherosclerotic lesion such as lipoprotein deposition). By analogy, restenosis lesions in general appear to progress fairly rapidly over the one to three month period after angioplasty, yet complete occlusions occurring rapidly after the onset of the return of a high grade stenosis are unusual, perhaps as a result of a potentially protective effect of a relatively high blood flow velocity on further propagation of the lesion when the latter is smooth, concentric, and has a tapered inlet and outlet (which is typical of most restenosis lesions) which favor laminar flow patterns. Although the possibility exists that achievement of relatively large luminal dimensions might, through this relationship with flow velocity, be associated with a greater loss of the initial gain, it might be erroneous to conclude that an intervention is less efficacious on this basis if the chronic result were nonetheless improved in terms of absolute minimum luminal diameter.

In view of the technology currently available for objective analysis of angiographic luminal diameter from digitized cine frames, it probably is no longer acceptable to use subjective visual methods to quantitate luminal dimensions. In 1983, we described for the first time the observation that, irrespective of modifications of all potentially relevant radiographic imaging parameters, each of a variety of computerized algorithms could be used to automatically locate the anatomic luminal boundary within the radiographic vessel image edge gradient from digitized cine frames, thereby validating the accuracy ($<100\,\mu$) of this approach [8]. It should be noted, however, that the concentration of contrast medium did affect diameter measurements (smaller diameter with decreasing concentration – a relationship which occurs also in subjective visual measurements), but this effect is a trivial one for a vessel well-filled ($>80\%$ concentration of a 37 g% iodine solution) with contrast medium.

Computerized edge tracking in digitized cine images undoubtedly increases the objectivity and reproducibility of luminal diameter measurements compared to visual estimates. However, caution should be exercised in comparing diameter measurements between different image processing laboratories, particularly for measurements of diameters $<1\,mm$, since a rigorous comparison between various systems has yet to have been performed. For example, a mean pre-PTCA minimum diameter value was found by Nobuyoshi et al to be 0.75 mm in 276 patients [1], while a mean value of 1.13 mm to 1.20 mm was found by Serruys et al in 342 patients [2], despite a close similarity in the mean size of the reference segment (approximately 2.8 mm). Mean pre-PTCA percent stenosis values therefore differed markedly between the two studies – 73% and 58%, respectively. Whether these differences resulted from patient selection or from the manner in which the films were analyzed is unknown, of course, but until comparisons are made between various image processing systems, interpretation of differences in the incidence of high grade stenoses (both pre- and post-PTCA) found in studies performed with different image processing techniques will be difficult.

When the geometry of the coronary lumen deviates from circular symmetry, diameter measurements may result in an underestimation of the severity of the area stenosis [9]. In this situation, which is probably uncommon for most restenosis lesions, a densitometric approach would therefore be potentially attractive for a more direct measurement of the relative luminal areas of the stenotic and adjacent reference segments. An assumption of a linear relationship between the film optical density (gray scale) and the thickness of contrast medium is made, and the area under a transverse densitometric scan across the vessel image, between luminal edges, provides an estimate of the relative quantity of contrast medium and, therefore, the relative anatomic area of the scanned segment. Under ideal conditions, a measurement of the relative area of non-axisymmetric lumina is then rotationally invariant in terms of the radiographic view. However, this approach is potentially problematic in the clinical setting for a variety of reasons. The above-discussed assumption of linearity is correct only for the midportion of the film characteristic curve (H & D curve) relating log relative exposure and film optical density. The full curve is sigmoidal in shape and is significantly affected by a variety of radiographic exposure settings, such as kilovoltage, as well as by variations in film processing. Further deviation from a linear relationship between contrast medium thickness and film optical density occurs as a result of beam hardening of the polyenergetic x-ray source, i.e., the relationship between relative exposure and thickness of any material is truly linear only for a monoenergetic beam. Although I developed a method some years ago for calibrating the relationship between film gray scale and contrast medium thickness during patient exposure with automatic brightness settings, the method requires specialized equipment (a rotating wedge) during the exposure [10]. The gray scale/contrast medium thickness relationship is more linear for video images, but the reduced resolution of the video image compared to cinefilm makes the use of video format for precise measurement of luminal dimensions less reliable than the use of cinefilm. Additional potential problems with measurement of densitometric area are listed in Table 1. A particularly limiting problem, which does not affect diameter measurements, is that the orientation of the vessel long axis with respect to the x-ray beam must be the same for the stenotic and reference segments, but this information can be obtained only by use of a second, preferably orthogonal, view.

Setting an Angiographic Goal

Before a goal is set for improving the long-term results of angioplasty, it is first necessary to define the severity of restenosis after PTCA. Despite the fact that PTCA was introduced in 1977, the extent of the restenosis problem remains debatable. Ideally, any analysis of restenosis should deal with the entire population of patients subjected to PTCA in whom full balloon inflation was achieved. In the NHLBI PTCA Registry, only 88% of patients had a successful angiographic result, defined as a 20% reduction in diameter stenosis severity, and the overall acute clinical success rate was 78% [11]. Acute closure accounted for 7% of these patients, so that there very likely was a significant subset of patients who had a residual stenosis >50% without acute closure. Likewise, Mabin et al [12] found that only approximately two-thirds of patients treated with PTCA an acute post-PTCA result of <50% diameter stenosis. Virtually all angiographic studies of restenosis to date have included only those patients who had successful angioplasty, so that patients with a residual high grade stenosis without acute closure have been excluded from the analysis. It may not be surprising that only 51% of patients in the NHLBI Registry in the year following the procedure were free of a cardiac event [11], including repeat PTCA and recurrence of angina, since all patients in whom PTCA was attempted were followed clinically, including those with acutely unsuccessful procedures. Patients in whom the acute angiographic result lies between a successful result as defined in restenosis studies and acute closure probably constitute 10 to 20% of the general PTCA population, yet this group has received remarkably little attention.

When only those patients having a successful PTCA result are followed angiographically with objective analysis of luminal diameter and a high degree of angiographic follow-up, the mean percent stenosis at 3 months was 47% with a mean minimum luminal diameter of 1.43 mm in the largest (n = 276) of several groups of patients studied by Nobuyoshi et al [1] while mean values of 38% and 1.77 mm were found, respectively, at this same period of time by Serruys et al [2] in a smaller group of patients (n = 93 lesions in 82 patients). If one uses a > 50% loss of the gain as a criterion of restenosis, the incidence of restenosis at 3 months after PTCA differs in the two studies, 43% and 33%, respectively. The results of Nobuyoshi et al suggest that the incidence of restenosis by this criterion will increase further by approximately 10% between 3 and 12 months after PTCA. Interestingly, the mean absolute loss in minimum luminal diameter over the 3 month period in the two studies was similar, 0.4 mm to 0.5 mm, as was the standard deviation of the mean minimum luminal diameter, 0.6 mm to 0.7 mm, at the time of follow-up. A recent report by King et al [13] suggests, however, that the population frequency distribution of diameter stenosis at the time of a 4 to 12 month angiographic follow-up may be bimodal, with approximately 2/3'ds of the patients demonstrating a mild stenosis and the remainder a severe stenosis; comparisons of various treatment strategies in terms of restenosis would then require non-parametric analyses if continuous variable measures of restenosis were used.

At a minimum, laudible goals related to the issue of restenosis would be, first, to reduce the incidence of an acute suboptimal result to <5% and, second, to improve the chronic mean minimum luminal diameter by at least 0.5 mm compared to that associated with PTCA. A loss in luminal diameter equivalent to roughly two standard deviations of the mean would therefore be required before a "critical" stenosis of approximately 1.0 mm is reached. In view of the possible bimodal distribution of restenosis, the improvement would probably not be normally distributed and would hopefully be greater for those patients having severe restenosis.

References

1. Nobuyoshi M, Kimura T, Nosaka H et al (1988) Restenosis after successful percutaneous transluminal coronary angioplasty: serial angiographic follow-up of 229 patients. *J Am Coll Cardiol* 12:616–23.
2. Serruys P W, Luijten H E, Beatt K J et al (1988) Incidence of restenosis after successful coronary angioplasty: a time-related phenomenon. *Circulation* 77:361–71.
3. Stehbens W E (1975) The role of hemodynamics in the pathogenesis of atherosclerosis. *Prog Cardiovasc Dis* 18:89–103.
4. Demer L, Gould K L, Goldstein, Kirkeeide R L (1988) Assessing stenosis severity: Coronary flow reserve, collateral function, quantitative coronary arteriography, position imaging, and digital subtraction angiography. A review and analysis. *Prog in Cardiovasc Dis* 33:07–322.
5. Holmes D R, Vlietstra R E, Smith H C et al (1984) Restenosis after percutaneous transluminal coronary angioplasty (PTCA): a report from the PTCA Registry of the National Heart, Lung, and Blood Institute. *Am J Cardiol* 55:77C-81C.
6. Beatt K J, Luijten H E, De Feyter P J, Van Den Brand M, Reiber J H C, Serruys P W, Ten Katen H J, Van Es G A (1988) Change in diameter of coronary artery segments adjacent to stenosis after percutaneous transluminal coronary angioplasty: failure of percent diameter stenosis measurement to reflect morphologic changed induced by balloon dilitation. *JACC* 12:315–234.
7. Reiber J H C (1991) An overview of coronary quantitation techniques as of 1989. In: J H C Reiber and P W Serruys (eds) *Quantitative Coronary Arteriography*. Dordrecht: Kluwer Academic Publishers, 55–132.
8. Spears J R, Sandor T, Al A V et al (1983) Computerized image analysis for quantitative measurement of vessel diameter from cineangiograms. *Circulation* 68:453–61.
9. Spears J R, Sandor T, Baim D S, Paulin S (1983) The minimum error in estimating coronary luminal cross-sectional area from cineangiographic diameter measurements. *Cathet Cardiovasc Diagn* 9:119–28.
10. Spears J R (1981) Rotating stepwedge technique for extraction of luminal cross-sectional area formation from single plane coronary cineangiograms. *Acta Radio Diag* 22:Fasc 3A.
11. Detre K, Holubkov R, Kelsey S. Bourassa M, Williams D, Holmes D, Dorros G, Faxon D, Myler R, Kent K, Cowley M, Cannon R, Robertson T, and coinvestigators of the National Heart, Lung and Blood Institute's Percutaneous Transluminal Angioplasty Registry (1989). One-year follow-up results of the 1985–1986 National Heart, Lung, and Blood Institute's Percutaneous Transluminal Coronary Angioplasty Registry. *Circulation* 80:421–428.
12. Mabin T A, Holmes D R, Smith H C et al (1985) Follow-up clinical results of patients undergoing percutaneous transluminal coronary angioplasty. *Circulation* 71:754–60.
13. King III S B, Weintraub W S, Tao X, Hearn J, Douglas Jr. J S (1991) Bimodal distribution of diameter stenosis 4 to 12 months after angioplasty: implications for definitions and interpretation of restenosis. *JACC* 17:345A.

1. Methodologic Aspects of Quantitative Coronary Angiography (QCA) in Interventional Cardiology

BRADLEY H. STRAUSS*, MARIE-ANGÈLE M. MOREL, ELINE J. MONTAUBAN VAN SWIJNDREGT, WALTER R.M. HERMANS, VICTOR A.W. UMANS, BENNO J.W.M. RENSING, PETER P. DE JAEGERE, PIM J. DE FEYTER and PATRICK W. SERRUYS

Introduction

Quantitative Coronary Angiography (QCA) has had a tremendous impact in the field of interventional cardiology. It has supplanted visual and hand-held caliper assessments of coronary arteriography due to its superior inter-observer and intraobserver variability [1–3]. Currently it is the gold standard to assess the coronary tree for research purposes although it has not gained widespread appeal for routine clinical use because of expense and time constraints. It has been particularly useful in interventional cardiology as the only reliable means to assess the short and long term effects of coronary interventions. In particular, the phenomenon of restenosis has been primarily described and researched most extensively on the basis of sequential QCA studies. At the Thoraxcenter in Rotterdam, we have been advocating the importance of QCA since the first publication by our group in 1982 [4]. The system developed at the Thoraxcenter by Johan Reiber and colleagues, the Coronary Angiographic Analysis System (CAAS), has been extensively and rigorously validated [5–7]. In our database, we have now collected information from over 1700 patients who have undergone several different forms of non-operative coronary revascularization (Fig. 1). We have had to adapt the principles of QCA, which were initially designed for diagnostic studies to assess the extent of coronary artery disease, to more complicated and complex situations related to either the device or the effect of the intervention on the angiographic appearance of a damaged vessel. The introduction of several newer devices in the past 4 years, has presented several unique and unforseen problems in our interpretation of important quantitative data. The purpose of this chapter is to highlight the basic features and information that can be obtained by our CAAS system and to discuss some of the benefits and limitations of this important method in the analysis of results from the devices of interventional cardiology. At the conclusion of the chapter, it is

*Dr. Strauss is a Research Fellow of the Heart and Stroke Foundation of Canada.

P.W. Serruys, B.H. Strauss and S.B. King III (eds), Restenosis after Intervention with New Mechanical Devices, 11–50.
© 1992 *Kluwer Academic Publishers. Printed in the Netherlands.*

INTERVENTION	PATIENTS	LESIONS
PTCA	1234	1452
STENTS	393	446
WALLSTENT	283	335
WIKTOR	91	92
PALMAZ-SCHATZ	19	19
ATHERECTOMY	105	114
DIRECTIONAL	95	103
ROTATIONAL	10	11
EXCIMER LASER	20	20
TOTAL	1752	2032

Figure 1. Inventory of quantitative cornary angiographic (QCA) results following various coronary interventions at the Thoraxcenter in Rotterdam.

hoped that QCA should be regarded as more than just setting up the cinefilm and returning 20–30 minutes later for the "perfect" data. Only close scrutiny of the results combined with ongoing communication between the angiographer, the analyst and the programmer ensures that meaningful and useful data emerge from the use of QCA.

Part A: The CAAS System – What Information Can We Learn?

The complexities of the algorithms essential for the operation of the CAAS system may intimidate the casual reader unfamiliar with physics. In this chapter, we do not wish to explain the series of complicated steps that convert a cinefilm to a digitized image that is amenable to computer asssisted analysis. For the expert, this has been described in the literature [5–7]. Rather we would like to focus more on the clinician's ability to assess data generated by QCA. The prime aim of QCA is to provide precise and accurate measurements of coronary anatomy. The CAAS system can provide this information by two different methods: (1) detection of lumen borders (so called edge detection), preferably in two orthogonal projections (to provide a three dimensional approximation of the diseased segment) which can then be converted into absolute values after calibration with a known diameter object such as the shaft of the guiding catheter and (2) densitometry, which is an approach that assesses the relative area stenosis by comparing the density of contrast in the diseased and "normal" segment. The method by which the relative area stenosis is converted to absolute area stenosis measurements will be explained later in the chapter. The advantage of the information acquired by the densitometry method is that meaningful data can be obtained by a single projection, even if the cross-sectional shape is highly irregular. In contrast, area measurements derived from edge detection data (and specifically from minimal luminal diameter values) by definition

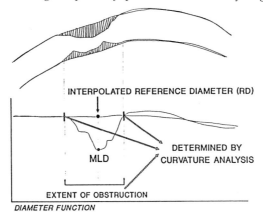

Figure 2. Diameter function curve derived from schematic coronary artery lesion. Minimal luminal diameter (MLD), interpolated reference diameter and the extent (or length) of the obstruction are determined by a curvature analysis. Reprinted with permission [26].

require an assumption of a circular cross-sectional shape in the diseased arterial segment, which is at odds with the observations of several pathologic studies [8, 9]. The limitations of both techniques will subsequently be discussed and discrepancies in the results of these two methods following coronary interventions will be presented later.

1. *Edge Detection*

The important parameters that can be obtained by edge detection are described below and in Figs 2–4:
  Direct Measurements
 i) minimal luminal diameter (MLD)

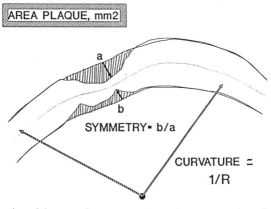

Figure 3. Determination of the area plaque, symmetry and curvature values. See text for details.

14   *B.H. Strauss et al*

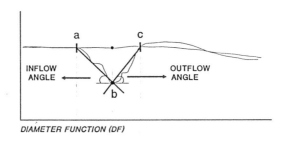

DIAMETER FUNCTION (DF)

INFLOW-ANGLE: AVERAGE SLOPE OF THE DF
                  BETWEEN (b) AND (a)

OUTFLOW-ANGLE: AVERAGE SLOPE OF THE DF
                  BETWEEN (b) AND (c)

Figure 4. Determination of inflow and outflow angles from the diameter function (DF). See text for details.

 ii) maximal luminal diameter
iii) mean luminal diameter
 iv) extent of the obstruction
    Interpolated Measurements
  i) reference diameter (RD) (the assumed "normal" segment of the vessel)
 ii) symmetry
iii) curvature
 iv) inflow angle/outflow angle
  v) area plaque
 vi) roughness
    Derived Measurements
  i) diameter stenosis (calculated from the MLD and RD)
 ii) area stenosis (assumes circular model)
    Hemodynamic Measurements
  i) theoretical transstenotic pressure gradient
 ii) calculated poisseuille resistance
iii) calculated turbulent resistance
    Contour detection is based on the use of first and second derivative function applied to the brightness distributions along scanlines perpendicular to the centerline of the vessel segment and using "minimal cost" edge detection techniques. The distances, in pixels, between corresponding left and right contour points, can be converted into absolute values by using the catheter as a scaling device. The direct measurements are derived from the "diameter function' which represents the size of the analysed vessel segment at intervals of approximately 0.1 mm as measured by the computed centerline (Figure 2). The diameter values are presented along the y-axis and the vessel length is represented along the x axis. The length of the lesion is specifically defined by a curvature analysis of the diameter function curve. To estimate the original diameter values over the obstructive region, the reference

diameter function is computed. To this end, a first degree least squares polynomial is determined through all the diameter values proximal and distal to the obstruction; this polynomial allows the vessels to taper. Next, the polynomial is translated upwards until 80% of the diameter values are below the polynomial. The resulting polynomial values are then assumed to be a measure for the normal size of the artery at the corresponding points; this polynomial function is denoted as the reference diameter function and displayed in the diameter function by the straight line. Thus, the reference diameter is taken as the value of the reference diameter function at the minimum position of the obstruction.

On the basis of the proximal and distal centerline segments and the reference diameter function, the reference contours over the obstruction region are determined in the following way. Vessel midpoints for the proximal and distal portions are found by averaging the coordinates of the left and right contour positions. For the obstructive region, the vessel midpoints are obtained by interpolation between the proximal and distal vessel midpoints with a second degree polynomial. The left and right reference contours are then obtained by centering the normal reference value for that position perpendicular to the local direction of the midline in each point. These computer-estimated predisease reference contours are superimposed in the image (Figure 3).

The area plaque is an interpolated value which is a measure of the atherosclerotic plaque (Fig. 3). This area is calculated as the sum of pixels between the computer-estimated predisease reference contours and the actual detected luminal contours of an obstructive lesion. Since measurement of area plaque is highly dependent on the length of the stenosis (which is subject to considerable variation) and the determination of the border of the artery in the presumed prediseased state, the usefulness of this parameter is debatable. The symmetry value is a measure of the eccentricity of a particular lesion. Unfortunately, this has not yet been validated with pathologic studies and thus the pathologist and angiographer may not be talking about the same feature. The curvature value is an attempt to assess the bend of the coronary vessel at a lesion site (Fig. 4). The view in which the vessel appears to be the least foreshortened (ie. the lesion length is longest) is chosen for the curvature analysis. The inflow and outflow angles are derived from the slope of the diameter function at the descending and ascending limb of the diameter function curve at the defined site of the obstruction.

The CAAS system has also attempted to convert information on angiographic parameters into functional significance based on well-known fluid-dynamic equations [6]. The calculated transstenotic pressure gradient over a particular stenosis derived from QCA describes the hemodynamic impact that a particular lesion would have under a range of flow conditions, within the range of "normal" aortic pressures. These calculations do not account for the effects of pulsatile flow or of curved and tapered vessels, more than one lesion in a vessel, the collateral circulation, or perfusion of areas of nonviable myocardium. The effects of the entrance and exit angle (along with the absolute lesion diameter, percent narrowing, length of stenosis, blood flow velocity, and inertial and frictional effects) are the important factors that determine the physiologic significance of a coronary stenosis [10]. The pressure gradient across a stenosis is determined by entrance effects, drag effects (frictional losses) and exit effects. Although the most important site of energy loss is at the exit of a stenosis where the separation of the fluid column occurs, neither the outflow nor inflow angle have yet been incorporated into the CAAS software package to calculate pressure gradients.

A Word of Caution in the Interpretation of Angiographic Data

The limitations of angiographic information in the evaluation of the extent of coronary artery disease has been well recognized [11]. After all, coronary angiography is really just a two-dimensional shadowgram of an opacified vessel. It merely demonstrates the effect of arterial wall disease on the contour of the arterial lumen. Moreover, atherosclerotic changes of the arterial wall are not reflected precisely enough by changes in the lumen. Due to the diffuseness of the atherosclerotic process which can narrow the entire lumen of a segment of a vessel smoothly and evenly, angiography may not detect its existence. This is reflected in many studies that have shown that coronary angiography frequently underestimates the severity of coronary artery lesions or even misses significant narrowings regarding the underlying extent of coronary disease [12–14]. Furthermore, depending on the radiologic view, elliptical or D-shaped lumens may result in either under or overestimation of stenosis [15]. The interpolated measurements reconstruct the "normal" segment of the vessel at the site of the lesion. Accordingly, these measurements may be underestimations of the true diameter value in the disease-free segment.

It is also important in interpreting the results of angiographic studies to know how the individual parameters were measured. Several angioplasty studies have identified multiple angiographic risk factors (e.g. lesion length (>10 mm), lesions on a coronary bend etc.) associated with a higher rate of restenosis [16–19]. However, the way in which lesion length and bend (curvature) may differ greatly depending on the type of system used.

Analyst-computer Interaction

The entire analysis can be derived by the computer. However the analyst can interact at several steps, hence the term "computer-assisted" analysis. The contours of the vessel detected by the computer can be manually adjusted by the analyst. This may be necessary when the angiogram is of poor technical quality, or in specific situations such as the presence of side branches which interfere with the edge detection programme or hazy vessel contours oc-

OSTIAL LESION

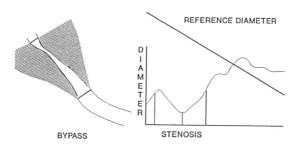

Figure 5. The computer-defined reference diameter is inaccurate in situations where there is no reliable proximal or distal boundary (e.g. ostial lesion or lesions located at the origin of a side branch). In this situation, the analyst must determine the reference diameter (user-defined).

casionally related to the presence of a dissection after an intervention. Excessive analyst interaction increases the risk of introducing bias and is discouraged. Thus, technically high quality angiograms are of paramount importance for reliable QCA. The second aspect of analyst-computer interaction is the definition of reference segment. Normally, the computer itself decides on the reference segment (ie. computer-defined). Occasionally, the analyst may decide to choose a different part of the vessel as the reference diameter. This may be necessary in situations where there is no reliable proximal or distal boundary such as lesions located at the ostia of a vessel or at the origin of side branches or in diffusely diseased vessels (Fig. 5). To obtain a reasonable value for the reference diameter by the CAAS algorithm, a prerequisite is comparable diameters proximal and distal to the lesion. The user-defined reference diameter may also be required when one wants to know the exact diameter at a specific location of the vessel segment. This has been useful in our validation studies of the intravascular echo (Fig. 6). Selection of the "user defined" reference segment will affect the determination of the interpolated and derived values but will not influence the direct measurement parameters.

2. *Densitometry*

The important parameters that can be obtained by densitometry are:
 i) % area stenosis
ii) minimal luminal cross-sectional area

As explained earlier, densitometry by itself can only provide relative measurements of area stenosis i.e. a ratio based on the relative differences in brightness (and thus density after appropriate transformations). For absolute measurements, the reference diameter must be determined from the edge detection data.

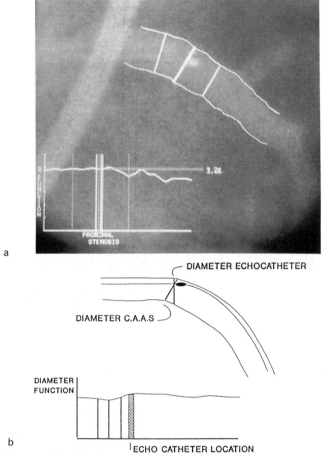

Figure 6. The user-defined reference diameter is also useful when the exact diameter is required at a specific location in the coronary artery. (a) In the validation studies of intravascular echo catheters, the tip of the echo-catheter is visible and the diameter of the segment (3.26 mm) has been determined by the CAAS analysis. (b) It is also clear from the schematic diagram, that different diameters are measured by the two methods when the intravascular echo catheter is placed in a bend in the coronary artery.

The following steps are used by the computer in the calculation of the minimal luminal cross-sectional area measurements from densitometry and edge detection obtained data:
1) Edge Detection obtained: Reference Diameter. The Reference Area (RA) can then be calculated by assuming that the reference (or "normal") segment has a circular cross-sectional configuration.
2) Densitometry obtained: Ratio (R) = Density of Reference Segment / Density of Obstruction Segment
3) Minimal Luminal Cross-Sectional Area = RA/R

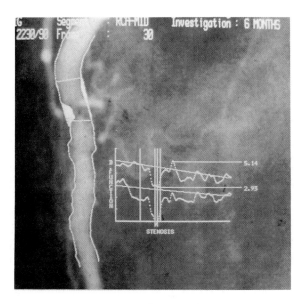

Figure 7. Densitometry measurements are affected and inaccurate in the presence of overlapping sidebranches. In this example, the upper curve (the diameter function) shows a minimal luminal diameter of 2.93 mm. However due to interference from side branches from the background subtraction, the densitometric determined minimal luminal cross-sectional area (MLCA) (lower curve) is a negative value.

In this method, no assumption is made about the cross-sectional shape of the lesion in the most severely diseased segment of the vessel. Although densitometry is extremely attractive on a theoretical basis, numerous technical problems have limited its use. The major limitation of this method is the strict requirement of a view that is perpendicular to the long axis of the vessel (i.e. to prevent oblique "cuts" which would lead to overestimate the luminal area) and absence of overlapping sidebranches in the segment (which would would interfere with the density of the lesion due to background subtraction) (Fig. 7). Densitometry is also more sensitive than edge detection to densitometric nonlinearities (x-ray scatter, veiling glare and beam hardening) and to incomplete contrast filling of vessels.

QCA and Coronary Interventions

Prior to a discussion of the various devices used for coronary intervention, the utility of the information generated by QCA in general (and the CAAS system specifically) must be addressed. The determination of anatomic information, such as minimal luminal diameter and percentage diameter stenosis, is the reliable information obtained by this system. The physiologic and clinical significance of any individual value can not be inferred although the

CAAS system can generate theoretical measures of resistance based on the lesion characteristics and assumed coronary flow rates. Angiographic features of a particular lesion which may be important to the clinical outcome such as ulceration or complex, ragged morphology have not been a focus of our research in the natural history of large populations undergoing coronary interventions. The long term variability of the CAAS system has previously been validated [5]. Specifically, we have found that a change in minimal luminal diameter greater than 0.72 mm represents angiographically detectable change. This does not infer physiologic significance but merely represents two times the standard deviation of measurements performed 3 months apart (ie. the 95% confidence interval). The physiologic significance will depend on the absolute minimal luminal diameter and other factors described earlier. For instance, if intervention A improves the MLD from 1.1 mm to 1.7 mm, and intervention B improves the MLD from 1.1 to 2.5 mm, a mean loss of 0.8 mm in the long term will be functionally more important to patients who have had intervention A. This lack of functional or physiologic significance in our definitions of restenosis of course applies to the other angiographic definitions (NHLBI 1–5) of restenosis. What QCA provides is an increased understanding of the natural history of lesions in populations of patients treated with a particular device, rather than aiding individual patient decisions.

Part B: QCA and Specific Coronary Devices

A. *Percutaneous Transluminal Coronary Angioplasty (PTCA)*

The largest experience in the Thoraxcenter databank has been with serial studies following angioplasty. These studies have demonstrated several important aspects of QCA. The reproducibility of the CAAS system for the analysis of large restenosis trials is extremely high (Fig. 8). In several large trials, comparable values have been obtained in the determination of minimal luminal diameter pre PTCA, post PTCA and at 6 month follow-up [20–22].

YEAR	N	PRE	POST	F\U
1988	88	1.13 ± .41	2.10 ± .40	1.69 ± .55
1990	309	0.99 ± .35	1.77 ± .34	1.46 ± .59
1991	261	0.98 ± .35	1.77 ± .34	1.49 ± .54

Figure 8. Minimal luminal diameter changes following PTCA. The reproducibility of QCA results by the CAAS system is seen in three different restenosis trials evaluated at the Thoraxcenter from 1988 (20), 1990 (21), and 1991 (22). In the two latter trials, data is presented only for the control patients. PRE = Pre PTCA, POST = Post PTCA, F%U = Follow-up

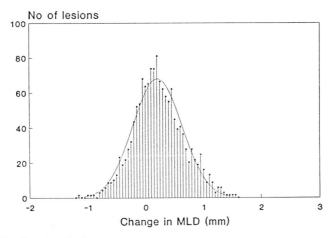

Figure 9. The Gaussian distribution of restenosis. The change in minimal luminal diameter (in mm) from post PTCA to follow-up is shown for 1234 patients from two restenosis trials approximately follows a normal distribution. Total occlusions at follow-up have been excluded. (Reprinted with permission (23))

Based on data obtained from these studies, we have learned that restenosis is not an all-or-nothing phenomenon as clinicians have been led to believe. Rather, the distributions of minimal lumen diameter pre angioplasty (1.03 ± 0.37 mm), post angioplasty (1.78 ± 0.36 mm), at 6 months follow-up (1.50 ± 0.57 mm) as well as the percentage diameter stenosis at 6 months follow-up (1.50 ± 0.57 mm) approximately follow a normal distribution [23]. Therefore restenosis can be viewed as the tail end of an approximately Gaussian distributed phenomenon, with some lesions crossing a more or less arbitrary cut-off point, rather than a separate disease entity occurring in some lesions but not in others (ie. a bimodal distribution) as suggested by the Emory group [24] (Fig. 9). This has quite profound significance in the design of trials (pharmacologic or specific devices) to inhibit the restenotic process since this is an underlying assumption for the use of parametric statistical tests (e.g. t-tail, analysis of variance).

To clarify conflicting data in the literature about the restenosis in diverse segments of the coronary tree, 1234 patients were studied with quantitative coronary angiography before PTCA, after PTCA and at follow-up [25]. No differences in restenosis rates were observed between coronary segments using a definition of either 50% diameter stenosis at follow-up or a continuous approach that compared absolute changes in minimal luminal diameter adjusted for the vessel size. These results suggested that restenosis is a ubiquitous phenomenon without any predilection for a particular site in the coronary tree. In a second study, relative gain in minimal luminal diameter at angioplasty (post PTCA-pre PTCA) adjusted for vessel size, lesion length ≥6.8 mm and total occlusions were independent predictors of restenosis [26]. Our interpretation of this data is that a too optimal result after PTCA, implying deeper arterial injury, adversely stimulates the fibroproliferative vessel reaction. No relationship was evident between the extent of elastic recoil at the time of PTCA and late luminal narrowing.

Insights into Mechanisms of Dilatation

The immediate result of percutaneous transluminal coronary angioplasty is influenced by both plastic (dissections, intimal tears) and elastic changes of the vessel wall. Experimental studies have shown that part of the angioplasty mechanism consists of stretching the vessel wall with a resulting fusiform dilation or localized aneurysm formation [27]. To evaluate elastic changes from our angiographic studies, we have defined elastic recoil as the difference between the minimal luminal diameter or area after angioplasty and the mean balloon diameter or cross-sectional area at the highest inflation pressure. We specifically have noted that elastic recoil after coronary angioplasty accounts for nearly 50% decrease in luminal cross-sectional area immediately after balloon deflation [28]. Further study showed that asymmetric lesions, lesions located in less angulated parts of the artery and lesions with a low plaque content showed more elastic recoil [29]. Furthermore, lesions located in distal parts of the coronary tree were also associated with more elastic recoil, probably related to relative balloon oversizing in these distal lesions.

However, CAAS analysis of the inflated balloon in addition to the lesion has increased our understanding of several important mechanisms of balloon dilatation such as stretch (theoretical maximal gain in diameter or area during the angioplasty procedure), elastic recoil (which appears to affect the immediate post-angioplasty result) and over or undersizing (which affects the incidence of dissection). In these assessments, the inflated balloon is used as a scaling device and presumed uniform along the entire balloon length at a diameter according to the manufacturer's specifications. However, we recently measured the balloon diameter over its entire length in 453 patients [30]. During an average inflation pressure of 8.3 ± 2.6 atm., we observed a difference of 0.59 ± 0.23 mm in diameter between the minimal and maximal balloon diameter (Fig. 10). This difference results in large variations in the calculated stretch, elastic recoil and balloon-artery ratio depending on the site of the balloon chosen for the assessment.

Several technical considerations have emerged from these large studies. The analyst determines the length of the segment analyzed as the distance between two major side branches. This enables the analyst to be certain of the location during follow-up studies. Sidebranches crossing within the segment require manual correction and increase the risk of analyst bias. The major limitation of edge detection (aside from the technical quality of the cinefilm) is the analysis of the post angioplasty result. Dissections are a frequent occurrence following PTCA and the resulting haziness, irregular borders or extravascular extravasation of contrast medium makes edge detection difficult (Fig. 11A,B). There is no ideal solution to this problem. We usually rely on

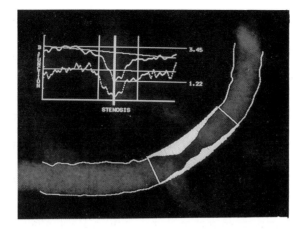

Figure 10(a).

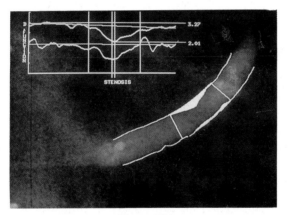

Figure 10(b).

manual corrections while accepting this limitation. Secondly, the computer generated interpolated measurements are unreliable for ostial lesions or lesions located at sidebranches due to a requirement in the algorithm for a particular length of the segment proximal and distal to the defined lesion (see Fig. 5). In this situation, the analyst can interact and make corrections so that there is a user defined reference diameter. Manual contour correction may also be necessary when the angiogram is of poor technical quality. In our large scale restenosis trials, only 0.9% of films have been rejected for analysis due to poor technical quality [23].

An additional important technical point for all serial studies is the requirement of comparable vasodilator use for every study. In a recent study [31], the mean diameter of a normal segment of a non dilated vessel pre PTCA, post PTCA and at follow-up in 202 patients was analyzed (Fig. 12). Thirty-

24   *B.H. Strauss et al*

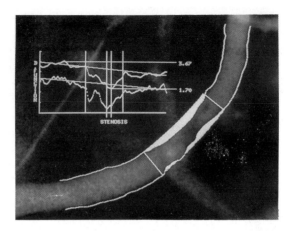

Figure 10. Non uniform balloon inflation during balloon angioplasty. Pre PTCA-minimal luminal diameter 1.22 mm (a). During balloon inflation with a 3.5 mm (manufacturer specification) balloon (b). The minimal balloon diameter is 2.01 mm and the maximal balloon diameter is 3.27 mm. Post PTCA (c). (reprinted with permission (30))

four of these patients did not receive intracoronary nitrates prior to post-PTCA angiography. In the group that did not receive the nitrates post-procedure, there was a decrease in diameter of 0.11 mm versus the small increase of 0.02 mm in the group that received nitrates post procedure. Lack of control of vasodilator therapy at follow-up angiograms may also partially explain an earlier observation from our group that there is significant deterioration in the mean reference diameter at four months post angioplasty since several subsequent studies that have controlled for this factor have not shown a loss of the reference diameter at follow-up [23, 32]. However, we still believe that in select patients, the reference segment is involved in the restenotic process and may contribute to the unreliability of an assessment of diameter stenosis at follow-up.

Densitometry may be more reliable than edge detection since it is theoretically independent of the projection chosen. In a study published in 1984, agreement between edge detection and densitometry was assessed by the standard deviation of the mean differrences of the % area stenosis, since absolute measurements of area by densitometry were not yet possible [33] (Fig. 13). Prior to PTCA, reasonable agreement existed between the densitometric percent-area stenosis and the circular percent-area stenosis (standard deviation of the mean difference was 5%). However, important discrepancies between these two types of measurements were observed after PTCA (standard deviation 18%). This discrepancy suggested the creation of asymmetric lesions after angioplasty, and an error in the circular assumption of cross-sectional area stenosis calculated from edge detection data.

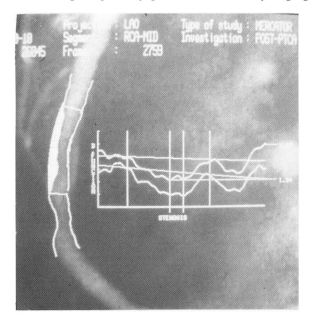

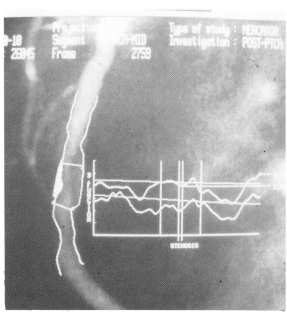

Figure 11. Edge detection of a lesion after PTCA has induced a large dissection. (a)Excluding dissection the minimal luminal dimater is 1.34 mm. (b) Including the dissection, the minimal luminal diameter is 2.53 mm.

INFLUENCE OF VASOMOTOR TONE ON QCA
MEASUREMENTS OF NON-DISEASED SEGMENTS

MEAN DIAMETER (MM)	WITHOUT NITRO POST-PTCA (N = 34)	WITH NITRO POST-PTCA (N = 168)
PRE-PTCA	3.12 ± 0.63	2.74 ± 0.63
POST-PTCA	3.01 ± 0.64	2.75 ± 0.59
F-UP	3.18 ± 0.55	2.82 ± 0.63
Δ POST-PRE	-0.11 ± 0.27 ⟷	+0.02 ± 0.21•)
Δ F-UP-PRE	+0.06 ± 0.22 ⟷	+0.07 ± 0.22••)

•) P < 0.001   ••) P = NS

Figure 12. Influence of vasomotor tone on QCA measurements of non-diseased segments. Thirty four patients did not receive intracoronary nitroglycerin post PTCA. In the non-diseased segments adjacent to the dilated site, these patients had a loss in the mean diameter of 0.11 mm compared with the pre PTCA values (where nitro had been given). This change was not seen in the group who recieved nitro post PTCA. The change in the mean diameter will affect the determination of percentage diameter stenosis.

B. *Stenting*

Three types of coronary stents have been implanted and followed with serial angiograms at the Thoraxcenter [34–38]. Two of these stents, the Wallstent and the Palmaz-Schatz stent are composed primarily of radiolucent stainless

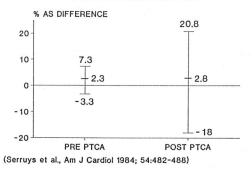

AGREEMENT BETWEEN DENSITOMETRIC PERCENT
AREA STENOSIS AND THE CIRCULAR PERCENT-
AREA STENOSIS POST PTCA

(Serruys et al., Am J Cardiol 1984; 54:482-488)

Figure 13. Agreement between densitometric percentage area stenosis and the circular (edge detection) percentage area stenosis pre and post PTCA. The mean difference (and standard deviation) for % area stenosis between the two methods was 2.3 ± 4.0% pre PTCA and 2.8 ± 18% post PTCA. Important discrepancies (ie. large standard deviation) between the two methods after PTCA are likely related to the non-circular, asymmetric configuration of the lesion after angioplasty.

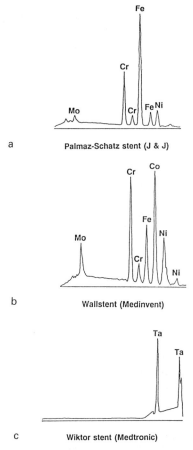

Figure 14. The metal composition according to X-ray energy dispersion spectrometry used in three currently investigated coronary stents. Ta = tantalum, Mo = molybdenum, Cr = chromium, Co = cobalt, Fe = iron, Ni = nickel. (reprinted with permission [40])

steel, whereas radiopaque tantalum is the principle constituent of the Wiktor stent (Fig. 14A,B,C).

Stainless Steel Stents

The main problem with these stents is their poor angiographic visibility (Fig. 15A,B). In particular, the Palmaz-Schatz stent which is the most difficult stent to visualize, can be dislodged from the balloon catheter and embolize distally without the stent operator's knowledge. Additionally, it can be quite difficult to ensure ideal placement of the stent across a lesion. For the analyst, this means that the stent boundaries may be uncertain at the time of implantation and the precise location of a late restenosis (within the stent or immediately adjacent) may be in some doubt. By carefully reviewing the

a

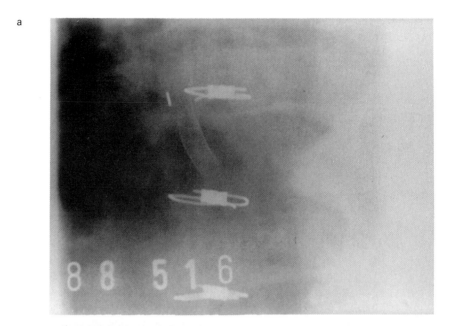

b

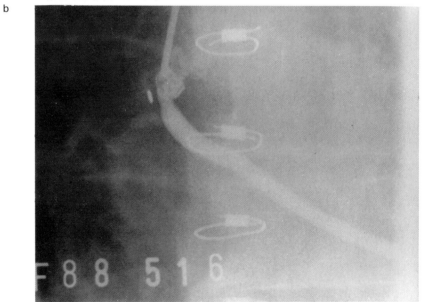

Figure 15. Wallstent (poor radiopacity) after implantation in a saphenous vein bypass graft. (a) in vessel without contrast. (b) in vessel filled with contrast.

angiograms done without contrast present, we usually can discern the position of the Wallstent for studies with contrast. In our follow-up reports of stenting, we have always included restenosis within and immediately adjacent to the stented segment to ensure restenosis is not underreported due to this problem [34].

A second problem with angiographic analysis of stented vessels is due to superior results immediately post stenting versus PTCA alone. Consequently, the "obstruction segment" may be completely corrected or in some cases overdilated in comparison to the reference diameter pre stenting. This causes problems specifically with the length of obstruction and the reference diameter. We arbitrarily define the length of the obstruction post stenting to be the actual length of the stent (which requires manual selection of the stent boundaries). Thus the extent of the stented segment is defined for future follow-up analyses. We perform each stent analysis either by stent or by vessel. In the former, the length of the lesion is the length of the stent as previously described. In the latter, there is no interaction with the choice of computer detected contours and the minimal luminal diameter may then be located outside the stent. In reporting our angiographic studies, we chose the pre and post PTCA frames to be analyzed by vessel, and the post stent and follow-up films according to the stent. This ensured that we could obtain the information related to the stent and its immediate adjacent segment rather than describing a more severe stenosis somewhere else in the coronary vessel.

Stenting has also taught us a limitation of the CAAS system in the measurement of the reference diameter in an overdilated segment. Theoretically, this should result in a negative value for diameter stenosis since the minimal luminal diameter (which we already mentioned was defined within the boundaries of the stent) was actually larger than the reference diameter which is determined according to the diameter of the proximal and distal segments (Fig. 16A,B). However, for reasons still unclear to us, a negative diameter stenosis never occurred and the reference diameter always remained larger than the minimal luminal diameter. A further confounding factor in the determination of the reference diameter post stenting is the marked vasospasm occasionally seen immediately proximal and distal to the stent which persists despite nitrate administration.

Tantalum Stents

The radiopacity of the Wiktor stent has greatly facilitated the implantation procedure (Fig. 17A,B). The stent can easily be visualized in a vessel with and without contrast. However, this particular property of the Wiktor stent severely limits the assessment of follow-up studies by the CAAS system. Several cases have now been documented in which the radiopaque stent wires are traced by the contour detection program instead of the arterial borders of the narrowed intrastent hyperplasia (Fig. 18). This invalidates the

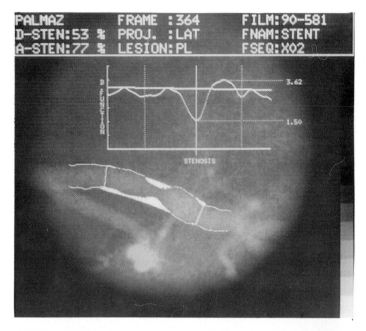

a

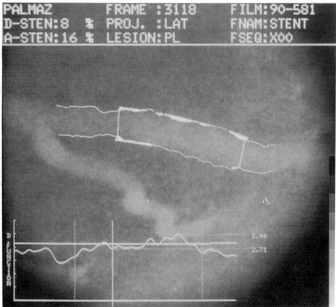

c

Figure 16. (a) Pre stent. (b) Post stent. Coronary segment overdilated by a Palmaz-Schatz stent. Although the minimal luminal diameter (MLD) in the stented segment should be greater than the reference diameter (which is determined by the smaller proximal and distal segments to the stented segment), the reference diameter remains larger than the MLD for unclear reasons and the diameter stenosis (8%) remains a positive value.

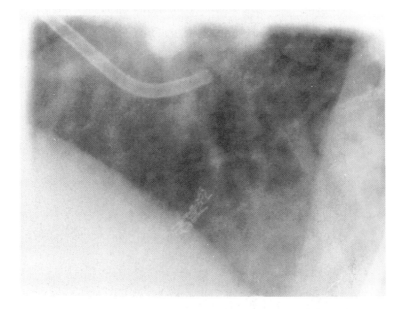

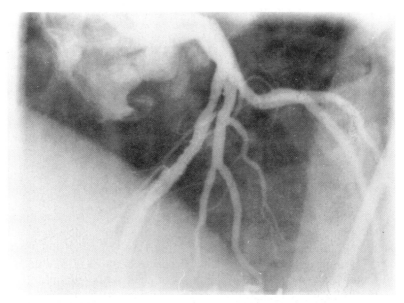

Figure 17. Wiktor stent after implantation in left anterior descending artery.
(a) in vessel without contrast. (b) in vessel filled with contrast, stent remains clearly visible.

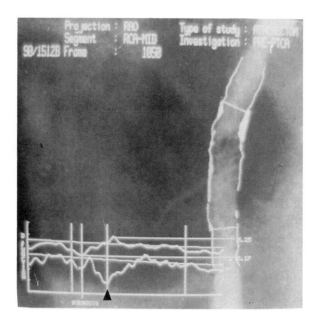

Figure 18. Restenosis within a coronary Wiktor stent not recognized by edge detection. Graph shows the diameter function (upper curve) and the densitometric area function (lower curve). Outside vertical lines on the graph and two horizontal lines in the angiographic image are lesion boundaries. The inner two vertical lines on the graph represent the minimal points on the diameter and densitometric graphs respectively. The minimal luminal diameter by edge detection is 2.17 mm. A discrepancy between the two functions is present and most severe at the vertical line which denotes the minimal densitometric value (arrowhead). The edge detection algorithm followed the outline of the stent and was unable to recognize the stenosis within the stent.(reprinted with permission (40))

computer derived data and requires manual selection of the contours by the analyst, which is also difficult in a segment containing radiopaque wires.

Densitometry

In contrast to the situation after PTCA, there is excellent agreement between minimal luminal cross-sectional areas determined by edge detection and densitometry after stent implantation with the Wallstent [39]. In 19 patients, the standard deviations of the mean differences between edge detection and densitometric determination of minimal luminal cross-sectional area were 0.51 mm² pre PTCA, 1.22 mm² after angioplasty and 0.79 mm² after coronary stenting (Fig. 19). This improvement is likely due to smoothing of the vessel contours by the stent and remodelling of the stented segment into a more circular configuration (Fig. 20). We concluded that both methods were appropriate to assess the immediate results post stenting. In a separate in-vitro study involving stents placed in known stenoses within plexiglass phantoms, we found that the Wallstent and Palmaz-Schatz stent had minor and likely

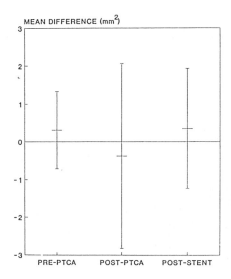

Figure 19. Mean difference (and 95% confidence intervals) between edge detection and densitometry before and after percutaneous transluminal coronary angioplasty (PTCA) and after stenting. Mean differences were slightly positive (0.31, 0.35 mm^2) before PTCA and after stenting, respectively and slightly negative (-0.38 mm^2) after PTCA. The widest 95% confidence interval was in the analysis after PTCA, indicating the poorest association between the two methods, compared with the analysis before PTCA and stenting. (reprinted with permission (39))

clinically insignificant contributions to the densitometric determination of MLCA within the known stenoses (Fig. 21A,B) [40]. Conversely, the radiopacity of the tantalum Wiktor stent increased the MLCA in these same narrowings by 10–56% depending on the concentration of contrast and specific stenosis (Fig. 21C). Therefore, the follow-up assessment of a lesion containing a Wiktor stent, is limited by both methods.

Directional Atherectomy

Few problems have been encountered in the analysis of patients treated with directional atherectomy [41]. The radiopacity of the device, particularly when the support balloon is inflated, allows the operator excellent visualization of the position of the eccentric cutting apparatus (Fig. 22A,B). The contours are typically smooth and much less ragged than after PTCA, facilitating the edge detection program. Despite the apparent smooth contours following atherectomy, similar discrepancy exist between analyses performed by edge detection or densitometry, as occurs post angioplasty (Fig. 23) [42]. This suggests that the vessel wall assumes a less circular configuration as a result of atherectomy. As Baim's group has suggested, this may be due to preferential expansion of the bases of the atherectomy cuts [43]. Furthermore, QCA of atherectomy-treated lesions has provided some insight into the mechanisms

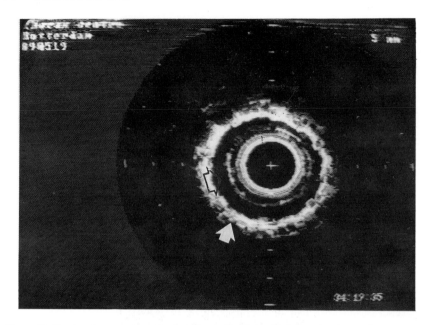

Figure 20. In vitro intravascular ultrasound examination of left anterior descending artery that was stented 24 hours earlier for a severe dissection during PTCA. (The patient died from intracerebral hemorrhage 12 hours after stenting.) The inner circle is due to the intravascular probe. The outer echodense pattern is due to the stent wires (large arrow). The lumen is the echo-free space inside the stent. The stent effectively tacked back the dissection and restored the circular configuration of the vessel. (reprinted with permission (39)).

of lesion improvement. Penny et al have shown that approximately 28% of the effect of atherectomy can actually be attributed to tissue removal, although the individual values had a wide range (7–92%) [43]. The correlation between the volume of tissue retrieved and the change in luminal volume was poor (r = 0.19). They concluded that the major component of luminal improvement was due to "facilitated mechanical angioplasty" resulting from the high profile of the device and the low pressure balloon inflations. Data from our angiographic core laboratory seems to support this hypothesis. In 10 patients that had QCA performed pre atherectomy, after crossing the stenosis with the device and after directional atherectomy, it was shown that the dottering effect of the device accounted for 65% of the luminal improvement [44].

Rotational Abrasion

The Thoraxcenter experience to date has been limited with this device (11 procedures) [45]. A unique feature of this particular device is its usefulness as a calibration unit. Usually we use the guiding catheter for this purpose. The tip (or shaft in the case of soft tip catheters) of the guiding catheter is

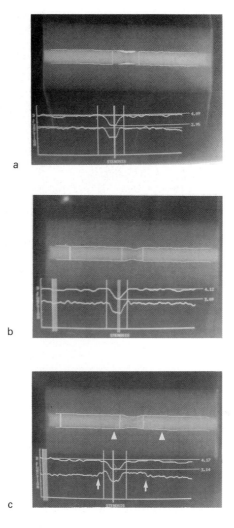

Figure 21. Control (a), Palmaz-Schatz containing (b), and Wiktor containing (c) plexiglass phantom (4x3 mm) filled with 50% iopamidol contrast reagent. Graphs show the diameter function (upper curve) and the densitometric area function (lower curve). Outside vertical lines on the graph and rightward two vertical lines on the phantom are lesion boundaries. The inner two vertical lines represent the minimal points on the diameter and densitometric graphs respectively. The multiple vertical lines in the left part of the graph and the leftward vertical line in the phantom represent the user defined reference segment. The numbers in the graph represent the maximum and minimum diameter. The boundaries of the Wiktor stent are visible in the phantom (arrowheads) and as a step-up in the densitometry graph (arrows). As a result of the Wiktor stent contribution to the densitometry values, the minimal cross-sectional area determination is overestimated compared with the control and Palmaz-Schatz containing phantom.(reprinted with permission (40)).

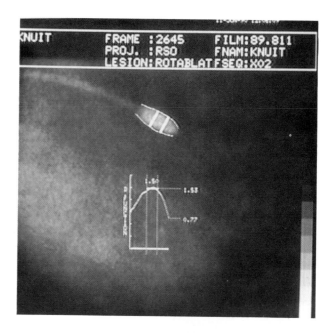

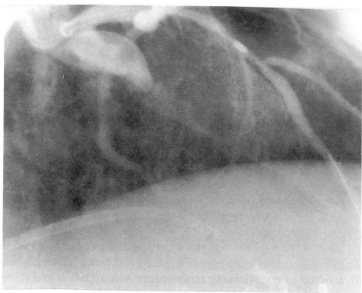

Figure 24. Rotational abrasion (Rotablator™) in a coronary artery. (a) without contrast. Since the burr is non deformable and of known diameter, calibration of the angiogram can occur at the site of the procedure in contrast to PTCA, stenting or directional atherectomy where we use the contrast-filled guiding catheter in one corner of the angiogram as the scaling device. In this case a 1.50 mm diameter burr was used. (b) in vessel containing contrast showing that the rotablator is clearly visible.

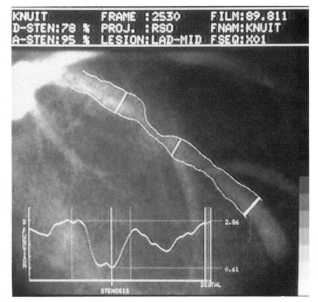

a

b

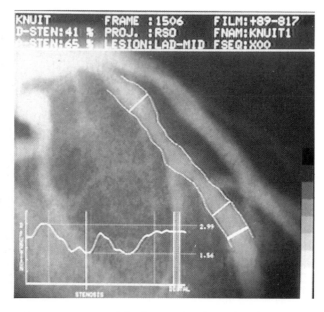

c

Figure 25. Due to intense vasospasm following rotational abrasion, it may be necessary to repeat the study 24 hours later to assess the maximal benefit. (a) Pre rotablator minimal luminal diameter (MLD) is 0.41 mm. (b) Immediately after the rotablator, MLD is 1.24 mm. (c) 24 hours later, MLD is 1.56 mm.

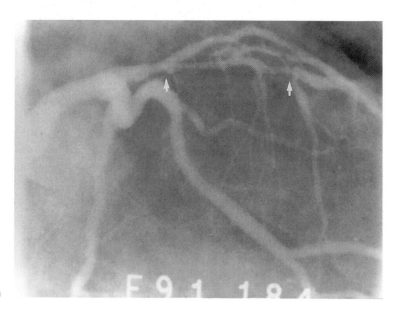

a

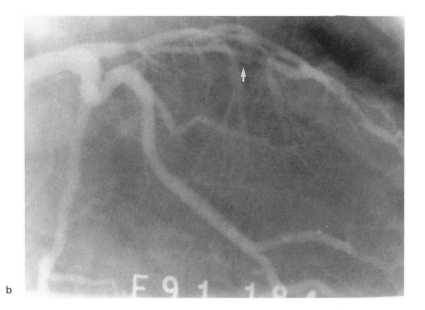

b

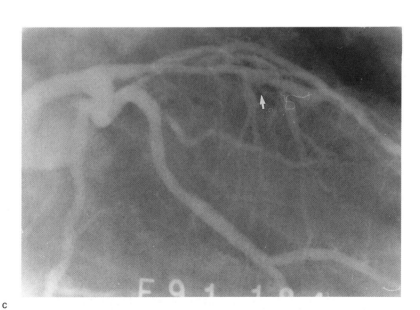

c

Figure 26. Excimer laser. (a) Pre laser, long narrowing in left anterior descending artery (between two arrows). (b) Post laser, roughened hazy appearance (arrow). (c) Post balloon, haziness still present (arrow).

How Should We Use QCA Data to Compare Interventional Devices?

We have now reached the stage where the safety and favorable immediate results for the various devices have been demonstrated by ourselves and other groups. The logical next step is the comparison of the devices to determine what specific features of a device or clinical situation may favor the use of a particular device.

1) *Immediate Results Post Procedure*: *The Expansion Ratio* (*Fig. 27A,B*).
The expansion ratio is a useful concept to assess the immediate results of an intervention [37, 48]. It relates the final effect of the device on the arterial diameter to the size of the catheter required to deliver this effect. A favorable ratio is best exemplified by a small catheter delivery system that is able to pass severely narrowed segments and yet optimally dilate the stenosis. However, the maximum effect of the device may be partially lost due to the elastic recoil of the vessel. The current interventional devices may have differential effects in these two areas: the acute result, when the device is initially used and then the partial loss of the initial gain after the device has been removed. We have attemped to separate these two effects by subdividing the expansion ratio into the *theoretical* expansion ratio, which is a measure of the effect while the device is operational, and the *functional* expansion ratio, which takes into account the elastic recoil phenomenon. For example, a 4 mm diameter balloon angioplasty catheter should achieve a vessel diameter of 4 mm at the time of balloon inflation but this is reduced immediately after deflation, primarily due to the elastic recoil of the vessel. Balloon angioplasty and stenting give extremely favourable theoretical and effective expansion ratios since they may be delivered on low profile catheters. The wide range for the theoretical and effective expansion ratios seen with balloon angioplasty is explained by the varying sized balloons (2.0–3.5 mm) used in the study from which this data was obtained. The atherectomy devices are more limited by the profile of the device that can be introduced into the coronary artery. The dimensions of the rotational atherectomy device and the excimer laser do not change while in operation and therefore both exhibit lower theoretical expansion ratios. However, by physically removing or vaporizing tissue, the potential elastic recoil effect is diminished by atherectomy and excimer laser devices.

2) *Late Results*
To date, no randomized trials have been reported that compare the various devices. In anticipation of this data, we have attempted to compare available data according to three methods. First, we have pre, immediately post and follow-up results in native vessels from separate studies of angioplasty [21], atherectomy and stenting [51] (Fig. 28).

Secondly, Kevin Beatt has devised 3 indices to assess the "utility" of each type of intervention [48]. This index can be subdivided into a dilating

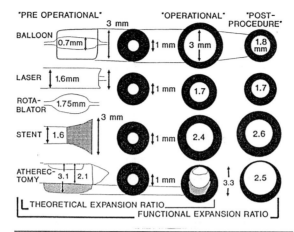

INTERVENTION	EXPANSION RATIO THEORETICAL	EXPANSION RATIO EFFECTIVE
BALLOON ANGIOPLASTY	2.2 - 4.1	1.4 - 2.6
STENT SELF EXPANDABLE	2.5 (1.6-3.8)	1.6
BAL. EXPANDABLE	2.1 - 2.4	1.5 - 1.7
ATHERECTOMY DIRECTIONAL	1.3 - 1.6	1.0 - 1.2
ROTATIONAL	1.0	0.9 - 1.1
EXCIMER LASER	1.0	0.9 - 1.1

EVS17-AUG'90

Figure 27. Comparison of various devices with the expansion ratio, which relates the final effect on the arterial diameter to the size of the catheter required to deliver this effect. (a) The far left column, pre operational refers to the relationship between the profile of the various device prior to the procedure and during the procedure. For example, balloon angioplasty catheter has a low profile (0.7 mm) but expands to a diameter of 3 mm in this case when it is fully dilated. The laser and the rotablator have the same profile prior to use and during use. The Wallstent is delivered on a 1.6 mm diameter catheter but can be expanded in this example to 3.0 mm (in fact it is possible to have a stent that expands to 6 mm). The directional altherectomy has a profile of 2.1 mm with balloon deflated and 3.1 mm with balloon inflated. The circles represent the diameter of the coronary artery pre procedure (far left), during activation of the device (center circle) and post procedure (far right). In this example, the pre procedure diameter was 1 mm. During activation of the device, the vessel diameter is expanded from 1.7 to 3.3 mm depending on the device. The post procedure results are based on the mean value of each procedure in the Thoraxcenter data bank. Elastic recoil is responsible for the immediate loss of 3 to 1.8 mm for balloon angioplasty and from 3.3 to 2.5 mm for directional atherectomy. The stent is an effective device against elastic recoil and due to the self-expanding property of the Wallstent, the vessel lumen continues to dilate (for at least the first 24 hours). Theoretical expansion ratio is the relation between the profile of the device and the maximal achievable diameter of the device. Functional (effective) expansion ratio represents the ratio between the post procedure result and the profile of the device and thus indicates not only the initial effect of the device but also the effect of elastic recoil, which is primarily responsible for the deterioration in the diameter from the maximal achievable diameter to the post procedure diameter.

INTER-VENTION	PTS	PRE	POST	FOLLOW-UP
PTCA	261	0.99 ±.35	1.77 ±.34	1.46 ± .59
WALLSTENT	166	1.17 ±.52	2.53 ±.53	*1.99 ± .81 **1.59 ±1.08
WIKTOR	62	1.09 ±.26	2.45 ±.35	1.71 ± .68
DCA	48	1.13 ±.40	2.52 ±.40	1.70 ± .58

* EXCLUDING IN HOSPITAL OCCLUSIONS
** INCLUDING IN HOSPITAL OCCLUSIONS

Figure 28. Results from the Thoraxcenter data bank for pre, immediately post and at follow-up in separate studies of angioplasty, stenting (Wallstent and Wiktor stent), and directional coronary atherectomy.

component and a restenosis component. The "dilating index" is the ratio between the gain in diameter during the intervention and the theoretically achievable gain i.e. the reference diameter. The "restenosis index" is the ratio between the loss at follow-up and the initial gain during the procedure. The net result at long term is characterized by the "utility index" which is the ratio between the final gain in diameter at follow-up and what theoretically could have been achieved. These indices are useful for studying the mean values for populations of patients who have undergone a particular intervention and have shown important differences between the initial effect of devices (atherectomy, stenting > PTCA) which are partially overcome by larger late losses in minimal luminal dimater. Recently we have used these indices to compare the results of balloon angioplasty and directional atherectomy (Fig. 29) [49]. The superior immediate results of atherectomy is shown in the dilating index, which is offset by the greater loss in MLD at late follow-up, resulting in a higher restenosis index. Thus the net effect at late follow-up is comparable ie. utility ratio was not different.

Thirdly, we have used "matched" lesions to compare interventions [50] (Fig. 30A-D). Matching is based on three principles: the angiographic dimensions of matched lesions are assumed to be "identical", the observed difference between the two "identical" lesions must be within the range of the CAAS analysis reproducibility of 0.1 mm (=1 SD), and finally that the reference diameter of the potentially "matched" vessels are selected within a range of ±0.3 mm (=3 SD; ie. 99% confidence limits) (Fig. 31 A,B). The

(b) the theoretcial and effective expansion ratio for various interventional devices. The range for expansion ratios is due to ranges in the profiles of the device depending on the size of the balloon or stent mounted on the balloon catheter.

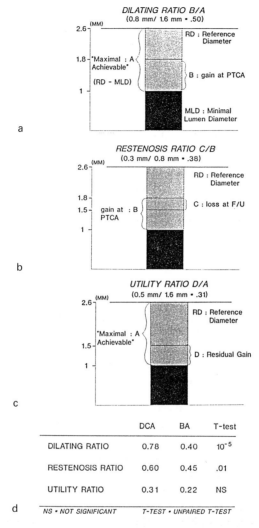

Figure 29. Example of new indices to compare the effect of directional atherectomy versus balloon angioplasty.(a) The dilating index is the ratio between the gain in diameter during the intervention and the theoretically achievable gain ie. the reference diameter. in this example, the minimal luminal diameter was 1 mm pre procedure, the gain at PTCA (B) was 0.8 mm and the maximal achievable gain in diameter (A) was 1.6 mm (RD-MLD). The dilating ratio was then calculated as 0.50 (B/A). (b) The restenosis index is the ratio between the loss at follow-up (BC), which was 0.3 mm in this example, and the initial gain during the procedure (B), 0.8 mm. This gave an overall restenosis ratio of 0.38 (C/B). The net result at long term is characterized by the utility index which is the ratio between the net gain in diameter at follow-up (D), ie. the difference between the initial gain and then the late loss due to restenosis which is 0.5 mm in this example, and the maximal theoretically gain possible (A) ie the difference between the pre procedure MLD and the reference diameter, which was 1.6 mm. The utility ratio is then calculated as 0.31 (D/A).(d) Comparison of directional coronary atherectomy (DCA) and balloon angioplasty (BA) for the three ratios in 30 matched patients with initially

	DCA	BA	P
REF-DIAM (mm)	3.03	3.07	NS
MLD (mm)	1.09	1.15	NS
D-Sten (%)	64	63	NS
A PLAQ (mm2)	9.5	8.4	NS
CURVATURE	15.9	22.2	< .02
SYMMETRY	0.6	0.5	NS
LENGTH (mm)	6.8	6.5	NS

a

	DCA	BA	P
RD (mm)			
PRE	3.03	3.07	NS
MLD (mm)			
PRE	1.08	1.15	NS
POST	2.61	1.92	10^{-5}
F-UP	1.69	1.57	NS
ΔIN MLD (mm)			
POST-PRE	1.53	0.77	10^{-5}
POST-F\U	0.92	0.35	10^{-3}

b

Figure 30. Matching lesions to compare interventions. (a) Matched pre procedural stenosis characteristics of patients. No significant differences exist between the two groups pre procedure except for a lower curvature value for lesions treated by DCA. Ref diam = reference diameter, MLD = minimal luminal diameter, D-Sten = diameter stenosis, A PLAQ = area plaque, length = length of lesion, P = probability (b) Quantitative comparison of the immediate and long-term results of directional coronary atherectomy (DCA), and percutaneous balloon angioplasty (PBA). Although there was a significant difference post procedure with larger MLD with directional atherectomy, this superior initial result was not maintained at late follow-up due to a greater loss in MLD at follow-up in the DCA group. RD = reference diameter, F-UP = follow-up.

appropriate lesions are selected by an independent observer who is unaware of the 6 month angiographic outcome.

3) *How Should Future Trials Be Designed to Compare Devices Using Angiographic Endpoints?*

In several large multicenter PTCA restenosis trials that have been analyzed by the CAAS system, we have used the mean difference in coronary diameter between post angioplasty and follow up angiograms as the primary angio-

---

successful treated lesions. Significantly higher dilating and restenosis ratios were seen with DCA in comparison to BA, suggesting that despite a superior immediate result with DCA, the late loss due to restenosis was much greater with DCA. As a result, there were no significant differences between the two procedures for the utility ratio which relates the immediate gain to the late loss.

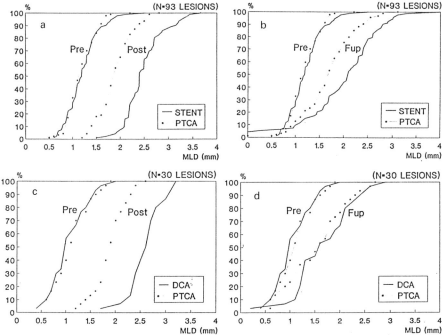

Figure 31. Comparison of results in native vessels from matched studies of balloon angioplasty, stenting and directional atherectomy using a cumulative curve. On the x-axis is the minimal luminal diameter (MLD) and on the y axis is the cumulative total. (a) Pre procedure and immediately post procedure results for PTCA and the Wallstent (93 lesions). (b) Pre procedure and follow-up results for PTCA and the Wallstent. (c) Pre procedure and immediately post procedure for PTCA and directional atherectomy (30 lesions). (d) Pre procedure and follow-up for PTCA and directional atherectomy.

graphic endpoint. However, this would be inadequate to compare various devices since atherectomy and stenting both result in superior initial results in addition to larger late losses than balloon angioplasty. We suggest that the important angiographic endpoint in these studies should be the minimal luminal diameter at follow-up provided that the lesions have comparable reference diameters and minimial luminal diameter prior to the initial intervention.

Conclusion

QCA remains the gold standard as the most objective and reproducible form of coronary artery disease. The Computer-Assisted Coronary Analysis System (CAAS) has been the most extensively studied form of QCA. This system, which has provided important information about the natural history of coronary artery disease, now enables researchers in the field of interven-

(approximately 1/2 hour per lesion for 2 views taken at any stage of the procedure).

References

1. Mancini G B J (1991) Quantitative coronary arteriographic methods in the interventional catheterization laboratory: an update and perspective. *J Am Coll Cardiol* 17:23B–33B
2. Zir L M, Miller S W, Dinsmore R E, Gilbert J P, Harthorne J W (1976) Interobserver variability in coronary angiography. *Circulation* 53:627–632
3. Goldberg R K, Kleiman N S, Minor S T, Abukhalil J, Raizner A E (1990) Comparison of quantitative coronary angiography to visual estimates of lesion severity pre- and post-PTCA. *Am Heart J* 119:178–184
4. Cherrier F, Booman F, Serruys P W, Cuillière M, Danchin N, Reiber J H C (1981) L'angiographie coronaire quantitative. Application à l'évaluation des angioplasties transluminales coronaires. *Arch Mal Coeur* 74.12:1377–1387
5. Reiber J H C, Serruys P W, Kooijman C J, Wijns W, Slager C J, Gerbrands J J, Schuurbiers J C H, den Boer A, Hugenholtz P G (1985) Assessment of short-, medium-, and long-term variations in arterial dimensions from computer-assisted quantitation of coronary cineangiograms. *Circulation* 71:280–288
6. Reiber J H C, Serruys P W, Slager C J (1986) *Quantitative Coronary and Left Ventricular Cineangiography; Methodology and Clinical Applications*. Martinus Nijhoff Publishers, Boston/Dordrecht/Lancaster
7. Reiber J H C, Kooijman C J, Slager C J, Gerbrends J J, Schuurgiers J C H, den Boer A, Wijns W, Serruys P W, Hugenholtz P G (1984) Coronary artery dimensions from cineangiograms: methodology and validation of a computer-assisted analysis procedure. *IEEE Trans Med Imaging* MI 3:131–141
8. Vlodaver Z, Edwards J E (1971) Pathology of coronary atherosclerosis. *Prog Cardiovasc Dis* 14:156–174
9. Saner H E, Gobel F L, Salomonowitz E, Erlien D A, Edwards J E (1985) The disease-free wall in coronary atherosclerosis: its relation to degree of obstruction. *J Am Coll Cardiol* 6:1096–1099
10. Marcus M L (1983) Physiologic effects of a coronary stenosis. In: Marcus M L (ed) *The Coronary Circulation in Health and Disease*. New York: McGraw-Hill Book Co, 242–269
11. de Feyter P J, Serruys P W, Davies M J, Richardson P, Lubsen J, Oliver M F (1991) Quantitative coronary angiography to measure progression and regression of coronary atherosclerosis. Values, limitations and implications for clinical trials. *Circulation* 84:412–423
12. Schwartz J N, Kong Y, Hackel D B, Bartel A G (1975) Comparison of angiographic and postmortem findings in patients with coronary heart disease. *Am J Cardiol* 36:174–178
13. Hutchins G M, Bulkley G H, Ridolf R L, Griffith L S C, Lohr F T, Piasio M A (1977) Correlation of coronary arterigrams and left ventriculograms with post mortem studies. *Circulation* 56:32–37
14. Arnett E N, Isner J M, Redwood D R, Kent K, Baker W P, Ackerstein H, Roberts W C (1979) Coronary artery narrowing in coronary heart disease. Comparison of cineangiograms and necropsy findings. *Ann Intern Med* 91:350–356
15. Thomas A C, Davies M J, Dilly S, Franc (1986) Potential errors in the estimation of coronary arterial stenosis from clinical arteriography with reference to the shape of the coronary arterial lumen. *Br Heart J* 55:129–139
16. Ellis S G, Roubin G S, King S B III, Douglas J S Jr, Cox W R (1989) Importance of stenosis morphology in the estimation of restenosis risk after elective percutaneous transluminal coronary angioplasty. *Am J Cardiol* 63:30–34
17. Leimgruber P P, Roubin G S, Hollman J, Cotsonis G A, Meier B, Douglas J S Jr, King S

B III, Gruentzig A R (1986) Restenosis after succesful coronary angioplasty in patients with single-vessel disease. *Circulation* 73:710–717

18. Myler R K, Topol E J, Shaw R E, Stertzer S H, Clark D A, Fishman J, Murphy M C (1987) Multiple vessel coronary angioplasty: classification, results, and patterns of restenosis in 494 consecutive patients. *Cathet Cardiovasc Diagn* 13:1–15
19. Vandormael M G, Deligonul U, Kern M J et al (1987) Multilesion coronary angioplasty: clinical and angiographic follow-up. *J Am Coll Cardiol* 10:246–252
20. Serruys P W, Luijten H E, Beatt K J, Geuskens R, de Feyter P J, van den Brand M, Reiber J H C, ten Katen H, van Es G A, Hugenholtz P G (1988) Incidence of restenosis after successful coronary angioplasty: a time-related phenomenon. *Circulation* 77:361–371
21. Serruys P W, Rutsch W, Heyndrickx G R, Danchin N, Mast E G, Wijns W, Rensing B J, Vos J, Stibbe J (1991) Prevention of restenosis after percutaneous transluminal coronary angioplasty with Thromboxane A2 receptor blockade. A randomized, double-blind, placebo controlled trial. *Circulation* 84:1568–80
22. The MERCATOR study group (1992) Does the new angiotensin converting enzyme inhibitor cilazapril prevent restenosis after percutaneous transluminal coronary angioplasty? (in press)
23. Rensing B J, Hermans W R M, Deckers J W, de Feyter P J, Tijssen J G P, Serruys P W (1992) Luminal narrowing after percutaneous transluminal coronary balloon angioplasty follows a near Gaussian distribution. A quantitative angiographic study in 1445 successfully dilated lesions. *J Am Coll Cardiol* 19:939–45
24. King S B III, Weintraub W S, Xudong T, Hearn J, Douglas J S Jr (1991) Bimodal distribution of diameter stneosis 4–12 months after angioplasty. Implication for definitions and interpretations of restenosis. (abstract) *J Am Coll Cardiol* 17:345A
25. Hermans W R M, Rensing B J, Kelder J C, de Feyter P J, Serruys P W (1992) Postangioplasty restenosis rate between segments of the major coronary arteries. *Am J Cardiol* 69:194–200
26. Rensing B J, Hermans W R M, Vos J, Beatt K J, Bossuyt P, Rutsch W, Serruys P W (1992) Angiographic risk factors of luminal narrowing after coronary balloon angioplasty using balloon measurements to reflect stretch and elastic recoil at the dilatation site. *Am J Cardiol* 69:589–91
27. Sanborn T A, Faxon D P, Haudenschild C G, Gottsman S B, Ryan T J (1983) The mechanism of transluminal angioplasty: evidence for aneurysm formation in experimental atherosclerosis. *Circulation* 68:1136–1140
28. Rensing B J, Hermans W R M, Beatt K J, Laarman G J, Suryapranata H, van den Brand M, de Feyter P J, Serruys P W (1990) Quantitative angiographic assessment of elastic recoil after percutaneous transluminal coronary angioplasty. *Am J Cardiol* 66:1039–1044
29. Rensing B J, Hermans W R M, Strauss B H, Serruys P W (1991) Regional differences in elastic recoil after percutaneous transluminal coronary angioplasty: a quantitative angiographic study. *J Am Coll Cardiol* 1734B–38B
30. Hermans W R M, Rensing B J, Strauss B H, Serruys P W (1992) Methodological problems related to the quantitative assessment of stretch, elastic recoil and balloon-artery ratio. *Cathet Cardiovasc Diagn* (In press)
31. Hermans W R M, Rensing B J, Paameyer J, Reiber J H C, Serruys P W (1992) Experiences of a quantitative coronary angiographic core laboratory in restenosis prevention trials. In: Reiber JHC and Serruys PW (eds) *Advances in Quantitative Coronary Arteriography*, Kluwer Academic Publishers, Dordrecht (in press)
32. Beatt K J, Luijten H E, de Feyter P J, van den Brand M, Reiber J H C, Serruys P W (1988) Change in diameter of coronary artery segments adjacent to stenosis after percutaneous transluminal coronary angioplasty: failure of percent diameter stenosis measurement to reflect morphologic changes induced by balloon dilatation. *J Am Coll Cardiol* 12:315–323
33. Serruys P W, Reiber J H C, Wijns W, van der Brand M, Kooijman C J, ten Katen H J, Hugenholtz P G (1984) Assessment of percutaneous transluminal coronary angioplasty by quantitative coronary angiography: Diameter versus densitometric area measurements. *Am J Cardiol* 54:482–488
34. Serruys P W, Strauss B H, Beatt K J, Bertrand M, Puel J, Rickards A F, Kappenberger

L, Meier B, Goy J J, Vogt P, Sigwart U (1991) Angiographic follow-up after placement of a self-expanding coronary stent. *New Engl J Med* 324:13–17

35. Serruys P W, Juilliere Y, Bertrand M E, Puel J, Rickards A F, Sigwart U (1988) Additional improvement of stenosis geometry in human coronary arteries by stenting after balloon dilatation. *Am J Cardiol* 61:71G–76G

36. Puel J, Juilliere Y, Bertrand M E, Rickards A F, Sigwart U, Serruys P W (1988) Early and late assessment of stenosis geometry after coronary arterial stenting. *Am J Cardiol* 61:546–553

37. Serruys P W, Strauss B H, van Beusekom H M, van der Giessen W J (1991) Stenting of coronary arteries. Has a modern Pandora's box been opened? *J Am Coll Cardiol* 17:143B–154B

38. Serruys P W, de Jaegere P, Bertrand M, Kober G, Marquis J-F, Piessens J, Uebis R, Valeix B, Wiegland V (1991) Morphologic change of coronary artery stenosis with the Medtronic Wiktor™ stent. Initial results from the core laboratory for quantitative angiography. *Cathet Cardiovasc Diagn* 24:237–245

39. Strauss B H, Julliere Y, Rensing B J, Reiber J H C, Serruys P W (1991) Edge detection versus densitometry for assessing coronary stenting quantitatively. *Am J Cardiol* 67:484–490

40. Strauss B H, Rensing B J, den Boer A, van der Giessen W J, Reiber J H C, Serruys P W (1991) Do stents interfere with the densitometric assessment of a coronary artery lesion? *Cathet Cardiovasc Diagn* 24:259–264

41. Serruys P W, Umans V A W M, Strauss B H, van Suylen R J, de Feyter P J (1991) Percutaneous directional coronary atherectomy: Short-term clinical and angiographic results. *Br Heart J* 66:122–129

42. Umans V A, Strauss B H, de Feyter P J, Serruys P W (1991) Edge detection versus videodensitometry for quantitative angiographic assessment of directional coronary atherectomy. *Am J Cardiol* 68:534–539

43. Penny W F, Schmidt D A, Safian R D, Erny R E, Baim D S (1991) Insights into the mechanism of luminal improvement after directional coronary atherectomy. *Am J Cardiol* 67:435–437

44. Umans V A, Haine E, Renkin J, de Feyter P J, Wijns W, Serruys P W (1992) On the mechanism of directional cornary atherectomy. *European Heart Journal* (submitted)

45. Laarman G J, Serruys P W, de Feyter P J (1990) Percutaneous coronary rotational atherectomy (Rotablator). *Netherlands J Cardiol* 6:177–183

46. Gijsbers G H M, Spranger R L H, Keijzer M, de Bakker J M T, van Leeuwen G, Verdaasdonk R M, Borst C, van Gemert M J C (1990) Some laser-tissue interactions in 308 nm excimer laser coronary angioplasty. *J Interven Cardiol* 3:231–241

47. Kalbfleisch S J, McGillem M J, Simon S B, Deboe S F, Pinto I M F, Mancini G B J (1990) Automated quantitation of indexes of coronary lesion complexity: comparison between patients with stable and unstable angina. *Circulation* 82:439–447

48. Beatt K J, Serruys P W, Strauss B H, Suryapranata H, de Feyter P J, van den Brand M (1991) Comparative index for assessing the results of interventional devices in coronary angioplasty. *Eur Heart J* 12[abstract supplement]:395

49. Umans V A W M, Strauss B H, Rensing B J W M, de Jaegere P, de Feyter P J, Serruys P W (1991) Comparative angiographic quantitative analysis of the immediate efficacy of coronary atherectomy with balloon angioplasty, stenting, and rotational ablation. *Am Heart J* 122:836–43

50. Umans V A W M, Beatt K J, Rensing B J W M, Hermans W R M, de Feyter P J, Serruys P W (1991) Comparative quantitative angiographic analysis of directional coronary atherectomy and balloon angioplasty: a new methodologic approach. *Am J Cardiol* 68:1556–63

51. Strauss B H, Serruys P W, Bertrand M E, Puel J, Meier B, Goy J-J, Kappenberger L, Rickards A F, Sigwart U (1992) Quantitative angiographic follow-up of the coronary Wallstent in native vessels and bypass grafts: The European experience March 1986–March 1990. *Am J Cardiol* 69:475–481

PART TWO

Intravascular Imaging

Introduction – Historical Aspects of Intravascular Imaging

KLAAS BOM, CHARLES T. LANCÉE,
WILMA J. GUSSENHOVEN and JOS R.T.C. ROELANDT

Today's strong interest in catheter tip echography is based on the fact that apparently the therapeutic interventional methods are not yet optimal, or cannot be optimal without further knowledge of the obstruction and the arterial wall itself. With ultrasound catheter tip systems, cross-sectional images can become available. It is with this in mind that intravascular echography has been stimulated to overcome the apparent limitations in present new interventional techniques.

In the early period of diagnostic ultrasound, one of the compelling reasons for the intraluminal approach was the low sensitivity of existing echo transducers and, therefore the need to bring the transducer close to the organs to be studied. A number of parameters further favoured the intraluminal approach. With higher frequency, the wavelength becomes shorter. As a result the acoustic element can be small, still yielding a sufficient acoustic aperture in wavelength and thus acceptable beam characteristics. The axial resolution depends on pulse length. Therefore, the higher the frequency the shorter the pulse and thus the axial resolution increases. In diagnostic echography always the following compromise has to be made. An improvement in axial resolution by increasing frequency will, unfortunately, decrease the penetration depth due to attenuation of the signal. Due to the close approach to the reflecting structure, however, the increase in attenuation with frequency does not create a serious problem. For intravascular echo application at a frequency between 20 and 30 MHz and an acoustic element diameter of 1 mm, the order of magnitude for the axial resolution is 0.1 mm. The lateral resolution, depending on the gain setting, will be in the order of 0.3 to 0.5 mm. With such detailed information present in an arterial cross-sectional image combined with the unsolved questions around interventional methods, the interest in high frequency intravascular echography can be easily explained today.

*This chapter is in part based on "Early and Recent Intraluminal Ultrasound Devices" by N. Bom et al (1989) *Int J Cardiac Imag* 4:79–88.

P.W. Serruys, B.H. Strauss and S.B. King III (eds), Restenosis after Intervention with New Mechanical Devices, 53–61.

Between 1956 and 1968 a variety of catheter tip ultrasonic measurement devices were described. These designs were based on one-sided single element methods for feasibility tests in the heart (Cieszynski, 1); measurement of left ventricular size and septal thickness (Kossoff, 2); a two-element cavity diameter method (Peronneau, 3) and a non-directional cylindrical element left ventricular diameter measurement system (Carleton, 4). These first systems all operated with frequencies below 10 MHz and were limited to distance measurement capabilities. No imaging could be obtained.

It was well known that frequency shift in reflected ultrasound waves may be used to measure blood velocity. With two transducer elements, one for transmission and one for reception, the so-called continuous wave Doppler technique was introduced. Already in 1967 Stegall (5) described a catheter for Doppler measurement of instantaneous phasic coronary blood velocity. Pulsed Doppler followed as described by Reid in 1974 (6). Measurements were made in coronary and femoral arteries in dogs. Smaller sizes such as 5F and high frequency were introduced by Hartley (7) in the same year. He suggested the use of an annular element, which allowed Sibley to combine this with a guide wire in 1986 (8) and Serruys (9) to suggest a further combination with dilatation balloon.

Although mechanical rotation for imaging was introduced earlier, Gichard (10) first described a catheter construction with a rotating echo element mounted on a flexible shaft for Doppler purposes in 1975. Diameter of the probe was 3 mm. Further concepts include work by Martin (11) to combine a forward looking Doppler with transverse vessel area measurement in order to calculate blood flow. In Fig. 1 the principal configurations as suggested by these early workers have been illustrated.

Today Doppler catheters are commercially available and have been shown to measure instantaneous blood velocity accurately. They have been of great value in studying coronary physiology and pathophysiology in man. However, because of uncontrollable factors affecting the measurements, care should be taken if treatment decisions are to be based on peak-to-resting velocity value as was concluded in a recent article by Hartley (12).

In Fig. 2, some of the early scientists who designed systems for cross-sectional intraluminal imaging have been schematically listed for the period from 1955 up to 1971. The first approaches were based on mechanically rotating transducers as described by Wild (13) in 1955 for rectal tumour location and Omoto (14) for study of cardiac structures. Ebina (15) developed a miniature concave transducer for rotation inside a rubber cuff in the oesophagus in 1964. Wells (16) designed a variation for intravenous ultrasonic cross-sectional imaging based on a rotating mirror in 1965. These systems were all based on mechanical rotation of the transducer itself or rotation of a mirror. Thereafter, an intermediate step based on rotation of a 4-element catheter for approximation of cardiac cross-section was suggested by Eggleton (17). The result of his system depended on a stable state of the heart, since he accumulated data over many beats for reconstruction of a cross-

INTRAVASCULAR DOPPLER

Stegall	1967	continuous wave	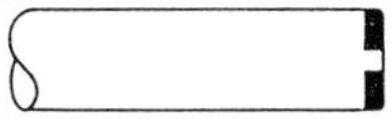	8 MHz Fr 7-8
Reid	1974	pulsed	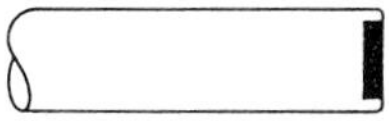	Fr 7
Hartley	1974	pulsed annular element		20 MHz Fr 5
Gichard	1975	rotating tip	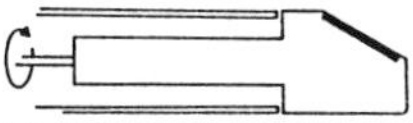	20 MHz
Martin	1975	vessel area and Doppler	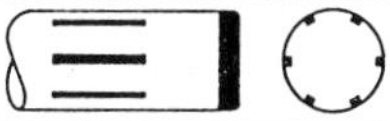	15 MHz Fr 7
Sibley	1986	with guidewire	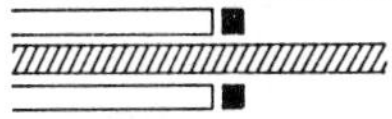	20 MHz Fr 3-4
Serruys	1988	with guidewire and balloon	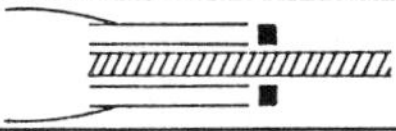	20 MHz Fr 3

Figure 1. Schematic display of early and more recent intravascular catheter tip Doppler systems (see refs. 5, 6, 7, 10, 11, 8 and 9).

section in a selected steady state. The first phased array multiple element approach for real-time cross-sectional imaging for intraluminal application was described by Bom in 1971 (18). A 32-element circular phased array with outer diameter of 3.2 mm mounted on the tip of a 9F catheter was constructed. With a frequency of 5.6 MHz and a frame rate of 190 frames/second, real-time cross-sectional images could be obtained without mechanical motion of the transducer elements.

INTRALUMINAL IMAGING

Wild	1955	echo-endoscope	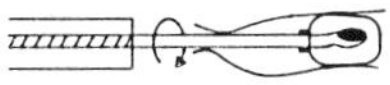	rectal tumour location
Omoto	1962	rotating probe C-scan	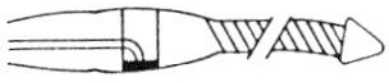	intracardiac tomography
Ebina	1964	transesophageal P.P.I. scanning	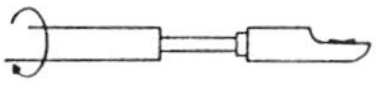	heart and vessels
Wells	1965	rotating mirror	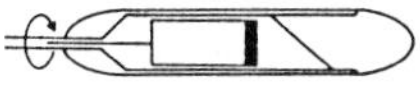	intravenous
Eggleton	1969	4-elements e.c.g. triggered	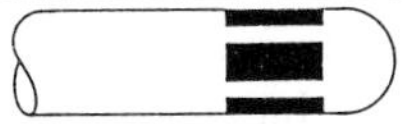	heart
Bom	1971	32-elements cylindrical phased array	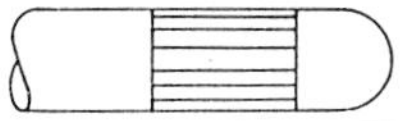	intracardiac tomography

Figure 2. Schematic display of early intraluminal imaging systems based on transducer rotation; mirror rotation and phased array principle (see refs. 13, 14, 15, 16, 17, 18).

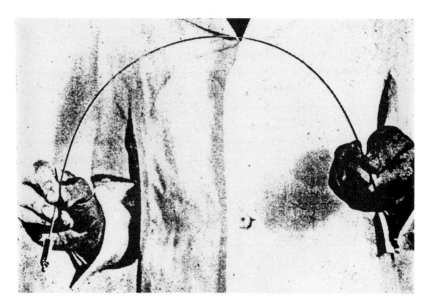

Figure 3. Intravenous probe with flexible shaft as described by Wells in 1966 (see ref. 16).

Today's intravascular imaging catheters are based on
1. a rotating tip system where a very flexible drive shaft contains the electric wire for the transducer and the transducer rotates together with this shaft;
2. an almost identical system which is based on a fixed acoustic element and a rotating mirror, or
3. an electronically switched phased array where a number of elements have been cylindrically mounted on the outer boundary of the catheter.

From Fig. 2 it can be seen that all three principles as quoted above had been incorporated already between 1955 and 1971. In the following, two examples of this early work are briefly described.

As illustrated in Fig. 3, Wells already described an intraluminal probe for intravenous application and he wrote "The probe must be of sufficiently small dimensions to permit easy insertion into the vein, and its driving rod must be flexible while possessing enough torsional rigidity to allow the probe to be rotated without excessive jerking or lagging" and "the idea is to use a transducer lying in the axis of the probe, and to deflect the beam radially through the shell by means of a reflector." He also stressed the need for an acoustically transparent dome as is presently used. In Fig. 4, an illustration of the 32-element's cylindrical phased array as developed by Bom in 1971 is shown. The outer diameter is 3 mm and the 32 elements were constructed by cutting a piezoelectric cylinder lengthwise by means of a wire saw. Fig. 5 shows a small part from the front of the wire saw, indicating the cylinder (arrow) in the cutting area. Tungsten wires with a diameter of 30 μm would yield an element separation width of 50 μm. The sawing procedure for a

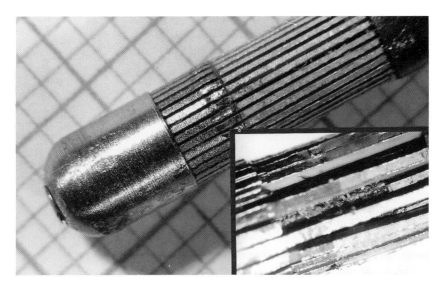

Figure 4. Phased array 32–element catheter tip after successful and unsuccessful (see insert) separation of elements with a wire saw (see ref. 18).

single catheter took 16 hours! Development of this cutting technique took in itself five years and was at first not always successful (see insert of Fig. 4). Obviously the fabrication method such as indicated with a wire saw is extremely complex and not fit for mass production. Today's approach is therefore based on cylindrical PVDF-foil where the elements are created by the electrodes only without cutting the material as such. Development of this phased array intraluminal probe was not based on the need to support interventional techniques which were not present at that time, but was based on the doubt that high quality non-invasive cardiac imaging would not work. History over the last decade has shown that these doubts were unrealistic.

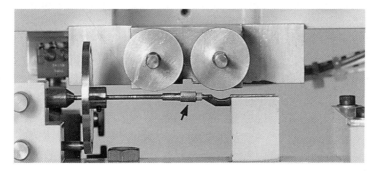

Figure 5. Close-up of the sawing area of the wire saw. Ceramic cylindrical element and single wire are indicated by the arrow (see text).

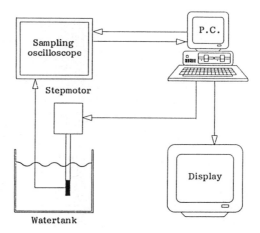

Figure 6. Schematic instrument set-up of first 40 MHz in vitro measurements in arterial segments obtained at autopsy.

When it became apparent that high frequency small catheter tip systems might indeed become of high diagnostic value to optimize therapeutic intervention in a number of laboratories, rather simple in-vitro test set-ups were developed. Parameters were: frequency 20–40 MHz; element diameter 1 mm; step motor rotation to build up cross-sectional images and sampling of the echo at 100 MHz for imaging in 512 × 512 8-bits video memory with

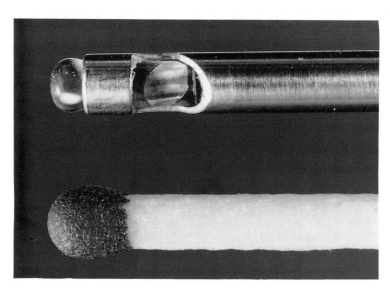

Figure 7. Close-up of the tip of a transducer holder with mirror as used in the set-up illustrated in Fig. 6.

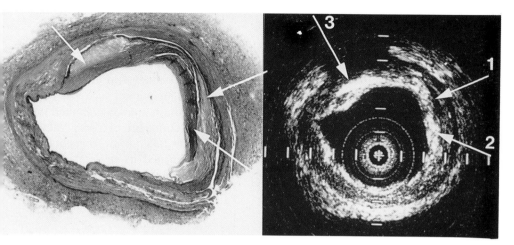

Figure 8. Comparison of histology and corresponding cross-sectional echo image as obtained in vitro.

many grey scales. The schematic diagram of such a test set-up is shown in Fig. 6. The stiff transducer holder with mirror is illustrated in Fig. 7.

Phased array catheter tip approach today incorporates image reconstruction software. Also much research has been devoted to the mechanical drive system. Rotation power from a proximally mounted motor is transferred via the flexible shaft to the rotating echo tip or mirror. In practice this tip does not identically follow the rotation of the motor which may create artifacts in the display. A compromise is necessary between the required low flexural rigidity and high torsional rigidity. A solution for this problem as suggested by Martin [19] was a two-layer helically wound coaxial drive. Similar approaches seem to have minimized this problem.

All this has led to today's high quality intravascular images. As an example an in-vitro observation as obtained with a 30 MHz intravascular catheter system (Du-MED) is illustrated in Fig. 8. The cross-sectional echogram and the corresponding histologic cross-section obtained in the superficial femoral artery is illustrated. Studies [20] have shown that the wall of a muscular artery presents as a typical three-layered structure: a hypoechoic media amidst the internal elastic lamina and the adventitia, both showing bright echoes whereas, conversely, an elastic artery is recognized by absence of this typical hypoechoic media. In Fig. 8, the typical muscular artery cross-section is shown, but in addition a hypoechoic area inside the lesion (arrow 1) indicates a large amount of lipid in the atheroma and a fibrous cap (arrow 2) and a calcified area with bright echoes prior to a shadow zone (arrow 3) can be recognized. Further diffuse intimal thickening as a zone of intermingled soft and bright echoes attached to the medial surface can be recognized.

Conclusion

Over the years many attempts to use intraluminal echography have been made. All these ideas from many early researchers in the field of diagnostic ultrasound have been a basis for the present developments in intravascular catheter tip echography. Only when interventional techniques such as PTCA were introduced and thus the clinical need arose, the researchers applied the vast amount of knowledge available to the development of these "new" exciting devices. For all new echo techniques, it has taken some years before the method became well known and one had learned its optimal clinical application. Intravascular echography will not be an exception.

Acknowledgements

Echo catheter research has been supported in part by The Interuniversity Cardiology Institute, the Netherlands Technology Foundation (STW, Grant RGN79.1257) and by Du-MED, Rotterdam, the Netherlands.

References

1. Cieszynski T (1960) Intracardiac method for the investigation of structure of the heart with the aid of ultrasonics. *Arch Immun Ter Dow* 8:551–557
2. Kossoff G (1966) Diagnostic applications of ultrasound in cardiology. *Australas Radiol* X:101–106
3. Peronneau P (1970) Catheter with piezoelectric transducer. U.S. Patent No. 3,542,014
4. Carleton R A, Sessions R W, Graettinger J S (1969) Diameter of heart measured by intracavitary ultrasound. *Med Res Engng* May/June:28–32
5. Stegall H F, Stone H L, Bishop V S, Laenger C (1967) A catheter-tip pressure and velocity sensor. *Proc 20th Ann Conf Eng Med Biol* 27:4 (abstract)
6. Reid J M, Davis D L, Ricketts H J, Spencer M P (1974) A new Doppler flowmeter system and its operation with catheter mounted transducers. In: RS Reneman (ed) *Cardiovascular Applications of Ultrasound*, North-Holland Publishing Co, Amsterdam/London, 183–192
7. Hartley C J, Cole J S (1974) A single-crystal ultrasonic catheter-tip velocity probe. *Med Instrum* 8:241–243
8. Sibley D H, Millar H D, Hartley C J, Whitlow P L (1986) Subselective measurement of coronary blood flow velocity using a steerable Doppler catheter. *J Am Coll Cardiol* 8:1332–1340
9. Serruys P W, Jullière Y, Zijlstra F, Beatt K J, De Feyter P J, Suryapranata H, Van den Brand M, Roelandt J (1988) Coronary blood flow velocity during percutaneous transluminal coronary angioplasty as guide for assessment of the functional result. *Am J Cardiol* 61:253–259
10. Gichard F D, Auth D C (1975) Development of a mechanically scanned Doppler blood flow catheter. *IEEE Ultrasonics Symp Proc*:306–309
11. Martin R W, Pollack G H, Phillips J (1975) An ultrasonic catheter tip instrument for measuring volume blood flow. *IEEE Ultrasonics Symp Proc*:301–305
12. Hartley C J (1989) Review of intracoronary Doppler catheters. *Int J Cardiac Imag* 4:159–168

13. Wild J J, Reid J M (1955) Ultrasonic rectal endoscope for tumor location. *Am Inst Ultrasonics Med* 4:59
14. Omoto R (1991) Intracardiac scanning of the heart with the aid of ultrasonic intravenous probe. *Jap Heart J* 8:569–581
15. Ebina T, Oka S, Tanaka M, Kosaka S, Kikuchi Y, Uchida R, Hagiwara Y (1965) The diagnostic application of ultrasound to the disease in mediastinal organs. Ultrasonotomography for the heart and great vessels. *Sci Rep Res Inst Tohoku Univ* 12:199–212
16. Wells P N T (1966) Developments in Medical Ultrasonics. *World Medical Electronics, Official Proceedings* Part 12
17. Eggleton R C, Townsend C, Kossoff G, Herrick J, Hunt R, Templeton G, Mitchell JH (1969) Computerised ultrasonic visualization of dynamic ventricular configurations. *8th ICMBE*, Palmer House, Chicago IL, July 1969, Session 10–3
18. Bom N, Lancée C T, Van Egmond F C (1972) An ultrasonic intracardiac scanner. *Ultrasonics* 10:72–76
19. Martin R W, Johnson C C (1989) Design characteristics for intravascular ultrasonic catheters. *Int J Cardiac Imag* 4:201–216
20. Gussenhoven W J, Essed C E, Frietman P, Mastik F, Lancée C T, Slager C, Serruys P, Gerritsen P, Pieterman H, Bom N (1989) Intravascular echographic assessment of vessel wall characteristics: a correlation with histology. *Int J Cardiac Imag* 4:105–116

2. Potential of Intravascular Ultrasound Imaging in the Evaluation of Morphology, Elastic Properties and Vasomotor Function of Coronary Arteries

NATESA G. PANDIAN, TSUI-LIEU HSU and ANDREW WEINTRAUB

Introduction

With rapidly evolving advances in the use of catheter-based interventional procedures for the management of coronary arterial disease, it has become important to delineate the coronary anatomy with much greater detail than has been possible to date by selective angiography. Besides many well known limitations of coronary angiography, an important problem has been the inability to visualize the arterial wall and the atheroma directly [1,2]. The morphology of a coronary atherosclerotic lesion is a major determinant of the clinical expression of coronary artery disease. In addition, the lesion morphology is a determinant of the primary success or failure of interventional procedures such as balloon angioplasty, mechanical atherectomy or laser ablation of atheromatous lesions. The composition and architecture of the atheroma before and immediately after an intervention also dictate the likelihood of complications such as acute total occlusion of the coronary artery treated. While the development of restenosis after an intervention is reduced by multiple factors, the size of the vessel following catheter-based treatments and the morphologic disruptions caused by those procedures are also important factors in the occurrence of restenosis. Elastic properties of the diseased arterial wall and vasoconstriction also play a role in the evolution of restenosis and its clinical expression. The increasing realization that coronary arterial morphology carries important therapeutic and prognostic implication has fueled the attempts to develop methods that could display the artery in a morphologic and morphometric fashion. Intravascular ultrasound is ideally suited to provide such information [3–10].

Intravascular Ultrasound Depiction of Coronary Atherosclerosis

A number of investigators, using both mechanical single-element ultrasound catheters and synthetic aperture array multi-element devices, have docu-

P.W. Serruys, B.H. Strauss and S.B. King III (eds), Restenosis after Intervention with New Mechanical Devices, 63–71.

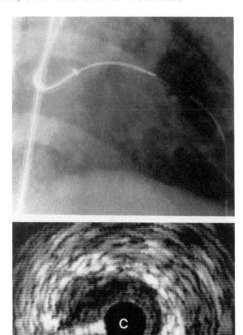

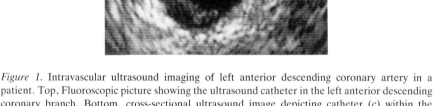

Figure 1. Intravascular ultrasound imaging of left anterior descending coronary artery in a patient. Top, Fluoroscopic picture showing the ultrasound catheter in the left anterior descending coronary branch. Bottom, cross-sectional ultrasound image depicting catheter (c) within the lumen, a discrete guide-wire signal and a soft atheromatous plaque from 6 o'clock to 11 o'clock.

mented that intravascular ultrasound imaging can provide detailed images in arterial circulation [11-16]. Both left and right coronary arteries can be imaged with ease and safety in humans in the catheterization laboratory (Figs. 1, 2). Recent advances in catheter technology allow for fabricating ultrasound catheters smaller than 4 F in size, allowing examination of not only proximal and mid-portions of the arteries but also of distal segments. Considerable in vitro and in vivo validation studies provide a morphologic background for quantitation of lumen area, wall thickness and atheroma size[17–22]. Importantly, intravascular ultrasound images of coronary arteries also allow characterization of the composition of atheromas. While a small intimal layer and a small hypoechoic medial layer are visualized in normal coronary arterial segments, atherosclerotic changes in diseased vessels display distinctly abnormal ultrasound patterns. (Figs. 3, 4) Calcific deposits produce very high intensity ultrasound signals with attenuation be-

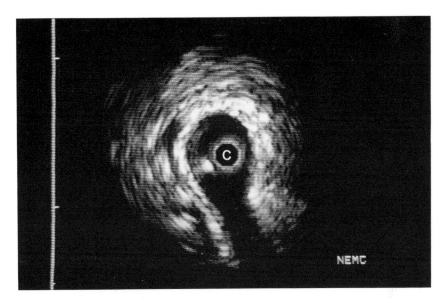

Figure 2. Intravascular ultrasound image of proximal left anterior coronary artery from another patient at the level of the origin of a diagonal branch. Except for the presence of a small, soft atheroma (8 o'clock to 10 o'clock position), the artery appears normal.

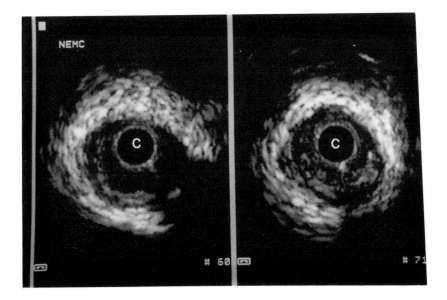

Figure 3. Intravascular ultrasound images of the left main coronary ostium (left) and the distal left main artery (right). In this patient with left main arterial stenosis, the lumen appears smaller in the left main caused by an eccentric atheroma which fills the major portion of the arterial cross-sectional area.

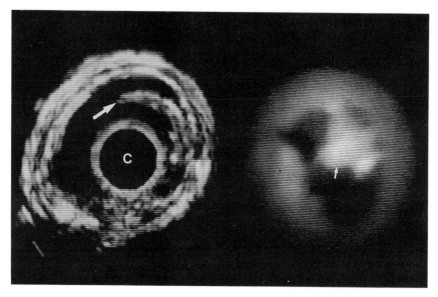

Figure 4. Intravascular ultrasound image (left) and fiberoptic angioscopic picture of a large intimal flap (arrow) protruding into the lumen.

yond the rim of calcium while predominantly fibrous atheromas result in bright ultrasound patterns without attenuation or shadowing. Predominantly soft atheromas, lipid deposits and intimal proliferation appear as less bright, soft patterns. Often there is a mixture of these various patterns since most atheromas encountered in symptomatic patients undergoing catheterization are rather advanced and complex. The unique strength of intravascular ultrasound technology in displaying lesion morphology overcomes the many drawbacks of coronary arteriography and points to a very useful potential in patients considered for interventional procedures and in the study of the problem of restenosis. The limitations of coronary arteriography are further compounded in the immediate post-angioplasty state by the disruptions in morphology caused by the dilation procedure. The edges of a lesion are often indistinctly seen in the post-angioplasty arteriogram thus precluding precise definition of the lesion morphology. The arteriographic criteria for identification of intimal flaps and thrombi are rather ambiguous [23–24]. Thus the arteriographic approach has been less than adequate and has been in use primarily for want of better techniques. It is now well known that the lesion morphology immediately after angioplasty is a major determinant of the likelihood of restenosis and also that the morphology of restenosis is different from primary atherosclerosis. It is in this area that intravascular ultrasound imaging has the potential to provide important morphologic information. The future approach to examining coronary arteries should include arteriography as a screening procedure and then intravascular ultrasound to examine the areas of interest in greater detail.

Study of the Mechanical Properties of Atheroma

A number of in vitro investigations of the atheroma and the arterial wall have demonstrated that both passive and active elastic properties of the wall change with the development of atherosclerotic plaques. Studies based on the morphologic findings suggest that the plaque rupture is believed to be the most important cause of acute coronary artery syndromes. However, the mechanism of plaque rupture remains unclear. When balloon angioplasty is performed, the stiffness of the atheromatous wall determines the likelihood and the pattern of intimal rupture, plaque cracks and luminal dilatation. The physical properties of atheroma are influenced by the composition of the atheroma. While one could intuitively postulate that calcific plaques are likely to be more stiff, a technique that could display the composition and architecture of the atheroma has not been available so far. A recent study by Lee et al explored whether intravascular ultrasound categorization of an atheroma based on the image appearance would correlate with its mechanical properties [25]. Fresh atheromatous caps obtained from 15 patients at autopsy were imaged by intravascular ultrasound and the atheromas were classified, based on their appearance on intravascular ultrasound, as predominantly fatty, fibrous or calcified. The stiffness (Young's modulus) of each atheroma was determined by an in vitro spectrometer set-up. Comparison of ultrasound image classification of the atheromas with the data on physical properties showed that fibrous atheroma caps demonstrated stiffness (in kilopascals) almost twice that of fatty caps and that calcific caps exhibited stiffness 6–7 times that of fatty caps. This study suggests that mechanical properties of human atherosclerotic tissue can be predicted by its appearance on intravascular ultrasound and that this imaging technology may be useful in understanding the mechanical stress in the plaque in vivo as well as in optimizing interventional strategies. Combined catheter devices that incorporate ultrasound elements within angioplasty, atherectomy and laser catheters would make imaging of a lesion easier not only before and after intervention but also during the actual procedure. Experience gained with these devices could not only help in guiding the procedure but also provide valuable knowledge on the actual in vivo mechanism of luminal dilatation.

Vasomotor Function of Normal and Atherosclerotic Coronary Arteries

Vasomotion and altered pharmacologic reactivity of the normal and diseased epicardial coronary arteries play an important role in the pathophysiology of coronary stenosis and its clinical expression. Furthermore, the early and late results of various interventional procedures are influenced by the vasoreactive state of the vessel treated. For the most part arteriographic methods have been employed to examine the effects of a variety of potent vasoactive substances which interact in the human coronary vascular smooth muscle. The pitfalls of angiography in interrogating vasoactive responses of coronary arterial circulation are well recognized. Some investigators use Doppler flow catheters to measure the coronary flow and flow reserve. This technique also has its inherent limitations [26]. Furthermore, it does not provide information helpful in understanding the relationship between vessel morphology and vasomotion. Intravascular ultrasound imaging may provide a new approach to the study of arterial pulsatility and distensibility in vivo and to examine vascular function at rest and following mechanical and pharmacological interventions. At this time, information on the morphologic basis for the functional alterations in the in vivo distensibility of atherosclerotic arteries is scant. To explore the impact of arteriosclerosis on arterial wall dynamics, Tutar et al analyzed the relationship between the presence and size of atheroma and the changes in regional and segmental arterial distensibility in humans [27]. From coaxial cross-sectional images, % segment wall expansion from a geometrically derived luminal center was measured along 3–4 radiants at multiple levels along the arterial long-axis. The % arterial distensibility was then correlated with the extent and composition of atheroma observed on the intravascular ultrasound images. The data from this study showed that % arterial distensibility was reduced in the presence of fibrous atheroma when compared to normal segments. Segments with calcific atheroma were almost adynamic. There was however no correlation between the thickness of the atheroma and arterial distensibility. This study yields in vivo information on the adverse impact of the composition of an atheroma on arterial wall dynamics. Gurley and associates, using a similar approach, examined the global and regional cross sectional area changes during the cardiac cycle in human coronary arteries [28]. They found a reduction in coronary vasomotion in patients with coronary atherosclerosis. In a well designed study, Sanzobrino and co-workers analyzed segmental vasoreactive response of diseased peripheral and coronary arteries to nitroglycerine in humans [29]. They noted that atheromatous quadrants exhibited markedly diminished vasodilatation while normal quadrants showed a good response. These investigations indicate that arterial pulsatility, distensibility and vasoreactivity are adversely affected by arteriosclerosis and that intravascular ultrasound technique is a potentially valuable approach to study dynamic arterial function in vivo in humans.

Three-Dimensional Intravascular Ultrasound Imaging

The ability to visualize a vessel in a three-dimensional orientation could have important diagnostic and therapeutic implications. Intravascular ultrasound provides an interesting and unique approach to such three-dimensional visualization. Sequential cross-sectional arterial images can be digitized, integrated into a three-dimensional matrix, volume-rendered and displayed maintaining quantitative accuracy and retaining gray scale information. The vessel can then be visualized in cross-sectional, longitudinal orthogonal and three-dimensional formats [30–31]. Attempts are also being made to develop on-line three-dimensional imaging. These developments could allow quick detailed examination of the arterial architecture of not only the vessel segment as a whole but also at any different level in any desired orientation. The cross-sectional and longitudinal size of atheromas, span of dissections and extent of thrombus could be assessed following an intervention. Importantly, such three-dimensional sizing of an atheroma could be extremely helpful in evaluating the progression and regression of atherosclerosis.

Conclusion

Using arteriography to assess the size, extent and shape of atheromatous coronary arteries is as refined or as crude as an orthopedic surgeon's observations on diseased or repaired bones. While selective arteriography will continue to play the vital role of identifying coronary arterial obstructions, intravascular ultrasound is likely to emerge as a critical adjuvant method to acquire structural, morphometric and functional information on the derangements associated with both primary and restenotic lesions. Ongoing refinements in ultrasound catheter technology and image processing underscore the availability of a valuable new tool that is likely to become the preferred vascular imaging method of the decade.

References

1. Pandian N G (1989) Intravascular and intracardiac ultrasound imaging: an old concept, now on the road to reality. *Circulation* 80:1091–1094
2. Yock P G, Linker D T (1990) Intravascular ultrasound. Looking below the surface of vascular disease. *Circulation* 81:1715–1718
3. Potkin B N, Bartorelli A L, Gessert J M, Neville R F, Almagor Y, Roberts W C, Leon M B (1990) Coronary artery imaging with intravascular high-frequency ultrasound. *Circulation* 81:1575–1585
4. Hodgson J M, Graham S P, Sheehan H, Savakus A D (1990) Percutaneous intracoronary ultrasound imaging: Initial applications in patients. *Echocardiography* 7:403–414
5. Tobis J M, Mallery J A, Gessert J M, Griffith J, Mahon D, Bessen M, Moriuchi M, McLeay L, McRae M, Henry W L (1989) Intravascular ultrasound cross-sectional arterial imaging before and after balloon angioplasty in vitro. *Circulation* 80:873–882
6. Yock P G, Linker D T, White N W et al (1989) Clinical applications of intravascular ultrasound imaging in atherectomy. *Int J Card Imaging* 4:117–125
7. Borst C, Rienks R, Mali W P T M, van Erven L (1989) Laser ablation and the need for intraarterial imaging. *Int J Card Imaging* 4:127–131.

8. Yock P G, Fitzgerald P J, Linker D T, Angelsen B A J (1991) Intravascular ultrasound guidance for catheter-based coronary interventions. *JACC* 17:(Suppl B) 39B–45B
9. Linker D T, Yock P G, Thapiiyal H V, Arenson J W, Johansen E, Gronningsater A, Lonstad H K, Angelsen B A J (1988) In vitro analysis of backscattered amplitude from normal and diseased arteries using a new intraluminal ultrasonic catheter. *JACC* 11:4A
10. Pandian N G, Kreis A, Brockway B, Isner J, Salem D, Sacharoff, Boleza E, Caro R (1988) Intraluminal ultrasound angioscopy of coronary arteries: in vitro (human) and in vivo (animal) studies. *Circulation* 78:11–84
11. Yock P G, Johnson E L, Linker D T (1989) Intravascular ultrasound: development and clinical potential *Am J Cardiac Imaging* 2:185–93
12. Pandian N G, Kreis A, Brockway B, Isner J M, Sacharoff A, Boleza E, Caro R, Muller D (1988) Ultrasound angioscopy: real-time, two-dimensional, intraluminal ultrasound imaging of blood vessels. *Am J Cardiol* 62:493–494
13. Hodgson J M, Graham S P, Savakus A D, Dame S G, Stephens D N, Brands D D, Sheehan H, Eberle M J (1989) Clinical percutaneous imaging of coronary anatomy using an over-the-wire ultrasound catheter system. *Int J Card Imaging* 4:187–193
14. Pandian N G, Kreis A, O'Donnell T (1989) Intravascular ultrasound estimation of arterial stenosis. *J Am Soc Echocardiography* 2:390–397
15. Gussenhoven E J, Essed C E, Lancee C T, Mastik F, Frietman P, Egmond F C V, Reiber J, Bosch H, Urk H V, Roelandt J, Bom N (1989) Arterial wall characteristics determined by intravascular ultrasound imaging: an in vitro study. *JACC* 14:947–952
16. Nissen S E, Grines C L, Gurley J C, Sublett K, Haynie D, Diaz C, Booth D C, DeMaria A N (1990) Application of a new phased-array ultrasound imaging catheter in the assessment of vascular dimensions. In vivo comparison to cineangiography. *Circulation* 81:660–666
17. Bartorelli A L, Potkin B N, Almagor Y, Keren G, Roberts W C, Leon M B (1990) Plaque characterization of atherosclerotic coronary arteries by intravascular ultrasound. *Echocardiography* 7:389–396
18. Nishimura R A, Kennedy K D, Warnes C A, Reeder G S, Holmes D R, Tajik A J (1990) Intravascular ultrasonography: image interpretation and limitations. *Echocardiography* 7:469–474
19. Pandian N G, Kreis A, Weintraub A, Motarjeme A, Desnoyers M, Isner J M, Salem D N (1990) Realtime intravascular ultrasound imaging in humans. *Am J Cardiol* 65:1392–1396
20. Nishimura R A, Edwards W D, Warnes C A, Reeder G S, Holmes D R, Tajik A J, Yock P G (1990) Intravascular ultrasound imaging: in vitro validation and pathologic correlation, *JACC* 16:145–154
21. Mallery J A, Tobis J M, Griffith J, Gessert J, McRae M, Moussabeck O, Bessen M, Moriuchi M, Henry W L (1990) Assessment of normal and atherosclerotic arterial wall thickness with an intravascular ultrasound imaging catheter. *Am Heart J* 119:1392–14
22. Tobis J M, Mallery J, Mahon P, Lehmann K, Zalesky P, Griffith J, Gessert J, Moriuchi M, McRae M, Dwyer M L, Greep N, Henry W L (1991) Intravascular ultrasound imaging of human coronary arteries in vivo: analysis of tissue characterizations with comparison to in vitro histological specimens. *Circulation* 83:913–926.
23. Pandian N G, Kreis A, Brockway B, Sacharoff A, Caro R (1990) Intravascular high-frequency two-dimensional ultrasound detection of arterial dissection and intimal flaps. *Am J Cardiol* 65:1278–1280
24. Pandian N G, Kreis A, Brockway B (1990) Detection of intraarterial thrombus by intravascular high-frequency ultrasound: in vitro and in vivo studies. *Am J Cardiol* 65:1280–1283
25. Lee R T, Richardson S G, Grodzinsky A J, Loree H M, Gharib S A, Tong L, Pandian N (1991) Prediction of mechanical properties of human atherosclerotic tissue by high-frequency intravascular ultrasound imaging. *JACC* 17:94A
26. White N W Jr, Yock P G (1989) Intravascular ultrasound: catheter-based Doppler and two-dimensional imaging. *Clin Cardiol* 7:525–535
27. Tutar A, Weintraub A, Chuttani K, Lee R, Pandian N (1991) Intravascular ultrasound study

of the impact of atherosclerosis on the in vivo regional and segmental arterial distensibility in humans: importance of atheroma composition. *JACC* 17:233A

28. Gurley J C, Nissen S E, Booth D C, Fischer C, DeMaria A N (1991) Reduction in global and regional coronary vasomotion: a descriptor of atherosclerosis by intravascular ultrasound. *JACC* 17:234A

29. Sanzobrino B W, Pachucki, Kiernan F J, Hirst J A, Primiano C A, Rinaldi M J, Pandian N G, McKay R G, Gillam L D (1990) Intravascular ultrasound assessment of reactivity of eccentrically diseased human arteries. (Abstract) *Circulation* 82:III–69

30. Burrell C J, Kitney R I, Rothman M T (1990) Intravascular ultrasound imaging and three-dimensional modelling of arteries. *Echocardiography* 7:475–484

31. Chandrasekaran K, Sehgal C M, Hsu T L, Katz S, Weintraub A, Mintz G, Elion J, Parisi A, Salem D, Pandian N (1991) Three-dimensional intravascular ultrasound imaging of arterial atherosclerosis and its complications: improved recognition of the atheroma bulk, the span of dissection and intimal flaps and the thrombus extent. *JACC* 17:233A

3. Intravascular Ultrasound Imaging Following Mechanical Coronary Interventions: Theoretic Advantages and Initial Clinical Experience

STEVEN E. NISSEN and JOHN C. GURLEY

Introduction

During the past decade, catheter-based mechanical interventions have emerged as the most frequently applied methods for revascularization in patients with coronary artery disease (CAD) surpassing bypass graft surgery in the number of procedures performed per annum. Although angioplasty has achieved widespread clinical acceptance, several problems continue to impede optimal application of catheter-based mechanical interventions. These include difficulty in selecting patients ideally suited for angioplasty, problems in assessing the adequacy of angiographic results, and limitations in predicting the long-term success of the procedure. Despite significant advances in the catheter equipment utilized for PTCA, technical developments have yielded little improvement in the incidence of restenosis.

Several of the limitations of catheter-based revascularization techniques can be directly or indirectly attributable to shortcomings of conventional radiographic imaging. Necropsy studies have demonstrated that the coronary stenoses are frequently complex and eccentric. Angiography portrays this complex coronary cross-sectional anatomy as a planar two dimensional silhouette of the vessel lumen. Current techniques for mechanical revascularization produce complex distortion of coronary intramural anatomy, a phenomenon that further impairs the accuracy of angiographic techniques. The advent of new interventional techniques such as atherectomy, laser ablation, and coronary stenting will present even greater challenges for coronary imaging.

Intravascular ultrasound generates detailed images of the lumen and arterial wall from a cross-sectional perspective. This tomographic orientation has the potential to offer important new insights into the mechanisms, complications and long-term results of mechanical interventions. However, there are important requisites for the acceptance of ultrasound as an alternative to radiographic coronary imaging. Clinical studies must demonstrate the safety and accuracy of intravascular ultrasound evaluation of the coronaries.

P. W. Serruys, B. H. Strauss and S. B. King III (eds), Restenosis after Intervention with New Mechanical Devices, 73–96.
© 1992 *Kluwer Academic Publishers. Printed in the Netherlands.*

Research must also overcome significant technical obstacles that impede routine application, particularly the large size and limited mechanical flexibility of the current devices. Ultimately, this new imaging modality must demonstrate the capability to significantly influence clinical decision-making.

Theoretical Limitations of Angiography in PTCA

During the initial decade of PTCA, cineangiography was the principle method used to select lesions suitable for treatment and to evaluate the results of interventional procedures. However, many investigators have questioned the accuracy and reproducibility of stenosis quantitation by angiography [1–9]. Several necropsy studies described important differences between angiographic and post-mortem stenosis severity, often reporting underestimation of lesion severity by radiographic methods [1–6]. Clinical studies have also repeatedly documented significant intra- and interobserver variability in the interpretation of coronary cineangiograms [7, 8]. More recently, studies have demonstrated major differences between the apparent angiographic severity of lesions and a physiologic measure of stenosis severity such as coronary hyperemic flow reserve [9].

Radiographic guidance of catheter-based revascularization has many theoretic and practical shortcomings. All mechanical revascularization procedures distort the coronary lumen creating complex fissures, cracks and dissections within the arterial wall. In the presence of complex alterations in luminal geometry, the planar orientation of angiography may significantly misrepresent the extent of luminal narrowing. Theoretically, two orthogonal angiograms should accurately reflect the severity of many lesions, but orthogonal views may be unobtainable because optimal imaging angles are unavailable because of overlapping sidebranches, disease at bifurcation sites and radiographic foreshortening. Even when orthogonal views are available, biplane angiography remains accurate only for relatively simple luminal shapes (Fig. 1A). Following mechanical interventions, no combination of angiographic views may accurately depict the extent of narrowing because of the complexity of the residual coronary lesion (Fig. 1B).

Traditional angiographic methods evaluate lesion severity by visual or computer assessment of the percent luminal area reduction. However, necropsy studies have demonstrated that coronary disease is usually diffuse and contains no truly normal segment from which to calculate percent stenosis [5]. In the setting of diffuse narrowing, angiographic assessment of percent luminal reduction will always underestimate lesion severity. In patients with atherosclerotic luminal encroachment, CAD also commonly produces "compensatory dilation" at other segments, a phenomenon known as "coronary remodelling" [10]. This outward expansion of the uninvolved vascular wall may lead to overestimation of the percent stenosis when an ectatic segment is used to determine luminal reduction for adjacent sites (Fig. 1C and D).

Lastly, angiography images only the vessel lumen - the intramural charac-

| Coronary Lumen | Tomographic Image | RAO Angiogram | LAO Angiogram |

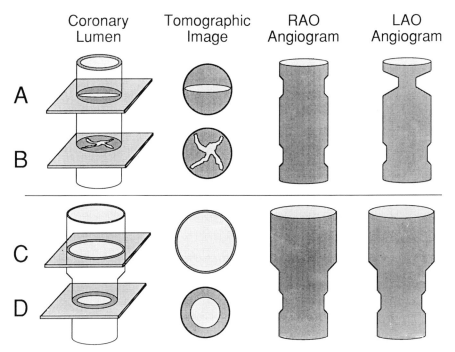

Figure 1. Schematic illustration of the differences between tomographic and silhouette imaging of the vascular structures. For elliptical narrowings (panel A), two angiographic views will provide accurate assessment of a stenosis. For complex lesions following PTCA, no angiographic projection will accurately depict the lesion (panel B). Ectasia of the coronary segment illustrated in panel C results in overestimation of the degree of stenosis for the adjacent segment in panel D.

teristics of atherosclerotic plaque are invisible to radiographic techniques. Thus, the true pathologic site of coronary atherosclerosis, the arterial wall, cannot be assessed by angiography before or after revascularization. Necropsy studies have demonstrated that plaque morphology is highly diverse and may involve a variety of tissue components including soft lipid accumulations as well as fibrous or fibrocalcific constituents [5, 11]. If the degree of luminal obstruction is similar, two morphologically different plaques will appear indistinguishable by angiography. It is likely that the natural history of atherosclerotic plaque is determined, at least in part, by their composition. Differences in plaques morphology may also be an important determinant of the response of the vessel to mechanical interventions.

Theoretical Advantages of Intravascular Ultrasound

Intravascular ultrasound has several theoretic and practical advantages in the evaluation of CAD following angioplasty. The tomographic perspective of intravascular ultrasound permits direct planimetry of the lumen area independent of the radiographic projection. Cross-sectional measurements should be accurate even when the coronary lesion is eccentric or the lumen distorted by mechanical revascularization. Tomographic imaging also permits evaluation of lesion severity for segments notoriously difficult to image radiographically, such as bifurcation sites and in arteries obscured by the presence of overlapping vessels. Ultrasound is also capable of imaging occult intramural atherosclerosis to identify diffuse coronary disease in angiographically "normal" segments.

The ability of ultrasound to penetrate tissue permits in vivo evaluation of the morphology of intramural atherosclerotic coronary plaques. Intravascular imaging provides quantitative measurements of normal and abnormal arterial anatomy, included the thickness and echogenicity of the vessel wall layers. Preliminary histologic studies have demonstrated significant differences in the acoustic impedance of the various plaque constituents thereby enabling classification of the morphology of vascular lesions [11–13].

Evaluation of the plaque characteristics within coronary lesions has the potential to provide unique insights into the pathophysiology and natural history of CAD. Ultrasound may enable identification of morphologic features that predict a high likelihood of plaque rupture and acute thrombotic occlusion. Similarly, it may be possible for characterization of lesion morphology to predict the propensity for restenosis following mechanical revascularization. Precise tomographic imaging of the anatomy of atherosclerotic plaques should also prove valuable in studies of atherosclerosis regression or progression.

Ultrasound Following PTCA: Technical Considerations

Many technical challenges have impeded development of intravascular ultrasound devices suitable for routine coronary imaging. The physical size of initial intravascular ultrasound devices (1.4 to 1.8 mm) is acceptable for peripheral vascular studies, but barely adequate for coronary evaluation. The normal first order coronary is 2–5 mm in diameter, but second-order vessels and atherosclerotic lumina exhibit diameters in the range of 0.1 to 2.0 mm. "Successful" angioplasty with a 2.0 mm balloon may leave a residual lumen of 1.5 mm or less. Thus, a practical coronary ultrasound device for post-PTCA imaging should be 1.0 mm or smaller in profile.

Safe imaging following PTCA requires a central lumen or monorail to enable "over-the-wire" exchange, a requirement that makes "down-sizing" more difficult. Intravascular ultrasound devices must also be flexible enough to permit safe passage through tortuous human coronaries without damaging the vessel endothelium. Mechanical flexibility also ensures that the catheter can be manoeuvered to a central and coaxial position in the vessel despite coronary tortuosity. Ease of positioning enhances image quality because the low acoustic power of intravascular ultrasound devices makes coaxial catheter position an important requisite of excellent images.

Most prototype intravascular ultrasound probes employ motorized rotation of the transducer or an acoustic mirror to achieve 360° cross-sectional images [14–18]. In clinical studies, we have utilized an alternative approach that employs a 20 MHz multi-element transducer array. (Endosonics Corp, Rancho Cordova CA) [19–21]. The device incorporates 64 annular elements within a 5.5 Fr (1.83 mm) transducer and contains no mechanical moving parts. The absence of a mechanical drive shaft enhances catheter flexibility and thereby improves trackability in tortuous coronaries. The catheter shaft is 4.5 Fr and accomodates a 0.014 inch central lumen guidewire to facilitate safe placement in the coronary. The device is sufficiently small to permit passage through a large lumen 8 Fr angioplasty guiding catheter.

Although multiple elements are used to reconstruct the image, the approach differs from the "phased-array" design commonly employed in transthoracic echocardiography. The transducer sequentially sends and receives ultrasound signals from each of the 64–elements. The resulting electronic signals are amplified and multiplexed by micro-miniaturized integrated circuits within the transducer assembly. The amplified signals are fiberoptically transmitted to a high-speed computer which performs image reconstruction using an algorithm known as a "synthetic aperture array". For pixels near the catheter surface, the computer reconstructs the gray value based upon data for only a few adjacent elements, whereas more distant targets utilize larger groups of elements. This variable aperture approach yields a device that remains dynamically focused from the surface of the catheter to infinity. The current computer enables real-time reconstruction of more than 1000 radial scan lines at 10 frames per second.

Safety of Coronary Intravascular Ultrasound

To achieve broad clinical acceptance, the safety of intravascular ultrasound must be demonstrated in a typical patient population undergoing routine diagnostic catheterization. Most investigators have limited coronary ultrasound to studies performed following interventional procedures such as balloon angioplasty [22]. In this setting, subselective coronary cannulation is performed for the purpose of angioplasty and intravascular ultrasound presumably does not constitute a major additional risk. Routine preinterventional coronary ultrasound requires safety data in patients in whom angioplasty is not a consideration.

We have now performed coronary intravascular ultrasound in more than 100 patients with CAD including 37 patients studied following balloon angioplasty. Because the current ultrasound catheter is 5.5 Fr (1.83 mm), we carefully avoided any potential reduction in coronary flow by restricting the study to vessels with a estimated diameter greater than 2.0 mm. The intravascular ultrasound probe was placed by a cardiologist thoroughly trained in interventional techniques. In initial studies, high-dose heparin (10,000 units) was administered, but subsequently, many patients were examined with a total dose of 3,000 units given at the start of the angiographic procedure.

The coronary was engaged with an 8 Fr large-lumen guiding catheter, a 0.014 inch angioplasty guidewire advanced into the distal coronary, and the ultrasound device passed over the wire subselectively into the vessel. The ability of the multi-element probe to accommodate a central lumen guidewire was advantageous, because handling and placement technique was similar to standard angioplasty methods. Some manipulation was employed to obtain optimal catheter positioning within the center of the vessel and orthogonal to the long axis.

Coronary intravascular ultrasound was well tolerated during routine catheterization. Occasionally, the device produced transient coronary occlusion when advanced into the distal vessel, but only one patient experienced chest pain. In each case, withdrawal of the catheter resulted in normal coronary flow. No other serious adverse effects were noted in this group except for transient coronary spasm in 6 patients, which responded promptly to sublingual or intracoronary nitroglycerin. A few patients developed groin hematomas at the sheath insertion site which may have been related to the requirement for an 8 Fr guiding catheter.

Subsequently, we expanded the indications for the procedure and studied patients admitted for acute coronary syndromes. A few patients were examined immediately (within 90 min) following acute myocardial infarction. Twenty-eight patients admitted for unstable angina were included, although most were stabilized with aggressive medical therapy prior to study. We also examined 12 patients with atypical chest pain and angiographically normal coronaries. The absence of serious complications in this diverse patient group establishes the safety of routine intravascular ultrasound imaging of coronaries performed during cardiac catheterization.

Coronary Dimensions and Stenosis Severity

In guiding interventional therapy, precise tomographic measurement of coronary dimensions represents an important potential application of intravascular ultrasound. Accordingly, comparative studies of angiography and ultrasound were performed to evaluate any systematic differences in the quantitation of coronary dimensions. For each patient, the intravascular device was positioned at a series of sites and ultrasound images continuously recorded on videotape. A cineangiogram was performed with the catheter in situ to document the precise coronary location of the ultrasound probe. This procedure yielded a series of ultrasound and angiographic images from identical sites for subsequent analysis.

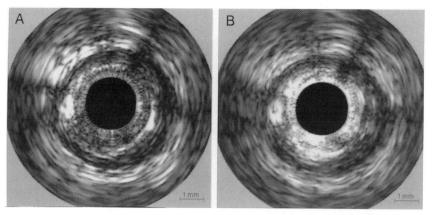

Figure 2. Intravascular ultrasound before (panel A) and after (panel B) injection of contrast. Luminal opacification aids in identifying the blood-intima interface.

For each examined site, vessel dimensions were determined for the angiographic projection demonstrating the minimum coronary diameter. To correct for radiographic magnification, the diameter of the guiding catheter was measured adjacent to the coronary ostium and compared with the known external dimensions of the catheter (2.67 mm). At stenosis sites, angiographic cross-sectional area reduction was calculated from diameter measurements.

Analysis of ultrasound images was performed using an array processor computer (Kontron Electronics) and custom software. This device contains 32 MB of video RAM permitting digitization and dynamic replay of 10 second intravascular ultrasound sequences. The minimum coronary diameter was measured with electronic calipers from a still-frame image. The interface between the lumen and vessel wall was planimetered to determine the cross-sectional area and perimeter of the lumen. Although measurements were performed using single digital stop-frames, the availability of a full motion sequence for review was an important adjunct to assist identification of luminal borders and confirm the location of vascular wall structures. In addition, injection of iodinated contrast media during imaging produced ultrasonic luminal opacification which assisted in the identification of the interface between lumen and vessel wall (Fig. 2).

Because atherosclerotic coronaries are frequently complex and eccentric, we anticipated that a tomographic imaging technique such as intravascular ultrasound might yield measurements that differed significantly from angiography. To test this hypothesis we compared angiographic and ultrasound dimension in subgroups of patients with and without coronary eccentricity as determined by intravascular ultrasound [23–25].

A standardized index of eccentricity, the circular shape factor, was utilized to classify the degree of deviation of the lumen cross-section from a perfect circle. The planimetered cross-sectional area was utilized to calculate a mean

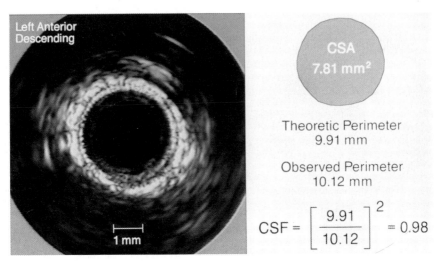

Figure 3. Coronary intravascular ultrasound and planimetered tracing of the lumen for a normal subject. Comparison of the theoretic and observed perimeters yields a measure of eccentricity, the circular shape factor (CSF). See text.

vessel diameter as $d = 2\sqrt{CSA/\pi}$ (where CSA = cross-sectional area). The perimeter for a perfect circle with this diameter was determined as $P = \pi d$ (where P = perimeter). This calculated perimeter was compared to the actual measured perimeter of the vessel lumen. This calculation yielded an index of eccentricity, the circular shape factor, defined as CSF = (calculated perimeter/observed perimeter)^2, where CSF = circular shape factor (Figure 3). This index yields a value of 1.0 for a perfect circle with smaller values indicating increasing eccentricity.

Subgroup analyses were performed for three patient cohorts–normal subjects, and CAD patients with concentric vs. eccentric lumens. In normals, we determined lumen shape (CSF) and compared measurements of lumen diameter by ultrasound and angiography. In these normal subjects, the circular shape factor averaged 0.92 ± 0.02, demonstrating that the lumen is nearly circular in the patients without coronary disease. In normals, the correlation between angiographic and ultrasound coronary diameter was close, r = 0.92, demonstrating concordance between planar and tomographic measurement for circular vessels.

In approximately two thirds of CAD patients, the lumen was concentric in shape (CSF > .92) and the correlation between ultrasound and angiography was also close, r = 0.93. However, the subgroup of CAD patients with an eccentric lumen (CSF < .92) demonstrated significant disagreement between angiographic and ultrasonic diameters, r = 0.78. We believe this reduced correlation is explained by the irregular, non-circular cross-sectional profile of the atherosclerotic vessels in CAD patients. These data demonstrate the potential superiority of a tomographic technique, such as intravascular ultrasound, in measurement of coronary dimension for the complex eccentric vessels commonly encountered in patients with atherosclerosis.

Focal luminal cross-sectional area reduction of 25% or greater was compared at 41 sites by cineangiography and 47 sites by ultrasound. For the lesions identified by both techniques, mean stenosis severity, expressed as percent luminal area reduction, was similar by cineangiography, $48.9 \pm 13.8\%$, and intravascular ultrasound, $52.3 \pm 16.3\%$ ($p = 0.10$). However, the correlation between percent stenosis by cineangiography and ultrasound was only moderate, $r = 0.63$. These data demonstrate major differences between ultrasonic and angiographic stenosis severity, presumably secondary to the limitations of angiographic measurements in complex lesions.

Minimum Luminal Diameter and Residual Stenosis Post-PTCA

Because of the differences between ultrasound and angiography observed in eccentric coronaries, we hypothesized that complex alterations in the cross-sectional profile of the coronary might significantly impair the accuracy of angiography. Therefore, in 27 patients, we compared luminal dimensions by angiography and intravascular ultrasound for residual lesions examined immediately following balloon angioplasty [26].

Post-PTCA, there was a very poor correlation between minimum luminal diameter by angiography and intravascular ultrasound, $r = 0.30$. Comparison of residual stenosis by angiography and ultrasound following angioplasty also revealed a poor correlation, $r = .54$. Similar findings have been reported by other groups for assessment of residual lesions following coronary angioplasty [22]. Because balloon dilation distorts the vessel lumen and wall, the reported differences between angiographic and ultrasonic measurements following angioplasty are not surprising. Theoretically, the tomographic perspective of intravascular ultrasound represents the more accurate approach.

The poor correlation between angiographic and ultrasonic dimensions post-PTCA has important clinical implications. In some cases, does "restenosis" sometimes represent a failure to adequately augment the lumen rather than late post-procedure proliferation of cellular elements? Can ultrasound assessment of the residual lumen predict early post-interventional complications and poor long-term results? Although large scale multi-center trials will be required to answer these important questions, our preliminary experience supports the promise of intravascular ultrasound to improve assessment of residual stenoses post-PTCA.

Normal Coronary Wall Morphology

Accurate interpretation of pathologic abnormalities in vessel morphology require a thorough understanding of normal ultrasound coronary anatomy. Significant alterations in ultrasound wall morphology are observed following removal and fixation of vessels [27]. Accordingly, we sought to determine anatomic features by imaging the coronaries in vivo for a cohort of normal subjects consisting of 12 patients with atypical chest pain in whom angiography demonstrated normal vessels. None of the normal subjects had a history of myocardial infarction, hypertension, diabetes, claudication, cerebral vascular events, valvular or congenital heart disease. None of the normal subjects had any physical findings of atherosclerosis.

Quantitative analysis of images for these normal vessels provided the basis for the recognition and classification of abnormal wall morphology in a larger group of patients with coronary disease. A total of 37 segments were available for analysis in the 12 normal subjects. Using digitized images, an electronic cursor was utilized to measure the maximal thickness of each of the characteristic vessel wall layers. The 95% confidence limits for each of these measurements provided a normal range from which to analyze coronary ultrasound images in the cohort of patients with CAD.

Subjects with normal coronaries exhibited characteristic wall morphology by intravascular ultrasound. A discrete linear ultrasonic reflectance was typically observed at the acoustic interface between the lumen and intima (Fig. 3). However, this layer was evident at only about two-thirds of the sites in the normals. Images frequently exhibited "drop-out" of endothelial reflections. Consequently, at nearly all the normal sites, any individual frame demonstrated a distinctly laminar structure of the vessel wall for only a portion of the circumference of the vessel.

For sites successfully measured, the maximum leading edge thickness averaged 0.18 ± 0.06 mm. A distinct sub-intimal sonolucent layer was also evident at a majority of sites with a maximal thickness averaging 0.11 ± 0.04 mm. This analysis yielded upper limits of 0.30 mm for the echogenic leading edge and 0.20 mm for the subintimal sonolucent zone. These wall morphology measurements demonstrate that the intimal leading edge and subadjacent sonolucent zones are thin and discrete in most normal subjects. Because of the minimal acoustic reflectance of normal intima, manipulation of the catheter and careful review of the dynamic imaging sequences were required to obtain optimal measurement of vessel wall structures.

Abnormal Wall Morphology: CAD Patients

In the coronary disease patients, a wall layer was classified as abnormal if its thickness was more than two standard deviations greater than the mean

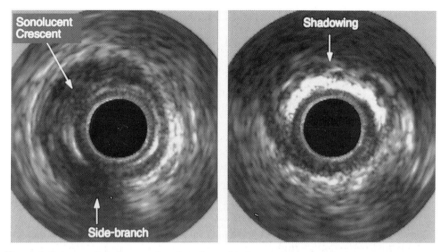

Figure 4. Intravascular ultrasound and angiographic images from two sites in the left anterior descending artery. In the top panels the arrows indicates the location of the ultrasound probe. In the bottom panels, the ultrasound images show a tri-laminar wall structure with a thick intimal leading edge and expanded sonolucent zone.

value obtained for normal subjects. Echogenicity of a wall layer was considered abnormal if the structure impeded transmission of ultrasound thus blocking visualization of underlying structures. Using these criteria, a variety of intravascular ultrasound abnormalities were documented at sites with apparent angiographic CAD.

Compared to normals, ultrasound "dropout" was less evident in diseased vessels, although severe atherosclerotic distortion of intramural anatomy precluded measurement of distinct vessel wall layers at every coronary site. In the coronary disease patients, both an intimal leading edge and a distinct subintimal sonolucent zone was measurable at more than 75% of sites. In segments with angiographic disease, the thickness of the intimal leading-edge was abnormally increased ($\geq$.30 mm) at more than 60% of measurable sites (Fig. 4). The maximal thickness of the sonolucent zone was abnormal ($\geq$0.20 mm) at more than 70% of CAD sites.

At segments containing an angiographic luminal irregularity, the most common morphologic appearance consisted of a crescentic sonolucent band encroaching upon the lumen (Fig. 4). Available evidence from in vitro studies suggests that these sonolucent crescents represent "soft", lipid-laden atherosclerotic plaque within the arterial wall [11–13]. Approximately 25% of diseased sites exhibited dense fibrocalcific intimal plaques that impeded ultrasound transmission thus shadowing underlying structures. These more echogenic "hard plaques" represent areas of greater intimal fibrosis with more specular ultrasound reflections [11–13]. In many patients, both lesions, thickening of the intimal leading-edge and broad sonolucent plaques, coexist at a single site or at different locations (Fig. 5).

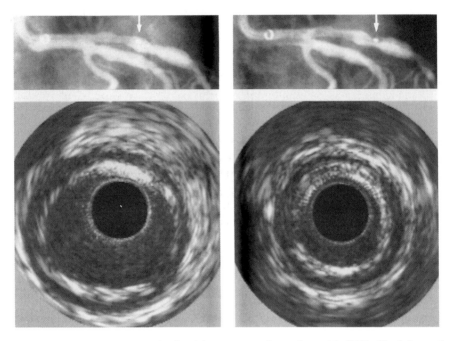

Figure 5. Two types of lesions in the right coronary of a patient with CAD. The left panel shows a large sonolucent crescent (soft plaque) while the right panel illustrates a fibrocalcific plaque that shadows underlying structures (hard plaque).

At some sites, the sonolucent band was thickened but symmetrical, lending a distinctive triple-layer appearance to the vessel (Fig. 5). This exaggerated tri-laminar appearance was not evident in any of the normal subjects. A third, deeper layer of the arterial wall was present at most coronary vascular sites and varied widely in appearance. A distinct interface at the trailing edge of this third layer was not apparent except within bypass grafts. Since this deeper layer likely represents the adventitia and other tissues encasing the vessel, the ambiguity of the trailing edge precludes measurement of total vessel wall thickness by intravascular ultrasound.

For segments with an angiographic luminal irregularity, more than 90% of sites demonstrated an abnormality of ultrasound wall morphology. These data demonstrate that intravascular ultrasound is a sensitive descriptor of coronary atherosclerosis. The high sensitivity of the technique makes ultrasound ideally suited for many research applications including regression-progression trials.

Wall Morphology: Angiographically Normal Sites

Because of the sensitivity of ultrasound in detecting abnormalities in patients with angiographic CAD, we sought to evaluate the utility of intravascular imaging in the detection of atherosclerotic disease at sites in which no lesion was present by angiography [28]. Using 95% confidence limits for thickness of wall structures in normal subjects, more than 75% of angiographically normal sites in CAD patients demonstrate abnormal wall thickness or echogenicity by intravascular ultrasound. In some patients with a few minimal luminal irregularities by angiography, intravascular ultrasound demonstrated CAD at nearly all other coronary sites.

The extraordinary extent of ultrasound abnormalities in angiographically normal vessels confirms the finding, previously reported from necropsy studies, that coronary disease is frequently more diffuse than apparent by angiography. In some cases, it was evident that preservation of angiographic lumen size was a consequence of compensatory remodelling of the vessel wall (Fig. 5). This finding confirms the observation that atherosclerosis can produce a variety of morphologic changes, including both luminal encroachment and luminal expansion [10]. Co-existing luminal expansion can obscure angiographic detection of CAD and impair accurate calculation of stenosis severity.

Wall Morphology Following Angioplasty

A diverse spectrum of morphologic findings were observed in patients following balloon angioplasty including complex cracks or splits in the vessel wall (Fig. 7). Measurements of luminal diameter and cross-sectional area following angioplasty were often smaller when determined by ultrasound in comparison to angiography ($p \leq .01$) [26]. These differences may represent an enhancement of the apparent angiographic diameter produced by extraluminal contrast within cracks or splits in the intima and/or media of the vessel wall. It is likely that a tomographic technique such as intravascular ultrasound is more accurate in determining the actual cross-sectional area following angioplasty.

Some investigators have speculated that intravascular ultrasound would be particularly valuable in detecting angioplasty-related complications such as dissection or intraluminal thrombus. Our angioplasty experience suggests that current technology does not yet provide this enhanced capability [26]. Following PTCA, it is difficult to distinguish therapeutic from pathologic dissection by intravascular ultrasound. Dissection planes may be difficult to differentiate from certain plaque features such as lipid laden plaques. In addition, the acoustic properties of intraluminal thrombus is similar to blood making it difficult to identify thrombi with certainty. Long-term studies to establish the relationship between ultrasound appearance and clinical outcome may resolve several of these ambiguities.

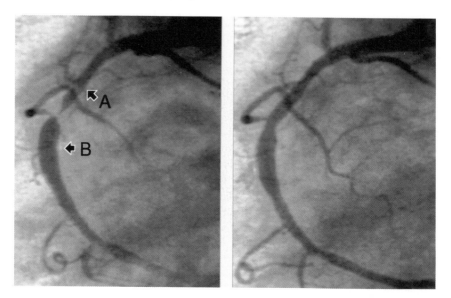

Figure 6. Right coronary artery before and after PTCA of a severe stenosis. The angiograms illustrate differences in lumen size for the segments proximal and distal to the lesion. See text.

Angioplasty Case Studies

Routine clinical application of intravascular ultrasound imaging will require demonstration of the value of the procedure in practical decision-making in the catheterization laboratory. From our initial experience with intravascular ultrasound following PTCA, several individual patient examinations clearly demonstrated the potential value of intraluminal imaging in guiding interventional therapy.

Case P.H. – Occult Diffuse Disease

Difficulty in determining optimal balloon size for angioplasty represents a common clinical problem in interventional practice. Figure 6 (left panel) illustrates the angiographic appearance of the right coronary artery prior to balloon angioplasty in a 51-year-old man admitted with unstable angina. Because of the severity of this stenosis, intravascular ultrasound with the current 5.5 Fr device was not feasible prior to PTCA. Accordingly, the operator (J.G.) determined appropriate balloon-sizing based solely upon the angiographic appearance of the vessel.

Quantitative analysis of the angiogram shown in Fig. 6 reveals a proximal, pre-stenotic coronary diameter of approximately 2.5 mm and a post stenotic lumen of 3.5 mm. There were two alternative possible explanations for the disparity in vessel size in the segments proximal and distal to the stenosis.

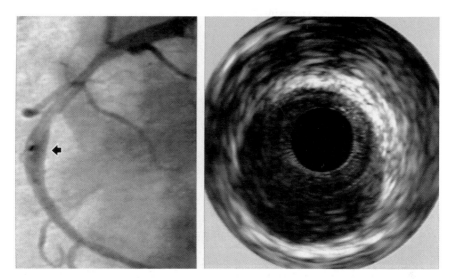

Figure 7. Angiography and intravascular ultrasound of the coronary distal to the dilated stenosis. The arrow indicates the ultrasound probe location. There is no atherosclerotic luminal encroachment. See text.

The large size of the post-stenotic vessel might represent coronary ectasia or, alternatively, the small size of the proximal vessel might represent diffuse disease. After consideration of this dilemma, the operator elected to dilate the lesion with a 2.5 mm balloon with the rationale that underdilation would represent a less potentially hazardous approach than overdilation.

After two inflations of the 2.5 mm balloon, the post-PTCA coronary angiogram in Fig. 6 (right panel) was obtained and interpreted as a satisfactory result. Following angioplasty, intravascular ultrasound was performed with the 5.5 Fr, 64-element probe. The ultrasound angiographic and ultrasound appearance of the post-stenotic vessel segment is shown in Fig. 7. The lumen exceeds 3.5 mm in diameter and demonstrates no atherosclerotic luminal encroachment. In the proximal vessel segment (Fig. 8), the ultrasound image demonstrates a large sonolucent plaque occupying approximately 50% of the lumen. Thus, the proximal segment utilized as the normal "reference" vessel for balloon sizing exhibits diffuse disease by intravascular ultrasound.

The angiographic and ultrasound appearance of the PTCA site is illustrated in Fig. 9. The ultrasound demonstrates a small lumen with a very large sonolucent plaque. The intimal leading edge is in contact with the external surface of the transducer, and the sonolucent plaque occupies nearly 75% of the lumen. Thus, at the site of this "successful" angioplasty, a large residual atheroma is evident in the ultrasound image. The short and long-term clinical implications of such residual lesions is unknown and therefore no further inflations were performed in this patient. However, the presence of

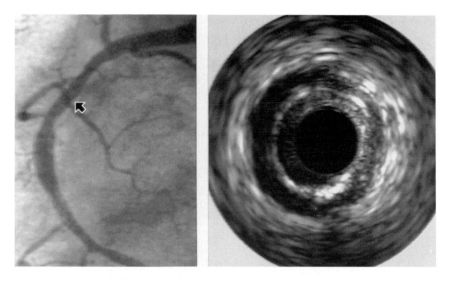

Figure 8. Intravascular ultrasound and angiography with the transducer in the proximal right coronary. The arrow indicates the site of imaging. The ultrasound image shows a large, concentric ultrasound plaque occupying more than 50% of the lumen. See text.

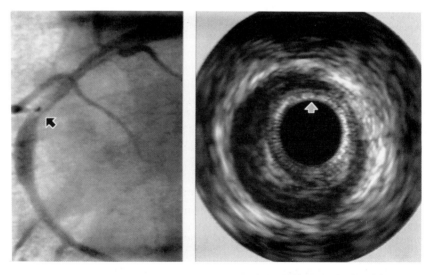

Figure 9. Angiography and intravascular ultrasound of the PTCA site in the right coronary artery. The black arrow indicates the site of imaging. The gray arrow identifies the intimal leading edge in close proximity to the surface of the catheter. The sonolucent atheroma occupies more than 70% of the lumen. See text.

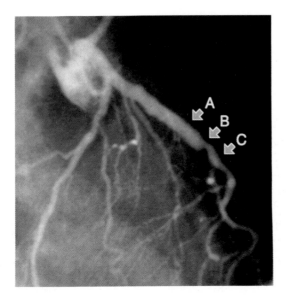

Figure 10. Angiogram of the left anterior descending in a patient referred for angioplasty. The stenosis (arrow B) is severe if percent luminal reduction is calculated using the proximal vessel (arrow A) as the reference segment. Comparison of the stenosis to the distal coronary (arrow C) yields a minimal percent reduction. See text.

such a large residual atheroma post-PTCA is disturbing and raises important questions regarding the adequacy of angiographic methods for evaluation of stenoses following mechanical interventions.

Patient F.W. – Pseudo-stenosis

Patient F.W. is a 54 year old female referred from an outside institution for balloon angioplasty of the left anterior descending coronary artery (LAD). Figure 10 illustrates an angiographic view of the LAD with a significant lesion graded as a 70% stenosis by the referring physician. However, the accuracy of the percent stenosis computation was problematic because of uncertainty whether the proximal pre-stenotic coronary (Site A) represents the true normal segment or is diffusely ectatic. If the post-stenotic coronary represents the "normal" segment (Site C), then the lesion may actually represent a minimal obstruction which appears more severe because of proximal ectasia.

Accordingly, intravascular ultrasound was performed prior to attempting PTCA. Figure 11 illustrates ultrasound images obtained from the proximal LAD and stenotic lesion. An abrupt reduction in the overall diameter of the external border of vessel is apparent near the site of the stenosis. This finding

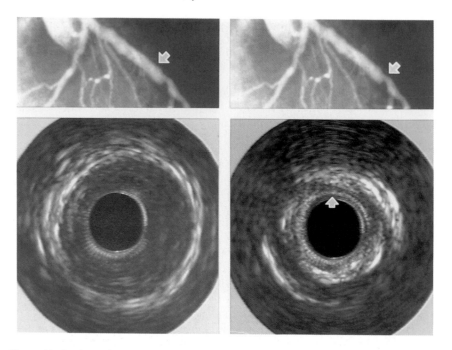

Figure 11. Angiography and intravascular ultrasound for the proximal LAD (left panel) and the tightest area of stenosis (right panel). The abrupt decrease in outer diameter of this vessel in the stenotic segment demonstrates that the proximal vessel is ectatic. Ectasia in the reference segment results in overestimation of stenosis severity.

provides strong evidence for ectasia of the proximal vessel since coronaries normally taper gradually from proximal to distal.

Advance of the ultrasound probe through the stenosis provided further confirmatory evidence of this phenomenon. Figure 12 illustrates ultrasound images obtained from the stenosis site and slightly distal to the lesion. The post- stenotic segment is nearly disease-free and when this site is utilized for comparative measurements, percent stenosis is less than 30%. Consequently, PTCA was not performed and measurement of trans-lesional gradient was performed under resting conditions and following induction of hyperemia with papaverine. The gradient was less than 10 mm Hg before and after papaverine, providing additional evidence of non-critical disease.

Case F.W. illustrates the difficulty in evaluating coronary disease by measurements of percent stenosis using angiographic luminal diameters. Atherosclerotic remodelling of the arterial wall may produce vessel ectasia as well

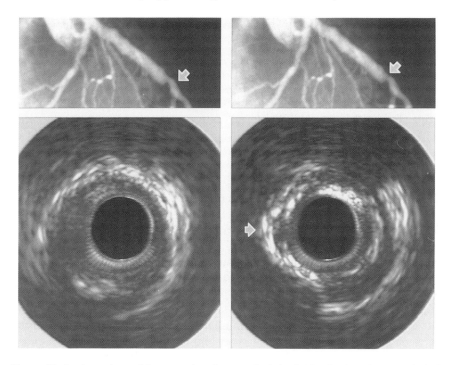

Figure 12. Angiography and intravascular ultrasound of the LAD distal to the stenosis (left panel) and within the stenosis (right panel). It is apparent from these ultrasound images that the degree of luminal area reduction is minimal for this lesion. See text.

as encroach upon the lumen. For any given segment, angiography is unable to discern the diameter of the "true normal" lumen and may therefore yield an erroneous impression of the extent of luminal narrowing.

Ultrasound Evaluation in PTCA: Current Status

Our initial experience supports an important potential role for intravascular ultrasound in the evaluation of PTCA results. Current ultrasound devices are sufficiently small to permit imaging of many, but not all, sites following successful angioplasty. The cross-sectional perspective of intravascular ultrasound is ideally suited for precision measurements of coronary luminal diameter and crosssectional area. Luminal size measurements post-procedure are often smaller and stenosis severity worse by intravascular ultrasound than angiography. These differences likely reflect augmentation of the "apparent" angiographic diameter by extra-luminal contrast within cracks, fissures or dissection planes. In the presence of complex alterations in the vessel wall, tomographic measurements by intravascular ultrasound are theoretically superior.

Identification of a truly normal reference segment for balloon sizing is a significant clinical problem in angioplasty. Intravascular ultrasound permits independent evaluation of the dimensions and extent of intramural disease in these "normal" segments and may prove a useful adjunct for balloon sizing. Images of atherosclerotic wall abnormalities provided by intracoronary ultrasound have the potential to greatly augment our understanding of anatomy and pathophysiology of CAD. Ultrasound is more sensitive than angiography in the detection of CAD and permits identification of the morphologic characteristics of plaques. Precision measurement of intramural atherosclerotic lesions may prove valuable in quantifying disease progression or regression.

The clinical value of routine ultrasound imaging following mechanical revascularization remains unproven. However, it seems likely that the morphology of the vessel wall following interventions will provide valuable insights into phenomena such as restenosis and abrupt occlusion. It also seems reasonable to anticipate that plaque characteristics will have some predictive value in defining the short-term and long-term results of revascularization procedures. However, a complete understanding of the relationship between intramural plaque morphology and complications such as restenosis will require careful long-term studies in large numbers of patients.

Current Artifacts and Other Ultrasound Limitations

All current intravascular ultrasound devices generate artifacts that may adversely affect image quality and/or quantitative accuracy. Mechanical transducers may exhibit cyclical oscillations in rotation speed caused by mechanical drag, particularly when the drive-shaft is bent by a tortuous coronary. The resulting non-uniform rotational velocity produces an unpredictable warping of the image. This distortion can be quite significant and may affect measurements of lumen size or alter the apparent location of structures.

High-amplitude ultrasound signals may obscure the near-field, a phenomenon known as transducer ring-down. Recent mechanical transducer designs employ a rotating acoustic mirror to permit a longer signal path from the ultrasound element to the vessel lumen. Electronic arrays must also eliminate ring-down, but the transducer elements are surface-mounted and it is therefore impossible to increase the signal path length. Our current multi-element device reduces ring-down by obtaining a reference image containing the ring-down artifact in a large vessel such as the aorta. The central portion of this reference image is subtracted in real-time from all subsequent frames to electronically remove the ring-down signal.

The physical size (5.5 Fr) of current devices does not permit imaging of small coronaries or tight stenoses and precludes examination of most lesions prior to balloon angioplasty. An additional limitation stems from the vulnerability of ultrasound techniques to distortion produced by imaging in a plane not orthogonal to the vessel walls. Thus, an artery with a circular lumen will appear elliptical when the transducer is obliquely oriented to the long axis of the vessel. This phenomenon can represent a significant confounding variable in quantitative measurements. It must also be emphasized that intravascular ultrasound relies upon differences in acoustic impedance of tissues to obtain images. Consequently, ultrasound can demonstrate the thickness and echogenicity of structures, but does not provide actual histology.

Current intravascular ultrasound devices employ very low acoustic power to produce images. Normal subjects often have an intimal leading-edge of minimal acoustic reflectance and this delicate interface may poorly reflect ultrasound, a phenomenon that leads to dropout of ultrasound signals. Although drop-out is frequently observed in normal segment, it is less prevalent in diseased vessels [23]. Heavily fibrotic or calcified intimal plaques can impede transmission of the low energy, high-frequency ultrasound signals utilized for intravascular imaging. The resultant "shadowing" by calcific plaque can obscure the underlying structure of the arterial wall. Shadowing plaques may also preclude measurement of atheroma area because the full thickness of the vessel wall is not imaged.

Future Research and Development

The technology for intravascular ultrasound examination of the coronaries is still rapidly evolving and future developments will likely expand the utility of intraluminal imaging following mechanical interventions. A new multi-element probe with a maximum diameter of 3.5 French (1.15 mm) is currently undergoing initial human testing. In vitro studies with this prototype device have yielded image quality as good or better than the current 5.5 Fr device.

Initial clinical testing is also currently underway using a combination device that incorporates both an angioplasty balloon and a 64-element transducer array. Preliminary experience indicates that ultrasound guidance of balloon dilation with this combination device is practical and convenient. Combined imaging and therapy devices have the potential to become the future standard for mechanical revascularization devices. Other current research projects include development of an imaging catheter that combines an ultrasound transducer with a Doppler flow probe to provide simultaneous cross-sectional area and flow velocity measurements. Such a device could provide continuous beat-to-beat assessment of coronary blood flow.

94   S.E. Nissen and J.C. Gurley

Summary and Conclusions

The development of small, flexible intravascular ultrasound devices permits routine assessment of the coronary lumen and vessel wall following mechanical interventions. Intraluminal coronary ultrasound is a safe procedure in clinically stable patients. The tomographic orientation of coronary ultrasound provides an advantageous perspective for measurement of the vessel dimensions. In diseased coronaries, lumen diameters by ultrasound frequently differ from angiographic measurements. These differences are particularly evident for eccentric vessels and for post-PTCA residual stenoses.

Intravascular ultrasound provides detailed images of coronary wall morphology not previously available in vivo. Normal subjects exhibit a thin intimal leading-edge (<.30 mm) and subadjacent sonolucent zone (≤.20 mm). CAD patients exhibit abnormal thickness of wall layers in both angiographically diseased and normal segments. The extent of intramural disease at angiographically normal sites demonstrates that intravascular ultrasound imaging is a sensitive descriptor of coronary atherosclerosis.

Cross-sectional anatomy following PTCA is highly complex, sometimes revealing fissures or dissection planes that impair the accuracy of angiographic measurements. Intravascular ultrasound often reveals large residual atheromata at the site of a "successful" angioplasty. Although the clinical importance of residual disease is unknown, our initial experience suggests an important role for intravascular ultrasound evaluation of the results of mechanical revascularization. Insights gained from studying angioplasty sites by intraluminal ultrasound have the potential to dramatically alter interventional practice.

References

1. Arnett E N, Isner J M, Redwood C R, Kent K M, Baker W P, Ackerstein H, Roberts W C (1979) Coronary artery narrowing in coronary heart disease: comparison of cineangiographic and necropsy findings. *Ann Intern Med* 1:350–356.
2. Grodin C M, Dydra I, Pastgernac A, Campeau L, Bourassa M G (1974) Discrepancies between cineangiographic and post-mortem findings in patients with coronary artery disease and recent myocardial revascularization. *Circulation* 49:703–709.
3. Blackenhorn D H, Curry P J (1982) The accuracy of arteriography and ultrasound imaging for atherosclerosis measurement: A review. *Arch Pathol Lab Med* 106:483–490.
4. Isner J M, Kishel J, Kent K M (1981) Accuracy of angiographic determination of left main coronary arterial narrowing. *Circulation* 63:1056–1061.
5. Roberts W C, Jones A A (1979) Quantitation of coronary arterial narrowing at necropsy in sudden coronary death. *Am J Cardiol* 44:39–44.
6. Vlodaver Z, Frech R, van Tassel R A, Edwards J E (1973) Correlation of the antemortem coronary angiogram and the postmortem specimen. *Circulation* 47:162–168.
7. Zir L M, Miller S W, Dinsmore R E, Gilbert J P, Harthorne J W (1976) Interobserver variabilty in coronary angiography. *Circulation* 53:627–632

8. Galbraith J E, Murphy M L Desoyza N (1981) Coronary angiogram interpretation: interob-server variability. *JAMA* 40:2053–2059
9. White C W, Wright C B, Doty D B, Hirtza L F, Eastham C L, Harrison D G, Marcus M L (1984) Does visual interpretation of the coronary arteriogram predict the physiologic importance of a coronary stenosis? *N Engl J Med* 310:819–24
10. Glagov S, Weisenberg E, Zarins C K (1987) Compensatory enlargement of human coronary arteries. *N Engl J Med* 316:1371–1375
11. Guessenhoven E J, Essed C E, Lancee C T, Mastik F, Frietman P, Van Egmond F C, Reiber J, Bosch H, Van Urk H, Roelandt J, Bom N (1989) Arterial wall characteristics determined by intravascular ultrasound imaging: an in vitro study. *JACC* 4:947–52
12. Potkin B N, Bartorelli A L, Gessert J M, Neville R F, Almagor Y, Roberts W C, Leon M B (1990) Coronary artery imaging with intravascular high-frequency ultrasound. *Circulation* 81:1575–1585
13. Nishimura R A, Edwards W D, Warnes C A, Reeder G S, Holmes D R, Tajik A J, Yock P G (1990) Intravascular ultrasound imaging: in vitro validation and pathologic correlation. *JACC* 16:145–154
14. Bom N, Lancee C T, Van Egmond F C (1972) An ultrasonic intracardiac scanner. *Ultrason-ics* 10:72–76
15. Yock P G, Johnson E L, Linker D T (1988) Intravascular ultrasound: development and clinical potential. *Am J Cardiac Imaging* 2:185–193
16. Pandian N G, Kreis A, Brockway B, Isner J M, Sacharoff A, Boleza E, Caro R, Muller D (1988) Ultrasound angioscopy: real-time, two-dimensional, intraluminal ultrasound imag-ing of blood vessels. *Am J Cardiol* 62:113–116
17. Roelandt J R, Bom N Y, Serruys P W (1989) Intravascular high-resolution real-time, two-dimensional echocardiography. *Int J Cardiac Imaging* 4:63–67
18. Bessen M, Moriushi M, McLeary L, McLeay L, McRae M, Henry W L (1989) Intravascular ultrasound cross-sectional arterial imaging before and after balloon angioplasty in vitro. *Circulation* 80:873–882
19. Nissen S E, Grines C L, Gurley J C, Sublett K, Haynie D, Diaz C, Booth D C, DeMaria A N (1990) Application of a new phased-array ultrasound imaging catheter in the assessment of vascular dimensions: in vivo comparison to cineangiography. *Circulation* 81(2):660–666
20. Hodgson J, Graham S P, Savakus A D, Dame S G, Stephens D N, Dhillion D, Brands DC, Sheehan H, Eberle M J (1989) Clinical percutaneous imaging of coronary anatomy using an over-the-wire ultrasound catheter system. *Int J of Cardiac Imaging* 4:187–193
21. Nissen S E, Gurley J C, DeMaria A N (1990) Assessment of vascular disease by intravascular ultrasound. *Cardiology* 77(5):398–410
22 Tobis J M, Mallery J, Mahon D, Lehmann K, Zalesky P, Griffith J, Gessert J, Moriuchi M, McRae M, Dwyer M L, Greep N, Henry W L (1991) Intravascular ultrasound imaging of human coronary arteries in vivo. *Circulation* 83:913–926
23. Nissen S E, Gurley J C, Grines C L, Booth D C, McClure R, Martin Berk M D, Fischer C, and Anthony N, DeMaria M D (1991) Intravascular ultrasound assessment of lumen size and wall morphology in normal subjects and coronary artery disease patients. *Circulation* (in press)
24. Nissen S E, Gurley J C, Booth D C, McClure R R, Berk M R, DeMaria A N (1991) Spectrum of intravascular ultrasound findings in atherosclerosis: wall morphology and lumen shape in CAD patients. *JACC* 17;2:93A
25. Nissen S E, Gurley J C, Grines C L, Booth D C, Fischer C, DeMaria A N (1990) Comparison of intravascular ultrasound and angiography in quantitation of coronary stenoses and dimensions in man: impact of lumen eccentricity. *Circulation* 82;4:III-440
26. Gurley J C, Nissen S E, Grines C L, Booth D C, Fischer C, DeMaria A N (1990) Comparison of intravascular ultrasound and angiography following percutaneous translumi-nal angioplasty. *Circulation* 82;4:III-72
27. Gurley J C, Nissen S E, Diaz C, Fischer C, O'Connor W N, DeMaria A N (1991) Is

the three-layer arterial appearance an artifact? Differences between in vivo and in vitro intravascular ultrasound. *JACC* 17;2:112A
28. Nissen S E, Gurley J C, Grines C L, Booth D C, Fischer C, DeMaria A N (1990) Coronary atherosclerosis is frequently present at angiographically normal sites: evidence from intravascular ultrasound in man. *Circulation* 82;4:*III*-459

4. Ultrasound Guidance for Catheter-based Plaque Removal and Ablation Techniques: Potential Impact on Restenosis

PAUL G. YOCK, PETER J. FITZGERALD, KRISHNANKUTTY SUDHIR, VICTOR K. HARGRAVE and THOMAS A. PORTS

In the past decade a variety of new catheter devices have been designed with the general goal of removing or ablating plaque from the vessel wall. As many as a dozen "atherectomy" or mechanical plaque removal devices are currently at some point in development, while at least seven companies have active laser catheter projects under way. All of these programs have been started in the hope of improving the results currently obtained with balloon angioplasty. Implicit in this hope is the concept that the elimination of plaque under controlled circumstances may help reduce the rates of abrupt closure and restenosis.

The ultimate goal for any of these devices is to be able to remove plaque effectively without damaging the underlying vessel wall. A high level of selectivity for plaque versus normal vessel, however, is difficult to achieve based on the angiogram alone. Recent experience with intravascular ultrasound imaging has shown that ultrasound is a highly effective means of discriminating normal and abnormal vessel wall components, and thus represents a promising guidance modality for atherectomy and laser treatment of plaque. The purpose of this chapter is to review the prospects for ultrasound as a guidance strategy for these devices.

Current Guidance Approaches

Each of the devices currently in clinical trials has some feature intended to confer selectivity for plaque versus normal vessel wall. The Simpson Atherocath [1, 2] (TM, Devices for Vascular Intervention, Inc., Redwood City, CA) is an intrinsically directional device, exposing the cutting element only on one side of the catheter. The device can thus be oriented rotationally to the portion of the vessel wall judged to have the deepest accumulation of plaque. Theoretically, if the opening of the housing is exposed to normal wall, the elasticity of the segment will cause it to stretch out of the way of the rotating cutter. The Rotablator [3, 4] (TM, Heart Technologies, Inc.,

P.W. Serruys, B.H. Strauss and S.B. King III (eds), Restenosis after Intervention with New Mechanical Devices, 97–110.
© 1992 *Kluwer Academic Publishers. Printed in the Netherlands.*

Bellevue, Washington) has selectivity for plaque based on the mechanical properties of the high-speed rotating burr which performs the ablation. The burr preferentially cuts material with low viscoelasticity, and so tends to remove fibrous and fibrocalcific plaque while sparing normal vessel wall. The TEC device [5, 6] (TM, Interventional Technologies, Inc., San Diego, CA) has sharp, rotating blades at the catheter tip that cut concentrically around a central guidewire. Selectivity for this device is accomplished in a limited sense by means of centering with the guidewire. To some extent normal vessel wall may be spared from the cutters by stretching away from the blades.

The excimer lasers currently in clinical trials also are concentric devices, relying on centering by the guidewire to keep the catheter away from normal vessel wall [7, 8]. An argon laser system developed by GV Medical, Inc (Minneapolis, MN) uses a balloon located immediately proximal to the laser fiber to further enhance centering within the lumen of the vessel [9]. One problem with all of the concentric devices is that plaque tends to be deposited in an eccentric fashion. In a classic pathologic study, for example, 74% of coronary artery segments containing critical plaque accumulations had normal vessel wall occupying an arc of at least 16 degrees of vessel circumference [10].

Direct visualization with angioscopy has been suggested as a potential guidance modality for the various plaque removal techniques. Current stand-alone angioscopy systems have overcome most of the logistical difficulties associated with direct visualization in a blood-filled environment. In one system [11] the combination of proximal balloon occlusion with intermittent saline flushes provides good-quality, intermittent views of the coronary circulation. The angioscopic images are particularly useful for discriminating thrombus from normal vessel wall or atheroma [12]. One limitation of the angioscopic approach to guide plaque removal, however, is the inability of the angioscope to judge the depth of plaque in any given direction. Different types of plaque (for example, fibrous versus fatty) can be discriminated by means of the surface appearance, but the thickness of the plaque accumulation is very difficult to ascertain.

A more sophisticated guidance principle for lasers — laser induced fluorescence — has undergone initial feasibility testing [13], but has not yet had a successful clinical implementation. This technology is based on the differing fluorescent patterns of plaque versus normal media. The same laser fiber used for treatment can be employed to carry a diagnostic beam of laser light to interrogate the material at the tip of the catheter. The light returning to the proximal end of the catheter includes the fluorescent signal from the plaque, which can be characterized by computer-assisted spectral analysis. Like angioscopy, however, laser-induced fluorescence has an important limitation in penetration. In the one system that reached clinical trials, the estimated maximum penetration was 100 microns [13]. This restricts the application of the system to an "out of bounds" detector — that is, the computer is capable only of signalling when the catheter is about to enter media. Unfortunately, in severely diseased vessels the media may be highly attenuated or absent altogether, leading to a major practical concern for a device that relies on sensing the medial layer for its stopping point. Several other potential fiberoptic-based technologies may have the potential to overcome the penetration problem. In-vitro work has been performed with fluorescent chromophores that are taken up by atheroma selectively [14, 15]. Other spectroscopic techniques including infrared, Raman and photoacoustic spectral analysis have potential for in-depth assessment of plaque, but have not yet undergone extensive development for catheter-based systems [16].

Each of the second generation devices has been associated with perforations in clinical trials. With increasing experience, strategies for minimizing the risk of perforation for the devices are evolving. The multicenter trial with directional atherectomy, for example, has indicated that branch points and segments which have been severely dissected by balloon angioplasty have a significant risk for perforation [17]. Bifurcation lesions have also been documented to have a greater chance of perforation with excimer laser treatment [7].

Wall Injury and Restenosis

In addition to the issue of perforation, there is concern that trauma to normal vessel wall by nonguided devices may increase the risk of restenosis. Early animal models of balloon angioplasty demonstrated that exposure of the media by deep dissection led to markedly enhanced platelet deposition and accelerated rates of restenosis [18]. Recently, Nobuyoshi and colleagues published a clinicopathologic study of restenosis as a function of the depth of dissection following balloon angioplasty [19]. These investigators found that the amount of myointimal proliferation was nearly double in arteries where the dissection reached media or adventitia, compared to arteries in which tears where confined to the plaque itself. In a similar post-mortem analysis, Waller and colleagues confirmed that the degree of intimal proliferation in restenosis was greater for lesions with medial involvement compared to lesions with intimal injury only [20].

The ability to retrieve and study samples from directional atherectomy has provided further insight into the potential relation between trauma to normal vessel wall and restenosis. In peripheral atherectomy, a clear association between restenosis and the presence of media or adventitia in the atherectomy specimens has been documented by Backa and colleagues [21]. Subintimal tissue was found in approximately 50% of cases; in these cases, restenosis averaged 80%, compared to 35% in the cases in which there was no media or adventitia present in the specimens.

Data from the various coronary directional atherectomy series have been conflicting concerning the frequency and sequelae of subintimal tissue resec-

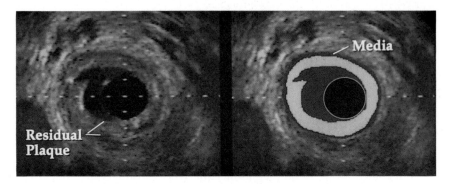

Figure 1. Post-atherectomy ultrasound imaging from a mid left anterior descending coronary artery. The media is seen as a thin dark band outlining the residual plaque accumulation. There is a small plaque tear seen at 10 o'clock. The neolumen following atherectomy measures 1.7 by 2.1 mm (calibration marks are 0.5 mm).

tion. In a report of the Sequoia Hospital experience [22], media was sampled in 44% and adventitia in 17% of 174 lesions. The incidence of perforation or pseudoaneurysm formation was 1.7% overall, but was 10.5% in the subgroup with adventitia present on histology. In a separate, preliminary report from this same group [23], penetration into media was not associated with increased levels of restenosis overall, although the subgroup of patients undergoing atherectomy for restenosis post PTCA did show a significant correlation between subintimal sampling and restenosis. In the Mayo Clinic experience, media was sampled in 51% and adventitia in 14% of cases [24]. Depth of resection had a significant relation to restenosis with rates of 42% for intima alone, 50% for media and 63% for adventitia [25].

Potential for Ultrasound Guidance

Ultrasound is unique in comparison to angiography, angioscopy and fluorescence detection in its ability to provide information beneath the luminal surface of plaque. In most circumstances the three layers of the arterial wall can be discriminated in a high-frequency ultrasound scan (Fig. 1). Because of a comparatively low content of elastin and collagen, the media of a muscular artery is poorly reflective of ultrasound compared to intima and adventitia, and therefore appears as a dark band. This medial layer defines the outer perimeter of any plaque accumulation (plaque is more echoreflective, and hence appears brighter on the ultrasound scan). In normal coronary vessels, some degree of intimal thickening is required before the intima can be clearly imaged. Studies from our laboratory suggest that the threshold for detection of intima at 30 MHz is approximately 150 microns thickness [26]. Prior pathologic studies have suggested that by age 20 the average intimal

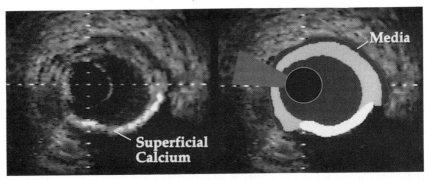

Figure 2. Post-atherectomy image from a proximal left anterior descending coronary artery. A rim of calcification is seen between three and 6 o'clock, producing shadowing of the deeper plaque. An approximate idea of the depth of the media in this sector is possible by locating the media in the adjacent, nonshadowed portions of the vessel wall. The superficial calcium limits cutting by the atherectomy device in this area.

thickness is 200 microns or more, indicating that the intimal layer should be detectable in a large proportion of the patients coming to catheterization or intervention [27].

Of greater concern than the ability to visualize normal intima, however, is the phenomenon of medial thinning under plaque. At 30 MHz the axial resolution of a catheter ultrasound system is in the range of 75–100 microns. This is easily sufficient for imaging normal media with an average thickness of 200 microns, but may be at the limit of resolution in diseased vessels, where the medial thickness can be 80 microns or less [28]. Fortunately, it is often possible to discriminate plaque from underlying vessel even in cases where media is not clearly defined, by virtue of the different speckle pattern of plaque and adventitia (see, for example, Fig. 4B). An additional practical point is that the catheter can be advanced or retracted a short distance from the level of interest in order to scan for media at these levels. Because the depth of plaque between two contiguous segments must be very similar, this scanning technique is effective for clarifying the anatomy at any given imaging plane.

Calcification presents the greatest single limitation of ultrasound imaging and guidance within vessels. As is the case with ultrasound imaging at lower frequencies, calcium is intensely reflective of ultrasound and shadows any tissues lying beyond the region of calcification (Fig. 2). Since calcium is present in a significant proportion of plaques, this is a potentially major limitation for ultrasound as a guidance modality for plaque removal. Fortunately, several factors mitigate the impact of this problem. First, in our experience the most common appearance of calcium within coronary plaque is as a thin rim deep at the base of the plaque, adjacent to the medial border. With this type of deep calcium deposit the distribution of the plaque and the depth of the media can be fairly well estimated on the ultrasound images. When calcium deposits occur in the body of the plaque or at the luminal

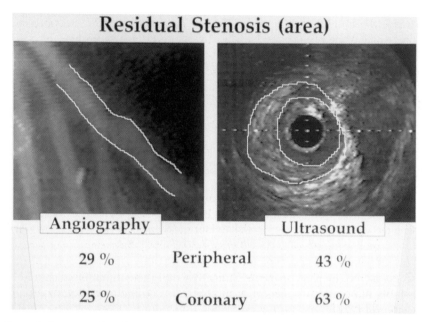

Figure 3. Summary of preliminary data [28, 29] on the comparison of percent area stenosis by angiography and ultrasound following directional atherectomy. See text for details.

surface, however, orientation may be more difficult. In these cases it is often possible to move the catheter a short distance forward or backward and establish the architecture of the vessel wall by continuity. Occasionally the amount and extent of calcium is so severe that it is extremely difficult to obtain a clear sense of the depth of plaque in any given direction. In these cases the operator is left to proceed with the expectation that at least the superficial layers of plaque can be removed without significant risk of violating media.

Clinical Experience with Guided Atherectomy

To date the largest experience with ultrasound guidance for atherectomy has been in association with the Simpson Atherocath. Initial studies from our group used stand-alone ultrasound imaging to analyze the plaque residual following directional atherectomy in peripheral vessels [29]. Although the mean percent area stenosis by angiography was only 29% (diameter stenosis of 17%), ultrasound imaging revealed that, on average, 43% of the available lumen was occupied by plaque at the end of the procedure (Fig. 3). Troughs cut by the atherectomy device were seen in many cases, and intimal fractures or dissections were seen in approximately one out of four cases. Similar qualitative results were obtained in an analysis of 41 patients undergoing coronary directional atherectomy [30]. Plaque fracture and dissections were again seen in the coronary cases (Fig. 1), although not as frequently as with balloon angioplasty. Troughs in the coronary arteries tended to be less pronounced than in the peripheral vessels, perhaps because of a closer match between catheter and vessel diameter. The plaque residual as measured by ultrasound was again significant, with a mean of 63% of the available lumen still occupied by plaque after the procedure had been taken to angiographic completion (Fig. 3).

The discrepancy between the angiographic and ultrasound assessment of residual stenosis is attributable to several factors. The most important of these is the fact that the angiographic measurement of percent stenosis is referenced to an angiographically "normal" segment of vessel which generally is not, in fact, free of plaque. Prior pathologic studies [31, 32] and recent catheter ultrasound studies [33, 34] have emphasized that angiographically normal segments of diseased vessels frequently have significant accumulations of plaque, accounting for as much as 30% of the potential lumen. Referencing the stenotic regions against these segments underestimates the actual plaque burden in the diseased regions. A second explanation for this discrepancy is the fact that the Atherocath has some "Dottering" or dilating effect on the vessel, which increases the lumen caliber without removing plaque. In a recent catheter ultrasound study Smucker and colleagues [35] estimated that as much as 2/3 of the effect of the Atherocath in increasing lumen area was due to expansion rather than tissue removal. Similar numbers have been derived from angiographic studies comparing the angiographic luminal improvement to the tissue weight removed with the device [36].

The potential effect of subintimal resection in increasing rates of restenosis has been mentioned above. At present there is no imaging study that has attempted to gauge the degree of penetration and follow patients for restenosis. In a preliminary study from our group [30], post-procedure images from patients who went on to have restenosis within a six month interval were compared to images from patients with open vessels at this same mean interval. There was no difference in these groups in terms of eccentricity/concentricity, lesion calcification, presence of dissection, deep troughs, or percent plaque residual. There was a significant difference in the groups, however, in the residual cross-sectional area by ultrasound. In patients who ultimately had restenosis, the mean post-procedure cross-sectional area immediately following the procedure was $4.6 \, mm^2$, compared to $9.2 \, mm^2$ in patients who had patent vessels at follow-up ($p < 0.01$). These data provide further evidence for a conclusion emerging from angiographic studies with second-generation devices, that risk of restenosis is inversely proportional to the size of the lumen at the end of the procedure [37].

Recently Keren and colleagues [38] have presented preliminary data comparing the intravascular ultrasound appearance of vessels following treatment with directional and excisional (TEC) atherectomy and rotational ablation. These investigators noted dissections with the atherectomy devices but described a smoother, more rounded lumen in the rotational ablation cases. Because of the concentric nature of cutting of the Rotablator and TEC catheters, the main advantage of ultrasound imaging when using these catheters is in attempting to size the catheter appropriately. If a successful pass has been made with the first catheter selected, the treatment segment can be imaged to assess the safety of employing a larger diameter tip. If there is a clear margin of plaque on all sides and no sign of dissection extending into media, it is reasonable to proceed with the larger catheter.

Guidance for Laser Ablation

The currently available laser catheters are concentric devices supplied in different diameters, so that the strategy outlined above for the coaxial atherectomy devices also applies — viz., stand-alone ultrasound scanning may be useful in helping to decide whether to choose a larger diameter catheter for a given lesion (Fig. 4). Because there is no clear selectivity in laser treatment for plaque versus normal wall, this type of assessment with ultrasound may be even more critical than in the case of the Rotablator.

Relatively little work has been done in attempting to evaluate the results of laser therapy by ultrasound imaging. In a preliminary report Linker and colleagues [39] demonstrated that laser bursts created a spontaneous contrast effect within the vessel lumen, which cleared quickly with cessation of discharge. The effect was attributed to the presence of particulate matter and/or "microbubbles" caused by the laser. Changes in the ultrasound appearance of tissue surrounding the laser site were also noted, and were shown to correspond to histologic changes including increased interstitial edema.

One of the potential applications for laser catheters — treatment of complete occlusions — could also potentially benefit from ultrasound guidance. Here the constraints on catheter design are different than for the "debulking" designs, however, since the most useful imaging format would be a forward-looking catheter. Although prototype forward-looking catheters have been developed, at present there is no in-vivo experience with such a device. The technical considerations for miniaturization of the forward-looking design appear to be even more formidable than for the conventional, side-directed format. One shortcut to miniaturization is to abandon the two-dimensional image format and use a single beam (A-mode format) of ultrasound to provide information about tissue properties as a function of distance from the catheter tip. The sensitivity and specificity of such an approach could potentially be improved by the application of tissue characterization techniques to the radiofrequency signal (see below).

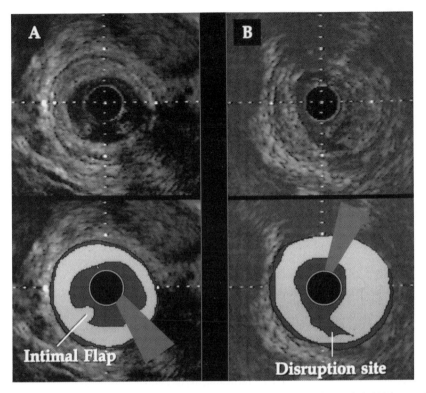

Figure 4. Ultrasound scans following treatment with an excimer laser. On the left (A) is a small intimal flap; on the right (B) is a more significant site of disruption. There is a relatively large margin of plaque remaining following the passage of the 1.6 mm device. Images provided by Edward B. Diethrich MD, Arizona Heart Institute, Phoenix, AZ.

Combined Imaging/Therapeutic Catheters

The desirability of combining ultrasound imaging with a means of plaque removal has been appreciated by several teams. Bom's group described an imaging catheter with a spark gap ablation device, which was tested in animal studies [40]. Our group has developed a combined ultrasound imaging/directional atherectomy device which we have tested on excised human vessels as well as in animal feasibility studies [41]. The device incorporates an ultrasound crystal within the body of the cutter, behind the cutting edge (Fig. 5). This provides a scan which is perpendicular to the long axis of the cutter housing. Because ultrasound does not penetrate through the housing of the device, images are obtained only through the open window — that is, only of the tissue that will be exposed to the cutter (Fig. 5, right image). The segment of the vessel that is being considered for a cut can then be scanned by retracting the rotating cutter from the forward position. Although feas-

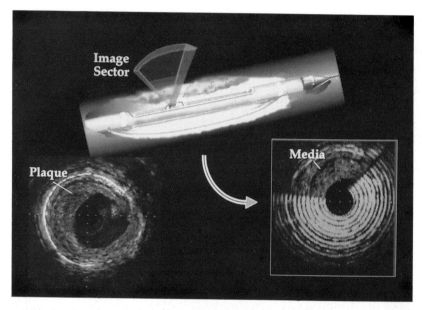

Figure 5. Schematic diagram and image from a prototype ultrasound imaging/atherectomy device [40]. The image is created from a beam originating immediately behind the cutter (see text for details). The image on the left is a full two-dimensional scan from a dedicated imaging catheter. The image on the right is from the combined device. The vessel wall is visualized through the opening in the housing (9 to 1 o'clock). The rings seen elsewhere in the image are ultrasound reverberations from the metal housing of the device.

ibility of this combination has been demonstrated by this prototype, considerable work remains in optimizing the imaging and cutting modalities.

Aretz and colleagues have reported on the combination of ultrasound imaging and radial laser ablation [42]. In order to allow miniaturization of the combined catheter system, this group has opted for a single transducer which is fixed on the catheter. An image is built up by manually moving the catheter within the segment of interest in both axial and radial scans, with the resulting ultrasound data being stored to progressively compile a three-dimensional representation of the segment in computer memory. In the beating heart this acquisition requires gating to the electrocardiogram in order to account for relative movement of the catheter and vessel wall. Once the image is accumulated, it can be displayed in either a standard cross-sectional view, or a longitudinal two-dimensional format. The information on plaque location and depth is then used to guide the firing of a laser which is directed perpendicular to the catheter tip. The axial location of the catheter is tracked by a position sensor mounted at the proximal portion of the catheter shaft. The rotational orientation of the catheter is measured to an accuracy of 1.5 degrees by means of an innovative external electromagnetic antenna. This complex but elegant system has recently been demonstrated to provide diagnostic images in the beating heart of a dog [42].

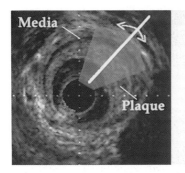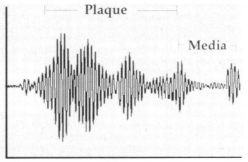

Figure 6. Example of the raw radiofrequency signal (right) from one scan line within an image of a diseased vessel segment. The depth of the plaque and thickness of the media can be accurately determined at this point from the information in the single beam.

Simplification of the catheter system for combined laser ablation with ultrasound sensing could also theoretically be achieved by means of "tissue characterization" (Fig. 6) [43–45]. In essence, ultrasound tissue characterization refers to a set of computer-based techniques for extracting information from the raw radiofrequency signals used to make the ultrasound images. This information is potentially more sensitive and precise in defining different tissue types than the image itself. Figure 6 shows a representation of a single beam of ultrasound and the corresponding radiofrequency signal. This signal, when properly interpreted by a computer, contains within it information about the type and depth of plaque as well as the thickness of media. The advantage of this approach is that it can be used with the ultrasound information from a single, nonrotating transducer, allowing for a simplified and potentially miniaturized catheter design.

Summary

Among the various potential guidance systems for the new generation of plaque removal and ablation catheters, ultrasound has an intrinsic advantage in being able to see beneath the surface of plaque. Images generated by stand-alone ultrasound catheters have provided useful information concerning the function of some of these new therapeutic catheters. Imaging is beginning to have clinical application in assessing the optimal position for directional atherectomy and the appropriate sizing for coaxial devices such as the rotational atherectomy catheters and lasers. Combined imaging/plaque removal catheters are in the prototype phase of development and show promise for providing truly "guided" treatment of plaque. There are preliminary data to suggest that if more aggressive debulking of plaque can be accomplished without creating subintimal trauma, reduced rates of restenosis may be possible.

Acknowledgements

Ultrasound images from various centers were generated using the Insight (TM) system from Cardiovascular Imaging Systems (CVIS) Sunnyvale, California. We gratefully acknowledge the skilled editorial assistance of Barbara Herz.

References

1. Simpson J B, Selmon M R, Robertson G C et al (1988) Transluminal atherectomy for occlusive peripheral vascular disease. *Am J Cardiol* 61:96G–101G
2. Hinohara T, Rowe M H, Robertson G C, Selmon M R et al (1991) Effect of lesion characteristic on outcome of directional coronary atherectomy. *J Am Coll Cardiol* 17:1112–1120
3. Hansen D D, Auth D C, Hall M, Ritchie J L (1988) Rotational endoarterectomy in normal canine coronary arteries: preliminary report. *J Am Coll Cardiol* 11:1073–1077
4. Buchbinder M, Warth D, O'Neill W et al (1991) Multicenter registry of percutaneous coronary rotational ablation using Rotablator. *J Am Coll Cardiol* 17:31A (abstr)
5. Stack R S, Quigley P J, Sketch M H, Newman G E, Phillips H R III (1990) Extraction atherectomy. In: Topol E J (ed), *Interventional Cardiology*, Philadelphia: W B Saunders Co, 590–602
6. Sketch M H, O'Neill W W, Galichia J P et al (1991) The Duke Multicenter coronary transluminal extraction-endarterectomy registry: acute and chronic results. *J Am Coll Cardiol* 17:31A (abstr)
7. Bresnahan J F, Litvack F, Margolis J et al (1991) Excimer laser coronary angioplasty: initial results of a multicenter investigation in 958 patients. *J Am Coll Cardiol* 17:31A (abstr)
8. Eigler N, Cook S, Kent K et al (1990) Excimer laser angioplasty of ostial coronary stenosis: results of a multicenter study. *Circulation* 82:III–1 (abstr)
9. Nordstrom L A, Casaneda-Zuniger W R, Young E G, Von Seggern K B (1988) Direct argon laser exposure for recanalization of peripheral arteries: early results. *Radiology* 168:359–364
10. Freudenberg H, Lichtler P R (1981) The normal wall segments in coronary stenosis: a postmortal study. *Z Kardiol* 79:863–869
11. Ramee S R, White C J, Collins T J et al (1991) Percutaneous angioscopy during coronary angioplasty using a steerable microangioscope. *J Am Coll Cardiol* 17:100–105
12. Sherman C T, Litvack F, Grundfest W et al (1986) Coronary angioscopy in patients with unstable angina pectoris. *N Engl J Med* 315:912–919
13. Leon M B, Lu D Y, Prevosti L G et al (1988) Human arterial surface fluorescence: atherosclerotic plaque identification and effects of laser atheroma ablation. *J Am Coll Cardiol* 12:94–102
14. Spears J R, Serur J, Shropshire D et al (1983) Fluorescence of experimental atheromatous plaques with hematoporphyrin derivate. *J Clin Invest* 71:395–399
15. Murphy-Chutorian D, Kosek J, Mok W et al (1985) Selective absorption of ultraviolet laser energy by human atherosclerotic plaque treated with tetracycline. *Am J Cardiol* 55:1293–1297
16. Leon M B, Geschwind H J, Selzer P M, Bonner R F (1990) Fluorescence-guided laser angioplasty. In: Topol E J (ed), *Textbook of Interventional Cardiology*, 713–723. Philadelphia, PA: W.B. Saunders Company
17. US Directional Coronary Atherectomy Investigator Group (1990) Complications of directional coronary atherectomy in a multicenter experience. *Circulation* 82:III–679 (abstr)
18. Steele P M, Chesebro J G H, Stanson A W et al (1985) Balloon angioplasty: natural history of the pathophysiological response to injury in pig model. *Circ Res* 57:105–112

19. Nobuyoshi M, Kimura T, Ohishi H et al (1991) Restenosis after percutaneous transluminal coronary angioplasty: pathologic observations in 20 patients. *J Am Coll Cardiol* 17:433–439
20. Waller B F, Pinkerton C A, Orr C M et al (1991) Morphological observations late (> 30 days) after clinically successful coronary balloon angioplasty. *Circulation* 83:I–2841
21. Backa D, Polnitz A V, Nerlich A, Hofling B (1990) Histologic comparison of atherectomy biopsies from coronary and peripheral arteries. *Circulation* 82(suppl III):III–34 (abstr)
22. Selmon M R, Robertson G C, Simpson J B et al (1990) Retrieval of media and adventitia by directional coronary atherectomy and angiographic correlation. *Circulation* 82:III–624 (abstr)
23. Hinohara T, Rowe M, Sipperly M E et al (1990) Restenosis following directional coronary atherectomy of native coronary arteries. *J Am Coll Cardiol* 15:196A (abstr)
24. Garratt K N, Kaufmann U P, Edwards W D et al (1989) Safety of percutaneous coronary atherectomy with deep arterial resection. *Am J Cardiol* 64:538–540
25. Garratt K N, Holmes D R, Bell M R et al (1990) Restenosis after directional coronary atherectomy: differences between primary atheromatous and restenosis lesions and influence of subintimal tissue resection. *J Am Coll Cardiol* 16:1665–1671
26. Fitzgerald P J, St.Goar F G, Kao A K et al (1991) Intravascular ultrasound imaging of coronary arteries: is three layers the norm? *J Am Coll Cardiol* 17:217A (abstr)
27. Waller B F (1989) The eccentric coronary atherosclerotic plaque: morphologic observations and clinical relevance. *Clin Cardiol* 12:14–20
28. Isner J M, Donaldson B S, Fortin A H et al (1986) Attenuation of the media of coronary arteries in advanced atherosclerosis. *Am J Cardiol* 58:937–939
29. White N W, Webb J G, Rowe M H, Simpson J B (1989) Atherectomy guidance using intravascular ultrasound: quantitation of plaque burden. *Circulation* 80(suppl II)II–374 (abstr)
30. Yock P G, Fitzgerald P J, Sykes et al (1990) Morphologic features of successful coronary atherectomy determined by intravascular ultrasound imaging. *Circulation* 82(suppl III):III–676 (abstr)
31. Vlodaver Z, Edwards J E (1971) Pathology of coronary atherosclerosis. *Prog Cardiovasc Dis* 14:256–274
32. Waller B F (1989) "Crackers, breakers, stretchers, drillers, scrapers, shavers, burners, welders and melters" — the future treatment of atherosclerotic coronary artery disease? A clinical-morphologic assessment. *J Am Coll Cardiol* 13:969–987
33. Nissen S E, Gurley J C, Grimes C L et al (1990) Comparison of intravascular ultrasound and angiography in quantitation of coronary dimensions and stenosis in man: impact of lumen eccentricity. *Circulation* 82:III–440 (abstr)
34. Tobis J M, Mallery J, Mahon D et al (1991) Intravascular ultrasound imaging of human coronary arteries in vivo. *Circulation* 83:913–926
35. Smucker M L, Scherb D E, Howard P F et al (1990) Intracoronary ultrasound: how much "angioplasty effect" in atherectomy. *Circulation* 82(suppl III):III–676 (abstr)
36. Sharaf B L, Williams D O (1990) "Dotter Effect" contributes to angiographic improvement following directional coronary atherectomy. *Circulation* 82:III–310 (abstr)
37. Kuntz R E, Safian R D, Schmidt D A et al (1991) Restenosis following new coronary devices: The influence of post-procedure luminal diameter. *J Am Coll Cardiol* 17:2A (abstr)
38. Keren G, Pichard A D, Satler L F et al (1991) Intravascular ultrasound of coronary atherectomy. *J Am Coll Cardiol* 17:157A (abstr)
39. Linker D R, Bylock A, Amin A B et al (1989) Catheter ultrasound imaging demonstrates the extent of tissue disruption of excimer laser irradiation of human aorta. *Circulation* 80(suppl II):II–581 (abstr)
40. Slager C J, Essed C E, Schuurbiers J C H et al (1985) Vaporization of atherosclerotic plaques by spark erosion. *J Am Coll Cardiol* 5:1382–1386
41. Yock P G, Fitzgerald P J, Jang Y T et al (1990) Initial trials of combined ultrasound imaging/mechanical atherectomy catheter. *J Am Coll Cardiol* 15:17A (abstr)
42. Aretz H T, Martinelli M A, LeDet E G (1989) Intraluminal ultrasound guidance of transverse laser coronary atherectomy. *Int J Cardiac Imag* 4:153–157

43. Landini L, Sarnelli R, Picano E, Salvadori M (1986) Evaluation of frequency dependence of backscatter coefficient in normal and atherosclerotic aortic walls. *Ultrasound Med Biol* 12:397–401
44. Barzilai B, Saffitz J E, Miller J G, Sobel B E (1987) Quantitative ultrasonic characterization of the nature of atherosclerotic plaques in human aorta. *Circ Res* 60:459–463
45. Fitzgerald P J, Connolly A J, Watkins R D et al (1991) Distinction between soft plaque and thrombus by intravascular tissue characterization. *J Am Coll Cardiol* 17:111A (abstr)

5. Intravascular Ultrasound: Potential for Optimizing Mechanical Solutions to Restenosis

JEFFREY M. ISNER, KENNETH ROSENFIELD, DOUGLAS W. LOSORDO and ANN PIECZEK

Introduction

The short-term results of percutaneous vascular recanalization, coronary as well as peripheral, have been conventionally assessed using contrast angiography. The fact that this time-honored approach provides facile and expeditious near-on-line analysis suggests that it will remain indispensable for assessment of vascular interventions. The limitations of contrast angiography for evaluating the vascular wall as well as lumen, however, have been well documented [1–11]. Because contrast media is injected into the vascular space, alterations of the vascular wall resulting from percutaneous interventions are appreciated only indirectly. While injection of contrast media directly into the vascular space is better suited to assess luminal diameter narrowing, this examination, too, is compromised by the fact that any single site of interest is evaluated only by comparison with adjacent, less-narrowed but nevertheless diseased sites.

Previous attempts to complement conventional contrast angiography with alternative imaging modalities during percutaneous vascular interventions in human patients have included fluorescence spectroscopy [12–13] and fiber-optic angioscopy [14–16]. Intra-operative investigations of coronary physiology and anatomy [17–19] demonstrated that high-frequency, epicardial ultrasound probes could be employed to generate high-resolution images of both the vascular wall and lumen. In vitro studies [20–24] established that the ultrasound image could be further enhanced by intravascular placement of the ultrasound probe. Subsequently, intravascular ultrasound (IVUS) imaging performed by a closed-chest, percutaneous approach was used to accomplish in vivo imaging of native coronary and peripheral arteries [25–28]. More recently, intravascular ultrasound has been applied as a means of assessing the results of percutaneous vascular recanalization in vitro [29–30] and in vivo [27].

Recent technological developments, as well as an expanding library of clinical experience with image interpretation, have facilitated the clinical

P.W. Serruys, B.H. Strauss and S.B. King III (eds), Restenosis after Intervention with New Mechanical Devices, 111–148.
© 1992 *Kluwer Academic Publishers. Printed in the Netherlands.*

applications of intravascular ultrasound. In this chapter, we review certain of these technological modifications as well as our clinical experience using intravascular ultrasound guidance for coronary and peripheral revascularition.

Clinical Experience in Patients Undergoing Peripheral Revascularization

Certain clinical data, including the degree of functional limitation [31] and the nature and site of the therapeutic intervention in the first 101 consecutive patients [32] in whom intravascular ultrasound examination was performed as an adjunct to percutaneous revasclarization, are listed in Table 1. All studies were performed using a 6.2 or 4.8 Fr. monorail-style, wire-guided IVUS catheter (Boston Scientific, Watertown, MA) with an imaging console adapted for 20 MHz operation and 360° scans (Diasonics, Milpitas, CA). The interventions for peripheral vascular disease included percutaneous transluminal (balloon) angioplasty (PTA) alone, PTA with implantation of an endovascular stent, directional atherectomy with or without PTA, and laser angioplasty with PTA and/or atherectomy.

As suggested by previous in vitro studies [29, 30], IVUS consistently provided exquisite detail regarding alterations in the arterial wall and subjacent plaque resulting from the barotrauma of balloon inflation. IVUS documented the presence of plaque cracks and/or dissections in most patients treated with PTA. The patterns of injury observed in these cases was markably similar to that which has been observed by light microscopy in patients studied at necropsy post-PTA [8]. It is not unreasonable to anticipate that improved definition of the site and extent of intraluminal flaps, cracks and/or dissections may ultimately improve attempts to retrieve failed interventions. Long-term follow-up of a larger group of patients studied by IVUS, however, will be required to confirm the appropriate interventional response to these qualitative fidings.

In contrast to IVUS findings post-PTA, IVUS images recorded post-atherectomy (Fig. 1) generally disclosed less extensive signs of arterial wall trauma; instead, the perimeter of the neolumen was typically smooth and uninterrupted. Signs of arterial wall trauma were most completely effaced on IVUS images recorded following delivery of an endovascular stent; the fact that extensive trauma was observed at these same sites post-PTA (pre-stent) suggests that stent implantation acutely ameloriates arterial wall pathology.

Observations in these patients confirm previous suggestions [29,30] regarding the potential utility of IVUS for assessment of post-procedural residual narrowing (Fig. 1). In a series of 17 patients reported previously [27], luminal cross-sectional area at the treatment site in five of 17 patients was < 69% of the cross-sectional area at an apparently normal site in the same artery; in all five patients, however, conventional angiography disclosed no apparent

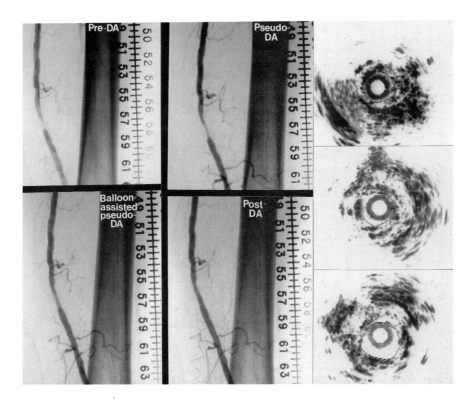

Figure 1. Use of intra-vascular ultrasound (IVUS) to quantify incremental luminal patency resulting from individual components of directional atherectomy (DA). *Top left* angiogram shows high-grade stenosis in superficial femoral artery (SFA), pre-DA. *Top right* angiogram shows improved luminal patency resulting from "Dotter" effect of advancing DA catheter through lesion (no balloon inflation, no atherectomy). *Bottom left* angiogram shows further improvement in luminal patency resulting from balloon inflation (2 atm) without activating cutter. *Bottom right* angiogram shows final result accomplished by activating cutter. Magnitude of serial improvement in luminal patency was determined by IVUS post-pseudo-DA (top: cross-sectional area {A} = 0.13 cm^2); post balloon-assisted pseudo-DA (middle: A = 0.16 cm^2); and post-DA (bottom: A = 0.20 cm^2).

residual luminal narrowing. The finding by IVUS of luminal narrowing at sites devoid of angiographic stenoses underscores the fact that angiographic assessment of luminal narrowing may be compromised by diffusely distributed intimal disease that allows determination of any focal stenosis only as a relative function of adjacent diseased, albeit less narrowed, sites [1–9]. On the other hand, in six of these 17 patients, luminal cross-sectional area post-procedure exceeded the luminal cross-sectional area of that artery arbitrarily identified as "normal." There are three possible explanations for this paradoxical outcome. In the two cases involving endovascular prostheses, it is likely that stent delivery resulted in "over-stretching" of the stented segments

Table 1. Clinical data for 101 consecutive patients in whom IVUS was used.

Pt	Sex	Age	Vessel	IQ	Intervention	Approach A vs R	C vs I	Guiding Catheter	IVUS Catheter	Catheter Pre	Post	IVUS in lieu of Angiography
1	M	54	RCI+REI-RCF	0	PTA	R	I	0	6.6	+	+	+
2	F	74	RCI	0	PTA+Stent	R	I	+	6.6	+	+	0
3	M	63	LCI+LEI	0	PTA+Stent	R	I	+	6.6	+	+	0
4	M	84	LCI+LEI	0	PTA	R	I	0	6.6	0	+	0
5	M	58	LSF	0	PTA+Atherectomy	A	I	0	6.6	0	+	0
6	M	61	RSF	0	PTA	A	I	0	6.6	+	+	+
7	F	63	REI	0	PTA	R	I	0	6.6	+	+	+
8	M	66	REI	0	PTA	R	I	0	6.6	+	+	+
9	M	67	REI+RSF+RPOP	0	PTA	R	C	0	6.6	0	+	0
10	M	53	LCF+LSF	+	PTA+Thrombolysis	A	I	0	6.6	0	+	0
11	M	77	LSF	+	PTA	A	I	0	6.6	0	+	0
12	M	69	RCI	0	PTA	R	I	0	6.6	+	+	+
13	M	72	LSF+LPOP	0	PTA	A	I	0	6.6	+	+	+
14	M	77	LSF+LPOP+LP+LAT	+	PTA	A	I	0	6.6	0	+	0
15	M	79	LCI+LEI	0	PTA	R	I	0	6.6	+	+	+
16	F	66	LEI	0	PTA	R	I	0	6.6	+	+	+
17	F	65	RCF+RPF+LCI+LEI+LGR	0	PTA	R	C	0	6.6	0	+	0
18	M	75	RSF+RTPT+RP+RAT	+	PTA	A	I	0	6.6	+	+	0
19	M	73	RSF	+	Laser probe+PTA	A	I	0	6.6	0	+	0
20	F	71	RSF	+	PTA	A	I	0	6.6	0	+	0
21	M	62	RCI	0	PTA	R	I	0	6.6	0	+	0
22	M	75	RSF+RPOP	0	Atherectomy	A	I	0	6.6	0	+	0
23	M	75	LSF+LPT	0	PTA+Atherectomy	A	I	0	6.6	0	+	0
24	M	67	RSF+RPOP	+	PTA+Atherectomy	A	I	0	6.6	0	+	0
25	M	46	LEI	0	Atherectomy	A	I	0	6.6	0	+	0
26	M	47	REI+LCF+LSF	0	PTA	R	C	0	6.6	+	+	+
27	M	56	LSF	0	Laser probe+PTA	A	I	0	6.6	0	+	0
28	M	55	RSF+RPOP	0	PTA	A	I	0	6.6	+	+	+
29	M	67	RSF+RPOP	+	PTA	A	I	0	6.6	0	+	0

No.	Sex	Age	Lesion		Treatment							
30	M	58	RSF+RPOP	0	PTA	A	I	0	6.6	0	+	0
31	M	66	LSF+LPOP	0	PTA	A	I	0	6.6	+	+	+
32	F	67	LSF	+	Laser probe+PTA	A	I	0	6.6	0	+	0
33	M	64	LEI+LCF	0	PTA	R	I	0	6.6	+	+	+
34	M	82	LSF	+	Laser probe+Atherectomy	A	I	0	6.6	0	+	0
35	M	63	RSF+RPOP+RTPT	+	PTA+Thrombolysis	A	I	+	6.6	0	+	0
36	F	67	LR	+	PTA	R	I	0	4.8	0	+	0
37	M	64	RCI+REI+RCF	+	PTA	R	I	0	6.6	0	+	0
38	M	79	LSF+LPOP	0	PTA	R	I	0	6.6	+	+	+
39	M	70	LSF	+	PTA	A	I	0	6.6	0	+	0
40	M	77	RSF+RPOP+RP	+	Ex. Laser+PTA	A	I	0	6.6	0	+	0
41	M	74	RDF	0	PTA	R	I	0	6.6	+	+	+
42	M	72	LCI+LEI	0	PTA	R	I	0	6.6	0	+	0
43	M	68	RP	+	Ex. Laser+PTA	A	I	0	6.6	0	+	+
44	M	55	RCI+REI+RCF	0	PTA	R	I	0	6.6	+	+	+
45	M	64	RCI+REI+RCF	0	PTA	R	I	0	6.6	+	+	+
46	M	45	REI+RCF	0	PTA	R	I	0	6.6	0	+	+
47	M	69	RCI	0	PTA	R	I	0	6.6	+	+	+
48	M	72	RSF	+	Ex. Laser+PTA+Thrombolysis	A	I	0	6.6	0	+	0
49	M	72	RSF	0	PTA	A	I	0	6.6	+	+	0
50	M	79	RCI+RCF+LCI	0	PTA	R	C	0	6.6	0	+	+
51	M	77	REI	0	PTA	R	I	0	6.6	0	+	0
52	F	74	RDF	0	PTA	R	I	0	6.6	0	+	0
53	M	55	RSF+RPOP	0	PTA+Atheretomy	A	I	0	6.6	+	+	0
54	M	66	REI	0	PTA	R	I	0	6.6	+	+	0
55	M	68	LSF	+	PTA	A	I	0	6.6	0	+	+
56	F	74	RDF	0	PTA	R	I	0	6.6	+	+	+
57	M	45	LCI+LEI	0	PTA	R	I	0	6.6	+	+	0
58	F	69	LDF	0	PTA	R	I	0	6.6	+	+	+
59	M	55	RVG+RSF	+	Ex. Laser+PTA+Thrombolysis					0	+	0

Table 1. (Continued).

Pt	Sex	Age	Vessel	IQ	Intervention	Approach A vs R	Approach C vs I	Guiding Catheter	IVUS Catheter	Catheter Pre	Catheter Post	IVUS in lieu of Angiography
60	M	52	REI	0	PTA	R	I	0	6.6	+	+	+
61	F	64	RSF+RPOP	+	PTA	A	I	0	6.6	0	+	0
62	M	72	LCI+REI	0	PTA	R	I	0	6.6	0	+	0
63	M	63	LP+LAT	+	Ex. Laser+PTA	A	I	0	6.6	0	+	0
64	F	37	LDF	0	PTA	R	I	0	6.6	+	+	+
65	F	69	LCI	0	PTA	R	I	0	6.6	+	+	+
66	M	46	LCI+REI	0	PTA	R	I	0	6.6	+	+	+
67	M	79	REI	0	PTA	R	I	0	BUIC	+	+	+
68	M	72	RCI+LCI+LEI	0	PTA	R	I	0	BUIC	+	+	+
69	F	67	LEI	0	PTA+Atherectomy	R	I	0	6.6	+	+	+
70	M	59	LSF+LPOP	0	Ex. Laser+Atherectomy	A	I	0	6.6	+	+	0
71	M	66	LDF	0	PTA	R	I	0	BUIC	+	+	0
72	F	67	RSF	0	PTA+Atherectomy	A	I	0	6.6	0	+	0
73	M	36	LCI	+	PTA	R	C	+	6.6	0	+	0
74	M	78	RSF+RPOP	+	Ex. Laser+PTA+Atherectomy	A	I	0	6.6	0	+	0
75	F	75	RDF	0	PTA	R	I	0	6.6	+	+	0
76	M	52	RPOP	+	Ex. Laser+PTA	A	I	0	6.6	0	+	0
77	M	59	LCI	0	PTA	R	I	0	BUIC	+	+	+
78	M	69	RSF	0	PTA	A	I	0	6.6	+	0	
79	M	76	RCI+REI+RCF+LEI	0	PTA	R	C	0	6.6	+	+	+
80	M	64	LCI	+	PTA	R	C	0	BUIC	0	+	0
81	M	49	REI+RCF	0	PTA+Atherectomy	R	I	0	4.8	+	+	+
82	F	67	LEI	0	PTA	R	I	0	6.6	+	+	+
83	F	78	REI+RCF	0	PTA	R	I	BUIC	0	+	+	+
84	F	70	LCI	0	PTA	R	I	BUIC	0	+	+	+
85	F	75	RDF	+	PTA	R	I	6.6	0	+	+	0

Pt	Sex	Age	Lesion		Procedure							
86	F	78	RSF	0	Atherectomy	A	I	6.6	0	0	+	0
87	M	58	REI	0	PTA	R	I	BUIC	BUIC	+	+	+
88	M	66	LSFA+LP+LPTP+LPT	+	Ex. Laser+Atherectomy	A	I	0	6.6	+	+	0
89	M	46	RSF	+	Ex. Laser+Atherectomy	A	I	6.6	0	0	+	0
90	M	63	RSF	+	Ex. Laser+PTA	I	0	0	6.6	0	0	0
91	M	73	LSF	0	PTA	A	I	6.6	0	+	+	0
92	F	52	LCI	0	PTA	R	I	BUIC	0	+	+	0
93	M	62	LEI+LCF+LGR+LP+LAT	+	PTA+Thrombolysis	R	C	4.8	0	0	+	0
94	F	61	RSF+RPOP	0	PTA	A	I	6.6	0	+	+	+
95	M	72	RSF	+	Laser probe+PTA+Atherectomy	R	I	6.6	0	+	+	0
96	M	56	LCI	+	PTA	R	I	BUIC	0	+	+	0
97	M	71	LEI+LPF	0	PTA	R	C	4.8	+	0	+	0
98	F	30	RP	0	PTA	R	I	4.8	0	0	+	0
99	F	79	REI	+	PTA	R	C	4.8	+	0	+	0
100	F	80	LR	+	PTA	R	I	4.8	0	0	+	0
101	F	55	RSC	0	PTA	R	I	4.8	0	0	+	0
102	M	69	LR	0	PTA	R	C	4.8	+	0	+	0
103	F	71	LR	+	PTA	R	I	6.6	0	+	+	0
104	M	74	RCI+REI+RPF	0	PTA	R	I	4.8	0	0	+	0

Abbreviations: A = antegrade; BUIC = balloon ultrasound imaging catheter; C = contralateral; Ex. = Excimer; F = female; I = ipsilateral; IVUS = intravascular ultrasound; Laser probe = hot tipped laser; LAT = left anterior tibial; LCI = left common iliac; LCF = left common femoral; LDF = left dialysis fistula; LEI = left external iliac; LGR = left graft; LP = left profunda; LPF = left peroneal; LPOP = left popliteal; LPT = left posterior tibial; LR = left renal; LSF = left superficial femoral; LTPT = left tibio-peroneal trunk; Post = following intervention; Pre = before intervention; Pt = patient; PTA = percutaneous transluminal angioplasty; R = retrograde; RAT = right anterior tibial; RCI = right common iliac; RCF = right common femoral; RDF = right dialysis fistula; REI = right external iliac; RP = right peroneal; RPF = right profunda; RPOP = right popliteal; RSC = right subclavian; RSF = right superficial femoral; RTPT = right tibio-peroneal trunk; RVG = right vein graft; TO = total occlusion.

[33]. Even without stent-implantation, "over-stretching" of the treated arterial segment has been considered a possible mechanism for balloon angioplasty-induced augmentation of luminal patency [34]; interestingly, five of the six patients in whom there was excessive post-procedural luminal dilation had undergone balloon dilation. Finally, it is possible that attempts to identify "normal" sites on the basis of absent calcific deposits and preserved three-layered appearance of the arterial wall failed to exclude occasional cases of diffusely diseased arterial segments.

These results also suggest that IVUS may provide a superior index for guaging the diameter of balloon, stent, laser probe, and/or atherectomy catheter appropriate for a proposed intervention. There are two reasons why IVUS may constitute an improvement in this regard. First, the opportunity to image the "normal" segment with a coaxially positioned calibration device (i.e. the ultrasound transducer) obviates the inherent difficulty of determining radiographic magnification using a calibration instrument (catheter) which may be positioned in a plane or angle different and/or remote from the target lesion. Second, IVUS may allow more certain determination that the arterial segment judged to be "normal" in terms of luminal dimensions is free of important "baseline" atherosclerotic disease.

Initial clinical applications of IVUS have also indicated certain limitations, some of which are generic to the technique, and others of which are related to the specific instrument employed by our group. Perhaps the most decisive limitation concerns the inability of currently available IVUS devices to consistently discriminate boundaries between the three layers of the arterial wall at sites of severe narrowing by atherosclerotic plaque. In normal arteries, or arteries mildly or moderately narrowed by atherosclerotic plaque, the media is typically observed by IVUS as an echolucent layer bounded internally by the internal elastic membrane and/or subjacent intimal deposits of plaque, and externally by the external elastic membrane and thin layer of connective tissue which constitutes the adventitia [21–27]. With more advanced degrees of atherosclerotic narrowing, however, these ultrasound patterns become blurred. This is due principally to two factors: first, emaciation of the media typically accompanies progression of the atherosclerotic process [35]. Second, extensive calcific deposits, because they are often blanketed across the intimal-medial boundary, and because they attenuate or "shadow" the ultrasound reflections from the deeper layers of the wall, further obscure the normal ultrasound depiction of the arterial wall. Ambiguity regarding the boundary between intimal thickening and media reduces the precision with which any given measurement of wall thickness can be determined to represent atherosclerotic plaque versus normal wall [36]. Consequently, in those instances in which such demarcation is not possible, certain of the most potentially attractive applications of intravascular ultrasound – including precise balloon sizing and determination of cross-sectional area narrowing by atherosclerotic plaque – are seriously compromised.

A second limitation of all currently available IVUS devices is that the design of these devices allows only for side-viewing. Because forward-viewing is not possible, IVUS cannot be currently employed to determine the composition – e.g., thrombus versus plaque – of a total occlusion prior to recanalization. For this particular aspect of percutaneous interventional therapy, angioscopy may have superior utility.

Clinical Experience in Patients Undergoing Coronary Revascularization

The potential utility of IVUS as an adjunct to percutaneous coronary revascularization (percutaneous transluminal coronary angioplasty, PTCA) is perhaps best appreciated from the standpoint of advantages related to quantitative analysis of post-interventional results. We have previously [36] studied, for example, a consecutive series of 13 patients in whom the results of balloon [10] or laser [3] angioplasty were quantified by both quantitative angiographic analysis and intravascular ultrasound. Minimal luminal diameter and cross-sectional area were calculated for interventional sites and nearby reference sites. Corresponding ultrasound frames from both interventional and reference sites were digitized and the minimal luminal diameter was measured directly; cross-sectional area was obtained by tracing the perimeter of the lumen. Luminal diameter for reference sites measured 3.9 mm by IVUS, versus 3.3 mm by quantitative angiography ($p < 0.05$). Regression analysis disclosed a correlation coefficient of 0.87. For cross-sectional area of reference sites, the absolute difference between ultrasound and angiography – 12.6 versus 9.6 mm^2 was also statistically significant ($p < 0.05$). Regression analysis disclosed a correlation coefficient of .92, similar to that calculated for analysis of luminal diameter. Luminal diameter for interventional sites measured 2.8 mm by IVUS, versus 1.8 mm by angiography ($p < 0.01$). Regression analysis disclosed a poorer correlation – .62 – than that calculated for reference sites. Similarly, for cross-sectional area of interventional sites, there was a highly statistically significant difference between absolute measurements made by ultrasound (6.9 mm^2) versus quantitative angiography (2.8 mm^2, $p < 0.01$); the corresponding correlation coefficient was .71.

Fig 2 and 3 illustrate one possible explanation for the poor correlation found between these two quantitative techniques. Shown in the ultrasound images of the interventional site, obtained during the procedure, is an extensive plaque fracture resulting from balloon angioplasty. Accurate analysis of this highly irregular lumen, which does not conform to any conventional or regular geometric pattern, would be difficult for quantitative angiography. Two different diameters can be measured: one diameter includes only the area medial to the flap; whereas, a second diameter includes the lumen behind the flap. It is obvious that angiographic analysis of luminal diameter, and the cross-sectional area derived from it, would be equally difficult. In contrast, direct planimetery of this non-geometric lumen using the IVUS image is straightforward. The potential advantages of IVUS versus quantitat-

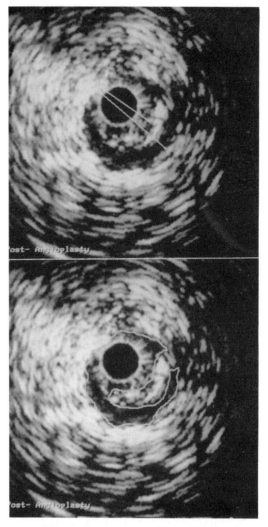

Figure 2. Measurement of luminal diameter (D, top) and cross-sectional area (XSA, bottom) by IVUS post-PTCA. Luminal D measument by IVUS, like angiography, is complicated by fact that D may be measured as a minimum value (internal to plaque fracture) or maximum value (external to plaque fracture). In contrast, luminal XSA may be determined *directly* by IVUS, rather than extrapolated from angiographic algorithms.

ive angiography in assessment of luminal dimensions post-intervention include the following. First, IVUS provides direct delineation of luminal borders, and thus obviates the need for multiple, including orthogonal views. Second, the ability to directly planimeter cross-sectional area eliminates dependence on generic algorithms, which make potentially incorrect assumptions regarding (uniform) luminal geometry. Third, with IVUS unlike angio-

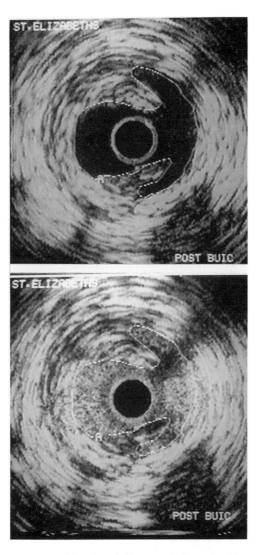

Figure 3. Irregular geometry resulting from balloon angioplasty (in this case performed using the BUIC to treat stenotic left common iliac, Table 2, patient 10). *Top:* planimetered cross-sectional area post-PTA. *Bottom:* injection of agitated saline confirms planimetry of luminal cross-sectional area.

graphy, the calibration instrument is by definition within the plane of measurement. Fourth, with IVUS, the region of interest wherein measurements are made occupies nearly the entire field of view. In contrast, for angiographic analysis, the region of interest involves only a small fraction of the cine frame.

Instruments for Combined Ultrasound Imaging and Percutaneous Revascularization

The concept of combining the elements responsible for intravascular imaging with those responsible for percutaneous revascularization has been investigated previously. Intravascular ultrasound [37] and angioscopy [14–16,38] were both recognized as potential solutions to the problem of arterial perforation which complicated early clinical trials of non-wire-guided laser angioplasty. One such catheter which was actually employed clinically included a dedicated lumen for vascular endoscopy in addition to the lumen housing the fiberoptic elements required to transmit laser light [39]. Although this catheter retained the advantage of angioscopy for forward-viewing, it also included the liability of requiring periodic evacuation of blood to record detailed images. Subsequent attempts to monitor laser ablation incorporated fluorescence spectroscopy in combination with a flash-lamp pumped dye laser [40]. This approach eliminated the requirement for a blood-free lumen, while preserving the ability to accomplish forward imaging.

More recently, attempts have been made to combine intravascular ultrasound imaging with balloon angioplasty and/or mechanical atherectomy. Mallery et al performed in vitro imaging with a 4.5 Fr balloon dilatation catheter fitted with an array of eight 20 MHz transducers mounted radially around the catheter [41]. The transducers were positioned within and midway between the two ends of a 3.0 cm polyethylene balloon; images were recorded perpendicular to the long axis of the catheter, through the balloon. Diameter measurements of pig aorta made by ultrasound reportedly correlated well with actual measurements of the aorta itself.

Yock et al investigated a prototype catheter which combined a 30 MHz transducer with a modified version of the Simpson directional atherectomy catheter [42]. Preliminary experiments performed in vitro and in vivo demonstrated that this device could be used to monitor the depth to which plaque was mechanically excised.

While these two prototype devices, like the catheter employed in the present trial, were designed so that ultrasound imaging could be performed on line, i.e. during balloon inflation or mechanical atherectomy, Hodgson et al [43] performed in vivo imaging in a series of normal canine coronary arteries with a balloon catheter on which a ring of modified phased array transducers were positioned proximal to the balloon. The design of this device was intended to permit pre- and post-dilation imaging without the requirement for multiple catheter exchanges.

Recent clinical investigation in our laboratory has confirmed that it is feasible to perform intravascular ultrasound imaging on-line during percutaneous revascularization, using a hybrid device that incorporates both diagnostic and therapeutic functions, imaging through polyethylene balloon material, the thickness of which is standard for peripheral angioplasty balloons [44]. The so-called balloon ultrasound imaging catheter (BUIC) [45], Boston

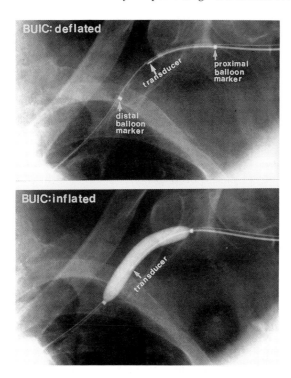

Figure 4. Design of balloon ultrasound inflation catheter (BUIC) used in the present study. Catheter is wire-guided with monorail design; wire enters distal to the tip of the catheter, then exits side-port, re-enters via dedicated port under balloon, and exits port 1 cm proximal to balloon. *Top*: cine frame of deflated BUIC illustrating distal transducer tip positioned midway between radiopaque balloon markers. *Bottom*: cine frame of BUIC fully inflated.

Scientific) which we have employed is illustrated in Fig. 4. The catheter was used with an imaging console capable of 20 MHz imaging and 360° scans (Diasonics) described previously in detail [27]. Briefly, the pulse repetition frequency is 10.2 KHz, the number of scans per second 10, and the number of vectors scanned in one revolution 1024. Vectors were converted, processed and displayed through a real time scan convertor with composite video output that allowed images to be archived on videotape or on a multiformat camera for later study.

Certain clinical data, including the site and extent of the therapeutic intervention performed in the first 10 patients in whom we investigated this device are listed in Table 2. In all 10 patients measurements were recorded from both the BUIC and a conventional (non-balloon) IVUS pre- and/or post-PTA and are listed individually in Table 3. In 8 of 10 patients images recorded from the BUIC were sufficiently satisfactory to permit quantitative analysis of minimum luminal diameter (D_{min}) and luminal cross-sectional area (XSA) pre-PTA. In the remaining 2 patients, artifacts resulting from

Table 2. Clinical data for 10 patients in whom BUIC was used to perform PTA.

Pt	Sex	Age	FCI	ABI	PTA Site	Approach	Sheath	BUIC Size (mm)	Pressure Gr(m) Pre	Pressure Gr(m) Post	Angio %DN Pre	Angio %DN Post
1.	M	79	3	.44	REI	R	10Fr.	8×40	7	0	72.1	2.4
2.	M	57	3	.42	LCI	R	10Fr.	8×40	27	6	100	4.3
3.	M	60	3	.34	LCI	R	10.5Fr.	7×40	2	0	52.3	22.3
4.	F	79	3	.39	REI	R	9Fr.	7×40	2	−2	98.9	9.8
5.	F	69	3	ND	LCI	R	9Fr.	7×40	4	2	76.7	0
6.	M	58	3	.51	REI	R	9Fr.	7×40	2	2	68.0	11.3
7.	M	66	NA	NA	LCV	R	10Fr.	8×40	90	10	75.0	24.8
8.	M	71	5	.33	RCI	R(k)	10Fr.	8×40	8	−2	52.9	0
9.	M	63	3	.58	LCI	C	9Fr.	7×40	15	−2	100	31.1
10.	F	53	3	.77	LCI	R	9Fr.	7×40	16	0	72.2	5.8

Abbreviations: ABI = ankle-brachial index; Angio = angiographic; BUIC = balloon ultrasound inflation catheter; C = contralateral; DN = diameter narrowing; F = female; Fr. = French; FCI = functional classification (Rutherford {44}); Gr = gradient; k = "kissing balloon" technique LCI = left common iliac; LCV = left cephalic vein; M = male; m = mean; NA = not applicable; ND = not done; Post = following angioplasty; Pre = before angioplasty; Pt = patient; PTA = percutaneous transluminal angioplasty; R = retrograde; RCI = right common iliac; REI = right external iliac.

Table 3. Measurements recorded from BUIC and IVUS Pre-, During, and Post-PTA.

Pt	Image Quality	Pre-PTA XSA (cm²) IVUS	BUIC	Δ	Dmin (cm) IVUS	BUIC	Δ	Balloon* Inflation XSA (cm²)	D (cm)	Post-PTA Image Quality	XSA (cm²) IVUS	BUIC	Dmin (cm) Δ	IVUS	BUIC
1.	S	.11	.09	+.02	.31	.30	+.01	.38	.70	S	.28	.25	+.05	.65	.59
2.	S	.05	.06	-.01	.29	.25	+.04	.50	.79	S	.47	.44	+.03	.64	.60
3.	P	.09	.09	0	.29	.38	-.09	.33	.63	S	.34	.33	+.01	.61	.63
4.	S	.09	.15	-.06	.38	.38	0	.33	.61	P	.17	.18	-.01	.45	.44
5.	S	.10	.10	0	.35	.36	-.01	.31	.66	P	.42	.30	+.12	.57	.60
6.	S	.09	.08	+.01	.33	.31	+.02	.32	.62	S	.25	.22	+.03	.55	.59
7.	S	.06	.07	-.01	.26	.31	-.05	.44	.75	S	.29	.25	+.04	.53	.58
8.	S	.15	.13	+.02	.33	.40	-.07	.42	.68	S	.36	.38	-.02	.66	.62
9.	P	.08	.22	-.14	.35	.35	0	.42	.72	S	.23	.26	-.03	.45	.46
10.	S	.10	.12	-.02	.36	.38	-.02	.34	.65	S	.31	.31	0	.56	.62

Abbreviations: Δ = mean difference; * = numbers listed here are maximum values among ≥1 balloon inflations listed individually in Table 4; BUIC = balloon ultrasound inflation catheter; IVUS = intravascular ultrasound (non-balloon catheter); P = poor; Post-PTA = post-balloon angioplasty; Pre-PTA = pre-balloon angioplasty; Pt = patient; S = satisfactory; XSA = cross-sectional area.

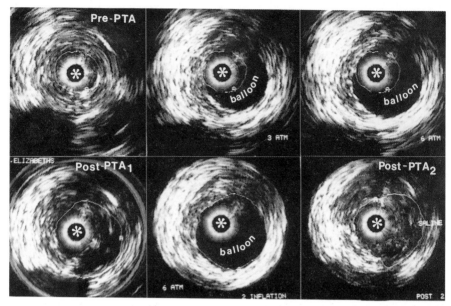

Figure 5. Typical sequence of images recorded from BUIC pre-, during, and post-PTA (pt. 10, Table 2). *Top left*: image recorded from BUIC (through balloon), immediately prior to first inflation demonstrates stenotic lesion of left common iliac artery. Top middle and right: images recorded from BUIC at 3 (middle) and 6 (right) atmospheres of inflation pressure; pre-inflation luminal cross-sectional area (A) is indicated by circle inscribed peripheral to ultrasound transducer (asterisk). Note asymmetric inflation of balloon towards less severely diseased portion of artery (2 to 6 o'clock). *Bottom left*: image recorded from BUIC immediately following balloon deflation; while luminal cross-sectional area has been augmented, there is loss of gain achieved at full balloon inflation (area, A, indicated by circle inscribed peripheral to transducer). *Bottom middle*: image recorded through balloon at full inflation #2; inscribed circle indicates planimetered balloon area (A). Balloon inflation is again asymmetric. *Bottom right*: image recorded immediately following deflation; injection of agitated saline has been used to confirm final luminal cross- sectional area indicated by inscribed circle.

subtotal evacuation of air from the angioplasty balloon and/or electrical interference compromised the diagnostic quality of the recorded image. In 9 of 10 patients, images recorded from the BUIC following the final balloon dilation were sufficient to permit quantitative analysis of post-PTA luminal XSA and Dmin. In the remaining patient, artifacts resulting from a small air bubble interfered with accurate assessment of arterial dimensions post-PTA.

As suggested from preclinical work performed in normal dogs and atherosclerotic microswine (J M Isner, D Gal, unpublished observations), the nature and mixture of material used to fill the balloon had a negligible effect on the quality of image obtained (Fig. 5). The exception to this was residual air within the balloon, which when present compromised detail required for quantitative analysis. When images recorded from the BUIC were not compromised by incomplete evacuation of air from the balloon, measurements of luminal cross-sectional area and minimum diameter were nearly indistinguishable from those recorded using a non-balloon ultrasound catheter (Table 3); measurements recorded from the latter have been shown to correlate well with measurements derived from quantitative angiographic analysis of native normal and diseased arteries [46–49].

All images recorded with the BUIC involved a 20 MHz transducer. While this frequency appeared satisfactory for qualitative and quantitative analysis both in the presence and absence of an inflation balloon, it remains to be determined whether frequencies investigated in other mechanical systems, specifically 30 [42] and 40 MHz [21] may yield superior results.

Assessment of recoil following balloon deflation constitutes a specific application of these quantitative findings. Recoil has long been inferred to constitute a mechanical reason for loss of gain achieved during balloon inflation [50–53]. More recently, several investigators have employed quantitative angiographic techniques to analyze the extent to which recoil complicates standard PTCA. Noboyushi performed coronary angiography routinely on 185 patients one day following PTCA [54]. "Restenosis" (>50% loss of gain in absolute diameter assessed by cinevideodensitomery) was already present in 27 (14.6%) of 185 patients or in 27 (11.4%) of 237 lesions by one day and was interpreted to represent evidence of elastic recoil. Stenosis diameter among these 185 patients decreased from 1.91 ± 0.53 immediately post-PTCA to 1.72 ± 0.52 mm one day post-PTCA (p <0.001).

Hjemdahl-Monsen et al derived pressure-diameter curves from videodensitometric meaurements made at incremental pressures (1–6 atmospheres) during PTCA of 29 lesions in 27 patients [55]. Recoil (balloon diameter at 6 atmospheres/post-PTCA luminal diameter >1.0) was observed in 25/29 lesions and ranged from 1.02 to 2.01 (m $\pm$ SD = 1.35 ± 0.33).

Rensing et al performed videodensitometric analysis on 151 lesions successfully dilated among 136 patients during balloon inflation, and directly after balloon deflation [56]. Mean cross-sectional area of the inflated balloon was 5.2 ± 1.6 mm^2, while mean (minimal) cross-sectional area of the dilated stenosis post-balloon deflation was 2.8 ± 1.4 mm^2. Thus, nearly 50% of the theoretically achievable cross-sectional area was lost immediately after balloon deflation. In contrast to the findings of Noboyushi et al, analysis of a subset of 16 patients (18 lesions) re-examined one day post-PTCA disclosed no further reduction in minimum luminal cross-sectional area.

Finally, Lehmann et al prospectively evaluated 114 lesions undergoing PTCA by quantitative angiography and found that recoil (percent loss of diameter gained during maximum balloon inflation) averaged $34 \pm 23.3\%$, reducing calculated post-PTCA cross sectional area from 5.65 mm^2 to 3.45 mm^2 (57).

Measurements recorded using the BUIC (Table 4, Fig. 6) confirm the preceeding observations made using angiographic techniques and establish that the phenomenon of recoil is common to peripheral as well as coronary angioplasty. Furthermore, because there is a nearly unavoidable delay be-

Table 4. Analysis of recoil from measurements recorded using BUIC.

Pt	Inflation #1 Full Inflation Dmin	XSA	Post-Deflation Dmin	XSA	% Recoil Dmin	XSA	Inflation #2 Full Inflation Dmin	XSA	Post-Deflation Dmin	XSA	% Recoil Dmin	XSA	Inflation #3 Full Inflation Dmin	XSA	Post-Deflation Dmin	XSA	% Recoil Dmin	XSA
1	.70	.38	.59	.23	16	39	.69	.38	.54	.25	22	34						
2	.47	.28	.49	.25	-4	11	.60	.34	.46	.39	23	-15	.79	.50	.60	.44	24	12
3	.62	.31	.62	.37	0	-20	.63	.32	.62	.39	2	-22	.63	.33	.62	.33	2	0
4	.56	.28	.39	.15	30	46	.61	.33	.44	.18	28	45						
5																		
6	.62	.27	.55	.28	11	-4	.61	.32	.48	.31	21	3						
7	.74	.44	.34	.17	54	61	.75	.44	.56	.27	25	39	.68	.38	.58	.25	15	34
8	.68	.42	.62	.38	9	10												
9	.62	.28	.31	.14	50	50	.72	.33	.39	.15	46	55	.71	.42	.46	.26	35	38
10	.65	.34	.61	.26	6	24	.62	.34	.59	.31	5	10						

Note: Recoil could not be accurately calculated in Pt. 5 in whom post-deflation images were unsatisfactory for measurements of Dmin and XSA.

Abbreviations: BUIC = balloon ultrasound inflation catheter; Dmin = minimum diameter; Pt = patient; XSA = cross-sectional area.

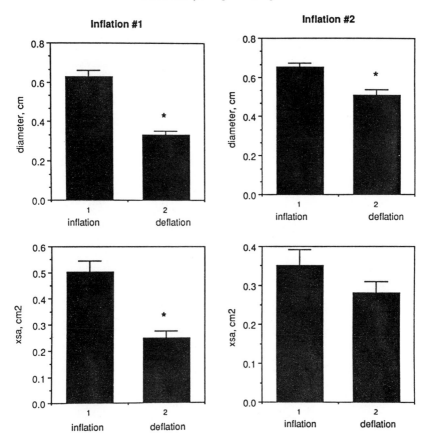

Figure 6. Magnitude of recoil measured by BUIC as function of minimum luminal diameter (Dmin) and cross-sectional area (XSA). For inflation #1 (n = 9), Dmin of vascular lumen immediately following balloon deflation (0.50 ± .04cm) was significantly less than diameter of fully inflated balloon (0.63 ± .03 cm, p = 0.03); XSA was likewise reduced from 0.33 ± .02 to 0.25.03 cm^2 (p = .03). For inflation #2 (n = 8), Dmin measured immediately post-deflation (0.51 ± .03 cm) was less than that measured for fully inflated balloon (0.65.02, p = .004); XSA was also reduced to 0.28 ± .03 from 0.35 ± .01 cm^2, although this difference did not achieve statistical significance.

tween balloon deflation and quantitative angiographic examination post-PTCA, Rensing et al had raised the possibility that platelet deposition and/or non-occlusive mural thrombus frequently observed at balloon angioplasty sites post-mortem could not be ruled out as the basis for apparent recoil observed angiographically [56]. The present series of observations, in which ultrasound analysis of recoil was accomplished immediately upon balloon deflation, establishes conclusively that such recoil is instantaneous. Interestingly, the single patient in this series ([7] Table 4) in whom clinical evidence of restenosis has thus far been observed was the patient in whom recoil was most severe (Fig. 7).

In five instances, measurements recorded with the BUIC disclosed "nega-

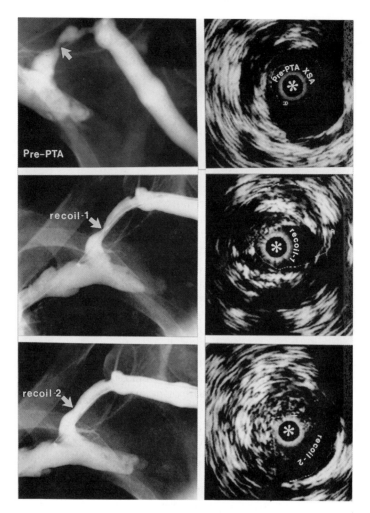

Figure 7. Most severe instance of recoil observed in present series of patients studied/treated with BUIC (pt 7, Table 2). *Top*: arrow in cine frame indicates stenosis in venous limb of arteriovenous dialysis fistula pre-PTA; image recorded from BUIC shows pre-PTA cross-sectional area (A) determined prior to balloon inflation superimposed upon area of fully inflated balloon. *Middle*: arrow in cine frame points to (deflated) BUIC ultrasound transducer positioned to measure luminal dimensions following balloon deflation #1; residual stenosis following PTA #1 of this site is apparent from contrast injection. Accompanying image recorded from BUIC demonstrates corresponding magnitude of cross-sectional area (A) measured following balloon deflation. *Bottom*: arrow in cine frame points to BUIC ultrasound transducer positioned to measure luminal dimensions following PTA #2; residual stenosis is evident by angiography. Accompanying image recorded from BUIC demonstrates corresponding cross-sectional area (A) measured following balloon deflation.

tive" recoil, i.e. luminal dimensions post-PTA exceeded those of the angioplasty balloon at maximum inflation. In one case, post-PTA diameter of the arterial lumen slightly exceeded that of the balloon, while post- PTA cross-sectional area was slightly less than that of the balloon. In the remaining four cases, while recoil varied fom 0 to 23% as a function of balloon diameter, when measured in terms of cross-sectional area luminal area post-PTA exceeded balloon area by 4 to 22%. Although not explicitly commented upon, inspection of findings reported previously by Hjemdahl-Monsen [55] and Lehmann [57] reveals several cases in which diameter measurements made by quantitative angiography were indicative of such "negative" recoil. Analysis of this phenomenon in the present series of cases suggests that it results from a relatively large (but non-flow limiting) plaque fracture; this has the previously noted effect of limiting elastic recoil.

Moreover, when a radial plaque fracture is associated with a circumferential extension, the resulting cross-sectional area may in fact exceed that of the inflated balloon, despite the fact that the post-PTA minimum luminal diameter, along a selected minor axis, is slightly less than that of the inflated balloon. Because intravascular ultrasound allows direct inspection of the often complex cracked and/or dissected post-PTA lumen, diameter and cross-sectional area may both be assessed directly and independently [46–49, 59,60]. Most algorithms developed for quantitative angiography calculate cross-sectional area as a function of measured luminal diameter, and previous studies have documented that the accuracy of such algorithms may be diminished in those cases in which satisfactory orthogonal views cannot be obtained [61]. Assessment of elastic recoil post-angioplasty may thus be more complicated than previously appreciated; it is in fact entirely possible that apparent recoil measured as a function of luminal diameter post-angioplasty is more frequently than previously appreciated associated with a paradoxical increase in luminal cross-sectional area.

Finally, on-line ultrasound monitoring of ballon inflation also facilitated identification of the initiation of plaque fracture (Figs. 8,9). On-line analysis of pressure-volume curves has been investigated previously as a means of characterizing the mechanism responsible for vascular dilation in vivo [62]. "Cracking," identified as sudden yielding of the balloon at a given inflation pressure, was less commonly observed than either patterns indicative of "stretching," or "compaction." The results of on-line ultrasound analysis of balloon inflation suggest that plaque "fracture" is proportionately more common than indicated by pressure-volume analysis, and this is further supported by post-hoc ultrasound analyses [27,49,59,60,63,] and previously reported necropsy studies [50]. Moreover, in at least one patient, ([3] Table 2; Fig. 10) we observed what graphically would appear to correspond to "sudden yielding of the balloon [and arterial wall] at a given inflation pressure" unaccompanied by evident plaque fracture during or post-PTA.

Images recorded from the BUIC disclosed that plaque fractures were initiated by dilatation at low (< 2 atmospheres) inflation pressures. This is

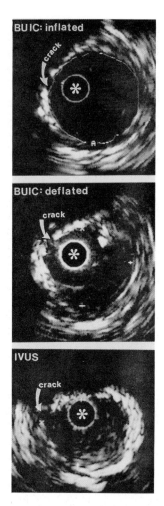

Figure 8. Example of fracture (crack) of heavily calcified plaque during PTA using BUIC. *Top*: crack near one end of calcific bar at full balloon inflation; inscribed circle denotes cross-sectional area (A) of balloon. *Middle*: appearance of the crack immediately following deflation of BUIC balloon. *Bottom*: confirmation of crack identified with BUIC by image recorded from IVUS.

consistent with previous clinical observations. Hjemdahl-Monsen et al, for example, found that most improvement in luminal size occurred at inflation pressures <2 atmospheres [55]. Likewise, Kahn et al observed that full balloon expansion as determined by fluoroscopic monitoring occurred in nearly 50% of patients at inflation pressures of 4 atmospheres or less [64]. These findings regarding the efficacy of lower inflation pressures supplement experimental data indicating a higher incidence of mural thrombus, dissection, and intimal hyperplasia as a result of higher inflation pressures. As suggested by Kleiman et al [65], any technique, whether it be pressure-volume or ultrasound analysis, that permits immediate, on-line recognition

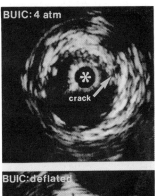

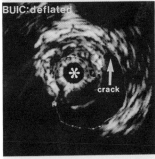

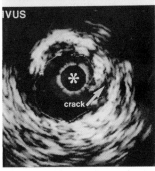

Figure 9. Example of plaque fracture (crack) observed during balloon inflation using BUIC. *Top:* image recorded at 4 atmospheres (atm) showing fully developed crack as seen during inflation. *Middle:* appearance of crack immediately following balloon deflation. *Bottom:* confirmation of crack identified with BUIC by image recorded from non-balloon intravascular ultrasound catheter (IVUS).

of plaque fracture might theoretically be employed to modify the remainder of the dilatation procedure in an attempt to prevent the development of a flow-limiting dissection.

Three-Dimensional Reconstruction

Comparison of individual segments examined by IVUS to adjacent or more distant segments requires repeated review of serially recorded images to

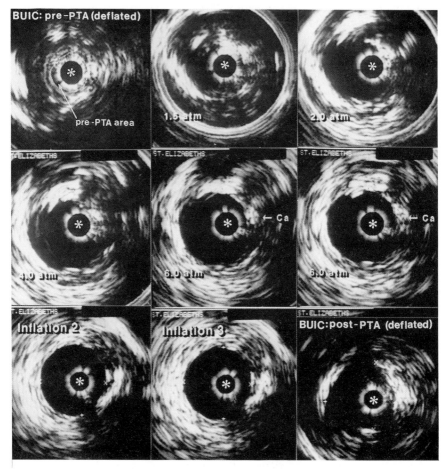

Figure 10. Serial images recorded from BUIC pre-, during, and post-PTA of common iliac arterial stenosis (pt 3, Table 2). *Top left*: image recorded from BUIC immediately prior to balloon inflation demonstrates pre-PTA cross-sectional area, indicated by inscribed circle. Subsequent images demonstrate serial expansion of balloon cross-sectional area recorded from BUIC during inflation #1 at 1.5, 2.0, 4.0, and 6.0 atmospheres (atm). The pair of images recorded at 6 atm demonstrates sudden yielding of arterial wall after several seconds at given inflation pressure; note movement of calcified (Ca) plaque towards arrow, position of which was not changed from first to second image recorded at 6 atm. *Bottom row* of images illustrates cross-sectional area of BUIC at full inflations #2 and 3, and final luminal cross-sectional area recorded from BUIC immediately post-balloon deflation.

reconstruct, in the mind's eye, the spatial relationship of the segments of interest. For example, while one tomographic image obtained during IVUS examination may offer high-resolution definition of a plaque fracture resulting from balloon angioplasty, details regarding the longitudinal distribution of the same plaque fracture at one site relative to proximal and distal sites cannot be displayed in a single image. In contrast, conventional angiography preserves the advantage of displaying each segment in longitudinal relationship to adjacent and more distant segments; once contrast media has opacified the artery of interest, any individual segment may be compared to adjacent and distant segments, limited only by the field of view. Three-dimensional reconstruction of serially recorded tomographic images represents a possible solution to the limited spatial display features characteristic of current IVUS imaging systems.

Original attempts to perform three-dimensional reconstructions in our laboratory involved the use of software (SigmaScan, Jandel Scientific, Corte Madera, CA) that required manual morphometric tracing of each serial tomographic image followed by computer-aided reconstruction [66]. The more detail intended, the more images were required, and consequently the more labor-intensive was the reconstruction. The principal liability of this approach, however, related to the fact that the modelling technique was based exclusively on boundary depiction and therefore allowed three-dimensional reconstruction of the lumen but not the arterial wall. Such an approach would clearly squander one of the chief assets of intravascular ultrasound, namely the capability to image the vessel wall and thereby evaluate characteristics of the native wall, as well as pathologic alterations resulting from interventional therapies.

Automated three-dimensional reconstruction of intravascular ultrasound images was investigated in a preliminary fashion by Kitney et al [67], using voxel modelling. This approach considers each voxel, or volume element, as an extension to three-dimensional space of the digital image element, or pixel (picture element). Voxel modelling is a particularly attractive option for three-dimensional reconstruction of the vasculature, because it allows representation of the arterial wall rather than simply surface features that would limit the reconstruction to the arterial lumen.

More recently [68–71] we have had the opportunity to perform three-dimensional reconstruction using a PC-based system (ImageComm Systems, Santa Clara, CA) and algorithms [72–74] designed specifically for analysis of images recorded during IVUS examination (Omniview, Pura Labs, Brea, CA). The software employs a surface rendering process predicated on segmented boundary formation, but includes interpolative algorithms designed to link boundary elements, and thereby preserve the capability of viewing the arterial wall as well as lumen.

Analysis of the three-dimensional reconstructions recorded in a preliminary series of 52 patients (Table 5) suggests that these three-dimensional images may in fact supplement analysis of conventional two-dimensional images. Use of the so-called sagittal format (Fig. 11) in particular not only facilitates comparative analysis of adjacent tomographic images, but offers the additional advantage of displaying the ultrasound data in a longitudinal profile-type format more familiar to the angiographer. While similar in orientation to an angiogram, sagittal reconstruction substantially augments information available from conventional angiography in two important ways.

Table 5. Clinical features, ultrasound examinations, and 3-dimensional reconstructions.

Pt	Sex	Age	Functional Status		Ankle Brachial Index		Vessel	Intervention	IVUS Catheter Size (Fr)	2-Dimensional Pre (#)		3-Dimensional Reconstructions Post (#)				On-line
			Pre	Post	Pre	Post				Pre	Post	Sag	Cyl	Sag	Cyl	
1	M	64	3	0	0.45	0	CIA	CIA	PTA	6.2	–	+	–	–	1	–
2	F	69	3	1	0.42	1.01	CIA	PTA	6.2	+	+	2	–	3	–	
3	F	53	4	0	0.75		CIA	PTA	6.2	–	+	1	4	1	1	
4	M	57	3	1	0.42	1.34	CIA	PTA	6.2	+	+	–	–	3	6	+
5	M	68	3	2	0.97		CIA	PTA	6.2	+	+	1	1	1	2	
6	F	69	3	0	0.80	0.87	CIA	PTA	6.2	+	+	3	1	5	1	+
7	M	80	4	2	0.54		CIA	PTA	6.2	+	+	2	–	1	–	
8	M	56	3	2	0.65		CIA/EIA	PTA	6.2	+	+	–	–	1	1	+
9	M	72	4	2		0.46	CIA/EIA	PTA	6.2	+	+	2	–	2	–	
10	M	56	3	1	0.63		CIA/EIA/CFA	PTA	6.2	+	+	1	–	2	–	
11	F	63	3	1	0.59	0.94	EIA	PTA	6.2	+	+	2	2	3	3	
12	M	67	3	1	0.69	0.92	EIA	PTA	6.2	+	+	1	–	1	1	
13	M	64	4	3	0.58	0.94	EIA	PTA	6.2	+	+	1	–	2	–	
14	F	66	5	2	0.23	0.61	EIA	PTA	6.2	–	+	–	–	1	–	
15	M	62	3	2	0.36	0.64	EIA	PTA, Stent	6.2	+	+	2	–	1	1	
16	M	54	3	3	0.71		EIA	PTA	6.2	+	+	2	3	3	3	+
17	M	79	3	2	0.44	0.52	EIA	PTA	6.2	+	+	1	1	2	1	
18	M	77	4	2	0.48	0.40	EIA	PTA	6.2	+	+	3	–	1	–	
19	F	79	4	1	0.39	0.57	EIA/CFA	PTA	6.2	+	+	2	–	1	–	
20	M	45	5	3	0.49	0.71	EIA/CFA	PTA	6.2	+	+	1	1	2	1	
21	M	71	3	2	0.39	0.82	EIA/Profunda	PTA	4.8	+	+	–	–	1	–	
22	M	59	5	3	0.45	0.90	SFA	PTA	6.2	–	–	4	–	7	7	
23	F	75	3	0	0.43	0.88	SFA	Laser, PTA	6.2	+	+	4	–	4	4	
24	M	52	3	2	0.60	0.82	SFA	Atherectomy	6.2	+	+	1	–	3	1	
25	M	56	3	1	0.49	0.48	SFA	PTA	6.2	–	+	1	–	1	–	
26	M	77	4	2	0.30	0.92	SFA/Pop A	Laser, PTA	6.2	+	+	1	–	2	–	
27	M	59	3	0	0.41		SFA/Pop A	Laser, Atherectomy	6.2	+	+		–	1	–	
28	M	63	3	2	0.40	0.77	SFA/Peroneal/Ant Tib	Laser, PTA	6.2	+*	–	1	1	–	–	

#	Sex	Age					Artery	Procedure								
29	M	67	3	0	0.76	1.20	Pop A	Laser. PTA	6.2	+	+	2	2	1	1	–
30	M	55	3	0	0.65	1.08	RSVG (Fem-Pop)	Lysis, Laser. PTA	6.2	+	+	–	–	3	3	–
31	F	55	NA	NA	NA	NA	Subclavian A	PTA	4.8	–	+	–	1	1	1	1
32	F	75	NA	NA	NA	NA	Dialysis Fistula	PTA	6.2	+	+	1	1	1	1	1
33	M	66	NA	NA	NA	NA	Dialysis Fistula	PTA	6.2	+	+	1	1	1	1	1
34	F	77	NA	NA	NA	NA	Dialysis Fistula	PTA	6.2	+	+	1	1	1	1	1
35	M	66	NA	NA	NA	NA	Dialysis Fistula	PTA	6.2	+	+	1	1	1	1	1
36	F	75	NA	NA	NA	NA	Dialysis Fistula	PTA	6.2	–	+	–	–	2	2	1
37	F	77	NA	NA	NA	NA	Renal Artery	PTRA	4.8	–	+	–	–	1	1	1
38	F	80	NA	NA	NA	NA	Renal Artery	PTRA	4.8	–	+	–	–	1	1	1
39	F	29	NA	NA	NA	NA	Renal Artery	PTRA	4.8	–	+	–	–	1	1	1
40	M	63	NA	NA	NA	NA	Renal Artery	PTRA	4.8	+	+	5	4	3	3	3 (+)
41	M	65	NA	NA	NA	NA	LAD	PTCA	4.8	–	+	–	–	1	1	–
42	M	65	NA	NA	NA	NA	LAD	PTCA	4.8	–	+	–	–	1	1	2
43	F	48	NA	NA	NA	NA	LAD	PTCA	3.5	–	+	–	–	2	2	2
44	M	69	NA	NA	NA	NA	LAD	PTCA	3.5	–	+	–	–	2	2	2
45	F	61	NA	NA	NA	NA	RCA	Laser, PTCA	4.8	–	+	–	–	1	1	1
46	M	64	NA	NA	NA	NA	RCA	PTCA	3.5	–	+	–	–	5	5	5
47	M	55	NA	NA	NA	NA	RCA	PTCA	4.8	–	+	–	–	2	2	2
48	M	48	NA	NA	NA	NA	RCA	PTCA	4.8	–	+	–	–	1	1	1
49	M	61	NA	NA	NA	NA	RSVG to RCA	Laser, PTCA	4.8	–	+	–	–	5	5	5
50	M	59	NA	NA	NA	NA	RSVG to RCA	PTCA	4.8	–	+	–	–	1	1	1
51	F	59	NA	NA	NA	NA	RSVG to LAD	–	4.8	+	NA	1	1	NA	NA	NA
52	M	52	NA	NA	NA	NA	RSVG to RCA/LAD	–	4.8	+	NA	2	2	NA	NA	NA

Abbreviations: = Rutherford class; # = number; † = 3-dimensional reconstruction and image generation during interventional procedure; – = not done; + = done; * = ultrasound examination on superficial femoral artery only; A = artery; Ant Tib = anterior tibial artery; CFA = common femoral artery; CIA = common iliac artery; Cyl = Cylindrical; EIA = external iliac artery. F = female; Fem-pop = femoro-popliteal graft. Fr = french; IVUS = intravascular ultrasound; LAD = left anterior descending coronary artery; Lysis = thrombolysis; M = male; NA = not applicable; PTA = percutaneous transluminal angioplasty; PTCA = percutaneous transluminal coronary angioplasty; PTRA = percutaneous transluminal renal angioplasty; Pop = popliteal; Profunda = profunda femoris artery; RCA = right coronary artery; RSVG = reverse saphenous vein graft; Sag = sagittal; SFA = superficial femoral artery.

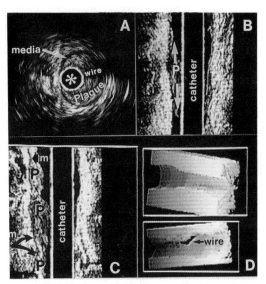

Figure 11. Atherosclerotic iliac artery: 3D reconstruction pre-TAA. (A) Representative IVUS image obtained from segment of diseased iliac artery, demonstrating eccentric plaque. Medial layer (m) remains intact. (B) Sagittal reconstruction of same vessel, with atherosclerotic plaque (P) that appears to be confined to center of vascular segment. (C) Sagittal view, obtained by revolving 60° about axis to IVUS catheter, demonstrating that eccentric plaque is not limited to central portion, but rather extends throughout entire length of this vascular segment. Media (m) is seen underlying plaque for its entire length. (D) Cylindrical reconstructions of two halves of hemisected vessel offer less detail than sagittal views in this example. Note shadowing artifact from guidewire.

First, limitless orthogonal views can be rendered by incremental rotation of the imaging plane around the reference catheter. Given the documented importance of orthogonal views in the assessment of luminal narrowing [61] on the one hand, and the logistical factors which frequently obviate the possibility of obtaining orthogonal views on the other, this feature may ultimately prove to be the principal advantage of three-dimensional reconstruction.

Second, information regarding pathologic alteration of the arterial wall is provided simultaneously with the conventional assessment of luminal diameter narrowing. Experience with several of the patients in the present series undergoing percutaneous revascularization indicates that certain features of arterial wall pathology are particularly well defined in such a longitudinal format. For example, three-dimensional reconstruction in the sagittal mode graphically demonstrated that recanalization of a lengthy total occlusion was achieved by tunneling a false lumen through calcified plaque (Fig. 12). Such a mechanism of recanalization has been previously described in vitro [75, 76] and is frequently inferred to occur in vivo [77], but, in the present case, definition equivalent to the reconstructed ultrasound image was absent from the completion angiogram. While the individual tomographic

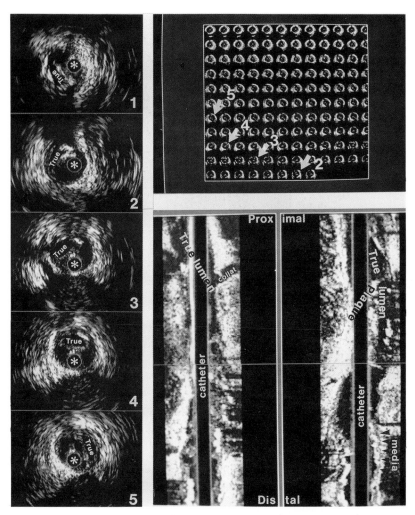

Figure 12. Three-dimensional reconstruction of recanalized superficial femoral artery (SFA). Left: 2D IVUS images obtained during pullback through recanalized, previously occluded segment of SFA show the IVUS catheter (asterisk) within dilated lumen. An apparent second lumen spirals around longitudinal axis of catheter; second lumen appears to be surrounded by three-layered wall, suggesting that it may represent true lumen, and that IVUS catheter has been advanced over wire positioned in a false (subintimal) channel, secondarily enlarged by balloon dilation. *Upper center*: tabloid showing 128 of the 256 digitized 2D images acquired and stored during IVUS pullback post-PTA; arrows point out frames corresponding to 2D images 2 through 5 in the left panel of this Fig. *Lower center*: sagittal 3D reconstruction from the stored image set explicitly demonstrate subintimal dissection tract; these two sagittal reconstructions represent orthogonal (biplane) views of the same segment of recanalized SFA, selected at approximately 90° of rotation from one another. In reconstruction shown at left, collateral (collat) branch is seen originating proximal to site of prior occlusion; there is residual narrowing of the recanalized segment. In sagittal view shown at right, IVUS catheter can be seen entering plaque, creating subintimal tract at the site of prior occlusion. Apparent *true* lumen is seen to right of catheter. Dense, apparently calcified plaque (note subjacent "shadowing" effect) located at origin of lesion, may have caused deflection of guidewire into the subintimal tract. Further distal in SFA, IVUS catheter is clearly seen to re-enter true lumen, bordered on both sides by 3–1ayered appearance reflecting media of arterial wall.

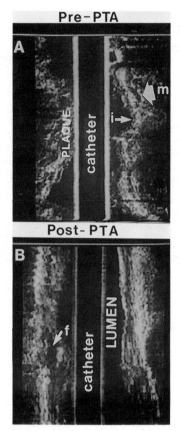

Figure 13. Sagittal reconstructions of iliac artery pre- and post-PTA. (A) Sagittal 3D reconstruction pre-PTA illustrates complex topography of arterial wall, extent of plaque, and relative degree of luminal narrowing. Intimal surface (i) and media (m) are irregular and discontinuous. (B) Sagittal image created from post-PTA IVUS pullback documents enhanced luminal patency and small, benign-appearing plaque fracture (f).

ultrasound images indicated creation of a "double-barrel" lumen, the full extent of pathologic disruption was more immediately apparent from inspection of the sagittal reconstructions. Similarly, sagittal reconstructions of balloon-dilated non-occluded vessels demonstrated the longitudinal distribution of barotraumatic injury (Fig. 13), otherwise evident as only local, isolated plaque fractures on the tomographic two-dimensional IVUS images.

Experience with the so-called cylindrical format (Fig.14) suggests that this mode of three-dimensional reconstruction – particularly when the reconstructed vascular segment is hemisected – is optimally suited for those cases in which direct inspection of luminal topography is of special interest, such as analysis of implanted endovascular prostheses (Fig. 14). Details of the "cobblestoned" neointima lining the stent cannot be appreciated angiographically or even by intravascular ultrasound, when viewed in standard video

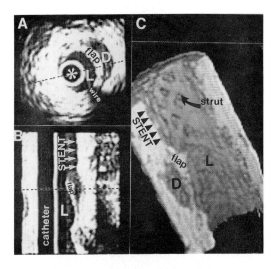

Figure 14. Three-dimensional reconstruction of endovascular stent. (A) Representative 2D IVUS image obtained post-PTA from non-stented portion of iliac artery immediately distal to stent. IVUS catheter (asterisk) is within the true lumen (L); as a result of balloon dilation, a large flap separates true lumen from dissection (D) tract in underlying vessel wall. Shadowing artifact is seen from wire. Dashed black line in (B) indicates the level of 2D image shown in (A). (C) Cylindrical reconstruction, with region of interest drawn to encompass a 180° hemisection of the same segment of iliac artery shown in (A) and (B); note "cobblestoned" appearance is imparted by stent struts. Adjacent dissection and intimal flap are seen below. The IVUS catheter has been eliminated from this image, using the mask function of software.

format [78]; the algorithms developed to accomplish the cylindrical reconstruction serve the dual functions of both joining together the series of adjacent elements representing the neointima, and then rotating the reconstructed image 90° to permit viewing of the endoluminal surface en face. The sagittal reconstruction supplements, the cylindrical format by facilitating analysis of arterial contour proximal and distal to the stent; such analysis is otherwise not feasible using the unassembled tomographic images.

Alternatively, the "third dimension" of the three-dimensional software may be used as a, temporal rather than spatial axis. We have utilized this option, for example, in conjunction with the BUIC, to summate composite balloon inflation and deflation within a single image (Fig. 15).

Certain limitations of current attempts to perform three-dimensional reconstruction must be acknowledged. First, it is apparent that the quality of the three-dimensional reconstructions can only be as good as the original two-dimensional images. Details which are absent from the original recordings will likewise be absent from the reconstructed images. In those instances when calcific deposits, for example, are observed on the two-dimensional images to attenuate echoes from the subjacent plaque and/or wall, these portions of the plaque and/or wall will not be incorporated into the reconstructed image.

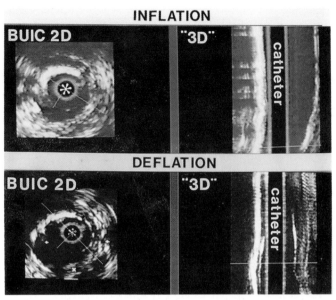

Figure 15. Composite depiction of balloon (BUIC) inflation and deflation summated by 3DR; third dimension in this case has been assigned to a temporal rather than spatial axis.

Second, "ring-down artifact", resulting from dead space in the acoustic transmission path and manifested on the two-dimensional image as a white halo immediately peripheral to the transducer, may obscure near-field structure in smaller, particularly stenotic vessels. In our preliminary work such artifact was routinely masked out of the three-dimensional reconstructions; in those cases in which reconstruction is applied to two-dimensional images with little or no lumen peripheral to the transducer, such masking could overestimate three-dimensional depiction of luminal patency. Current attempts by the manufacturers of mechanical transducer systems to eliminate such artifact will hopefully resolve this issue.

Third, while major branch points, such as the aortic bifurcation, are accurately depicted in the three-dimensional reconstruction, the two-dimensional images are otherwise reassembled as a straight tube; sharp bends in the artery are not faithfully reconstructed on either the two- or three-dimensional images. While this is typically not a severe liability in evaluation of the peripheral and renal circulations, it may become more significant in the assessment of the more tortuous coronary circulation.

Fourth, three-dimensional reconstruction shares with conventional intravascular ultrasound imaging the difficulty of matching the rotational orientation of the ultrasound transducer to that of the imaged vessel. Furthermore, if the ultrasound probe is inadvertently twisted during the pullback recording, the three-dimensional reconstruction will reflect this rotational event.

Fifth, in all studies performed to date, the two-dimensional images have been acquired during a slow (approximately 0.25 cm/sec), timed catheter pullback; this strategy is intended to optimize the number of acquired images over a given segment length and provide equal representation for each portion of the artery in the reconstructed image. Such catheter pullback, however, is entirely operator-dependent and small variations in the rate of pullback may ultimately influence the three-dimensional representation. For example, if the catheter withdrawal rate is slowed during pullback through an abnormal segment of vessel, and subsequently accelerated through a more normal segment, the abnormal segment will occupy proportionally more than its true length of the resulting reconstruction. This phenomenon is particularly likely to occur when there is a tendency for the operator to slow catheter movement through abnormal segments to achieve closer inspection of morphologic disruptions. To minimize this variable in the present investigation, the sole focus of the operator performing the pullback was to observe the catheter as it was withdrawn through the sheath or guiding catheter; analysis of two-dimensional ultrasound image registration was performed before and/or after the pullback recording. This acquisition technique is currently being modified to include automated image registration that will be less operator-dependent. One such potential modification is to alter the acquisition mode such that it be based on regular distance intervals, in contrast to the current system of time-interval based image acquisition.

Beyond these limitations, the extent to which three-dimensional reconstruction will be employed clinically is principally dependent on two factors: the time required for reconstruction and the prognostic implications of the resulting images. With regard to the former, image processing time has been reduced considerably through a combination of modifications in software and memory expansion. Whereas early reconstructions typically required 20 to 40 min to assemble, current reconstructions are routinely completed within 20 sec of completing the two-dimensional pullback recording. Preliminary work [31] with yet another iteration of software has generated both sagittal and cylindrical reconstructions within 30 sec of completing the pullback recording. It is thus realistic to expect that the time required to reconstruct and review the reconstructed images will be comparable to that currently required to review the video playback of a contrast angiogram. While reconstructions accomplished on-line in the current series were not used for the purpose of guiding therapeutic decisions, this strategy should be feasible in the future.

The extent to which three-dimensional reconstructions of two-dimensional intravascular ultrasound images will alter interventional or other therapy remains to be determined. The same, of course, remains true of the two-dimensional images as well. While the quality of the two-dimensional images has evolved to the point that they are in fact being used to make on-line decisions regarding the nature and extent of percutaneous revascularization [59, 79], prognostic implications associated with specific findings will require clinical and/or angiographic follow-up studies [80]. In the case of a dissection resulting from attempted balloon angioplasty, for example, it is conceivable that the geometric disposition of the dissection might determine whether it is likely to lead to early occlusion, later restenosis, or, in other cases, heal in a benign fashion. At present, such information cannot be adequately determined by conventional angiography, which provides too little detail regarding the plaque and/or arterial wall. Three-dimensional reconstruction of the two-dimensional examination should facilitate evaluation of the latter's prognostic utility by providing a comprehensive recapitulation of the sequentially recorded tomographic images. Ultimately, however, the utility of three-dimensional reconstruction as an adjunct to interventional procedures will need to be evaluated in prospective studies.

Finally, preliminary algorithms have already been developed to augment the utility of three- dimensional reconstruction in two important respects. First, an automated edge-detection scheme has been incorporated which will permit automated quantitative analysis of cross-sectional area from the cylindrical reconstructions. Second, characterization of plaque composition, long an elusive goal of vascular imaging, may be facilitated by three-dimensional reconstruction. Preliminary applications of intravascular ultrasound suggest that it is more sensitive than conventional fluoroscopy for detection of vascular calcific deposits and, furthermore, is capable of distinguishing predominantly fibrotic from predominantly fatty plaque. While manual morphometric assessment of each two-dimensional frame recorded during an intravascular ultrasound examination is an impractical means by which to analyze tissue composition, preliminary applications suggest that computer-aided analyses of reconstructed three-dimensional images may make such qualitative assessment feasible.

References

1. Vlodaver Z, Frech R, Van Tassel R A, Edwards J E (1973) Correlations of the antemortem arteriogram and the postmortem specimen. *Circulation* 47:162–169
2. Grondin C M, Dyrda I, Pasternac A, Campeau L, Bourassa M G, Lesperance J (1974) Discrepancies between cineangiographic and postmortem findings in patients with coronary artery disease and recent myocardial revascularization. *Circulation* 49:703–708
3. Pepine C J, Feldman R L, Nichols W W et al (1977) Coronary arteriography: potentially serious sources of error in interpretation. *Cardiovascuiar Med* 2:747–752
4. Arnett E N, Isner J M, Redwood C R et al (1979) Coronary artery narrowing in coronary heart disease: comparison of cineangiographic and necropsy findings. *Ann Int Med* 91:350–356
5. Isner J M, Kishel J, Kent K M, Ronan J A, Jr., Ross A M, Roberts W C (1981) Accuracy of angiographic determination of left main coronary arterial narrowing: angiographic-histologic, correlative analysis in 28 patients. *Circulation* 63:1056–1064
6. Spears J R, Sandor T, Baim D S, Paulin S (1983) The minimum error in estimating coronary luminal cross-sectional area from cineangiographic diameter measurements. *Cath Cardiovasc Diag* 9:119–128
7. White C W, Wright C B, Doty D B et al (1984) Does visual interpretation of the coronary arteriogram predict the physiologic importance of a coronary stenosis? *N Engl J Med* 310: 819–24

8. Isner J M, Donaldson R F (1984) Coronary angiographic and morphologic correlation. *Cardiology Clinics* 2:571–592
9. Gould K L (1985) Quantification of coronary artery stenosis in vivo. *Circ Res* 57:341–353
10. Zijlstra F, van Ommeren J, Reiber H C, Serruys P W (1987) Does the quantitative assessment of coronary artery dimensions predict the physiologic significance of a coronary stenosis? *Circulation* 75:1154–1161
11. Marcus M L, Skorton D J, Johnson M R, Collins S M, Harrison W, Kerber R E (1988) Visual estimates of percent diameter coronary stenosis: "a battered gold standard." *J Am Coll Cardiol* 11:882–885
12. Clarke R H, Isner J M, Gauthier T D et al (1988) Spectroscopic characterization of cardiovascular tissue. *Lasers Surg Med* 8:45–59
13. Deckelbaum L I, Stetz M L, O'Brien K M et al (1989) Fluorescence spectroscopic guidance of laser ablation of atherosclerotic plaque. *Lasers Surg Med* 9:205–214
14. Spears J R, Marais H J, Serur J et al (1983) In vivo coronary angioscopy. *J Am Coll Cardiol* 1:1311–1314
15. Jakubowski A, Hickey A, Glick D, Litvaik F, Grundfest W, Forrester J S (1989) Angioscopy. In: Isner J M, Clarke R H (eds) *Cardiovascular Laser Therapy*, Raven Press, New York, 201–212
16. White G H, White R A (1989) Percutaneous angioscopy as adjunct to laser angioplasty in peripheral arteries. *Lancet* 2:99 (letter)
17. Sahn D J, Barrett-Boyers, Graham K et al (1982) Ultrasonic imaging of the coronary arteries in open-chest humans: evaluation of coronary atherosclerotic lesions during cardiac surgery. *Circulation* 66:1034–1044
18. McPherson D D, Armstong M, Rose E et al (1986) High-frequency epicardial echocardiography for coronary artery evaluation: in vitro and in vivo validation of arterial lumen and wall thickness measuments. *J Am Coll Cardiol* 8:600–606
19. McPherson D D, Hiratzka L F, Lamberth W C et al (1987) Delineation of the extent of coronary atherosclerosis by high-frequency epicardial echocardiography. *N Engl J Med* 316:304–309
20. Pandian N G, Kreis A, Brockway B, Isner J M, Sacharoff A, Boleza E (1988) Ultrasound angioscopy: real-time, two-dimensional, intraluminal ultrasound imaging of blood vessels. *Am J Cardiol* 62:493–494
21. Gussenhoven W J, Essed C E, Lancee C T et al (1989) Arterial wall characteristics determined by intravascular ultrasound imaging: an in vitro study. *J Am Coll Cardiol* 14:947–952
22. Meyer C R, Chiang E H, Fechner K P, Fitting D W, Williams D M, Buda A J (1988) Feasibility of high-resolution, intravascular ultrasonic imaging catheters. *Radiology* 168:113–116
23. Yock P G, Linker D T, Thapliyal H V et al (1988) Real-time, two-dimensional catheter ultrasound: a new technique for high resolution intravascular imaging (abstr). *J Am Coll Cardiol* 2:130A
24. Hodgson J, Eberle, Savakus A (1988) Validation of a new real-time percutaneous intravascular ultrasound imaging catheter (abstr). *Circulation* 168:727–731
25. Mallery J A, Tobis J M, Gessert J et al (1988) Evaluation of an intravascular ultrasound imaging catheter in porcine peripheral and coronary arteries in vivo. *Circulation* 78:11–21
26. Pandian N, Kreis A, Desnoyers M et al (1988) In vivo ultrasound angioscopy in humans and animals: intraluminal imaging of blood vessels using a new catheter-based high resolution ultrasound probe. *Circulation* 78:II-22
27. Isner J M, Rosenfield K, Losordo D W, Kelly S, Palefski P, Langevin R E, Razvi S, Pastore J O, Kosowsky B D (1990) Percutaneous intravascular US as adjunct to catheter-based interventions: preliminary experience in patients with peripheral vascular disease. *Radiology* 175:61–70
28. Hodgson J M, Graham S P, Savakus A D et al (1989) Clinical percutaneous imaging of coronary anatomy using an over-the-wire ultrasound catheter system. *Intl J Card Imaging* 4:187–193

29. Tobis J, Mallery J, Gessert J et al (1988) Intravascular ultrasound visualization before and after balloon angioplasty (abstr). *Circulation* 78:II-84
30. Graham S, Brands D, Savakus A, Hodgson J (1989) Utility of an intravascular ultrasound imaging device for arterial wall definition and atherectomy guidance (abstr). *J Am Coll Cardiol* 13:222A
31. Rutherford R B, Flanigan D P, Guptka S K et al (1986) Suggested standards for reports dealing with lower extremity ischemia. *J Vasc Surg* 14:80–94
32. Isner J M, Rosenfield K, Pieczek A, Harding M, Razvi S, Langevin R E, Kosowsky B D (1991) Clinical experience with intravascular ultrasound as adjunct to percutaneous recanalization in 101 consecutive patients. *J Am Coll Cardiol* 17:125A
33. Palmaz J C, Richter G, Noeldge G et al (1988) Intraluminal stents in atherosclerotic iliac artery stenosis: preliminary report of a multicenter study. *Radiology* 168:727–731
34. Chokshi S K, Meyers S, Abi-Mansour P (1987) Percutaneous transluminal coronary angioplasty: ten years experience. *Prog Cardiov Dis* 30:147–210
35. Isner J M, Donaldson R F, Fortin A H, Tischler A, Clarke R H (1986) Attenuation of the media in coronary arteries in advanced atherosclerosis. *Am J Cardiol* 58:937–939
36. Rosenfield K, Voelker W, Losordo D W, Ramaswamy K, Kosowsky B D, Pastore J O, Isner J M (1991) Assessment of coronary arterial stenoses post-intervention by quantitative angiography versus intracoronary ultrasound in 13 patients undergoing balloon and/or laser coronary angioplasty (abstr). *J Am Coll Cardiol* 17:46A
37. Webster W W. Catheter for removing arteriosclerotic plaque. United States patent 4,576,177 (Issued March 18, 1986)
38. Ramee S R, White C J, Collins T J, Mesa J E, Murgo J P (1991) Percutaneous angioscopy during coronary angioplasty using a steerable microangioscope. *J Am Coll Cardiol* 17:100–105
39. Lee G, Lkeda R M, Stobbe D, Ogata C, Theis J, Hussein H, Mason D T (1983) Laser irradiation of human atherosclerotic obstructive disease: simultaneous visualization and vaporization achieved by a dual fiberoptic catheter. *Am Heart J* 105:163–164
40. Leon M B, Almagor Y, Bartorelli A L, Prevosti L G, Teirstein P S, Chang R, Miller D L, Smith P D, Bonner R F (1990) Fluorescence-guided laser-assisted balloon angioplasty in patients with femoropopliteal occlusions. *Circulation* 81:143–155
41. Mallery J, Gregory K, Morcos N C, Griffith J, Henry W (1987) Evaluation of ultrasound balloon dilatation imaging catheter (abstr). *Circulation* 76-IV:371
42. Yock P G, Fitzgerald P J, Jang Y-T, McKenzie J, Belef M, Starksen N, White N W, Linker D T, Simpson J B (1990) Initial trials of a combined ultrasound imaging/mechanical atherectomy catheter. *J Am Coll Cardiol* 15:105A
43. Hodgson JMcB, Cacchione J G, Berry J, Savakus A, Eberle M (1990) Combined intracoronary ultrasound imaging and angioplasty catheter: initial in vivo studies (abstr). *Circulation* 82:III-676
44. Isner J M, Rosenfield K, Losordo D W, Rose L, Langevin R E Jr, Razvi S, Kosowsky B (1991) Combination balloon-ultrasound imaging catheter for percutaneous transluminal angioplasty validation of imaging, analysis of recoil, and identification of plaque fracture. *Circulation* 84:739–754
45. Crowley R J, Couvillon L A, Abele J E. Acoustic imaging catheter and the like. United States Patent 4,951,677 (Issued August 28, 1990)
46. Hodgson J, Eberle M, Savakus A (1988) Validation of a new real-time percutaneous intravascular ultrasound imaging catheter (abstr). *Circulation* 178:II-21
47. Nissen S E, Grines C L, Gurley J C, Sublett K, Haynie D, Diaz C, Booth D C, DeMaria A N (1990) Application of a new phased-array ultrasound imaging catheter in the assessment of vascular dimensions. In vivo comparison to cineangiography. *Circulation* 81:660–666
48. Davidson C J, Sheikh K H, Haison J K, Himmelstein S I, Leithe M E, Kisslo K B, Bashore T M (1990) Intravascular ultrasonography versus digital subtraction angiography: a human in vivo comparison of vessel size and morphology. *J Am Coll Cardiol* 16:633–636
49. Gurley J C, Nissen S E, Grines C L, Booth D C, Fischer C, DeMaria A N (1990) Comparison

of intravascular ultrasound and angiography following percutaneous transluminal coronary angioplasty (abstr). *Circulation* 82:III-72

50. Waller B F (1986) Pathology of new interventions used in the treatment of coronary heart disease. *Curr Prob Cardiol* 11:666–760
51. Liu M W, Roubin G S, King, III S B (1989) Restenosis after coronary angioplasty: potential biologic determinants and role of intimal hyperplasia. *Circulation* 79:1374–1387
52. Sanders M (1985) Angiographic changes thirty minutes following percutaneous transluminal coronary angioplasty. *Angiology* 36:419–424
53. Powelson S, Roubin G S, Whitworth H, Gruentzig A R (1987) Incidence of early restenosis after successful percutaneous transluminal coronary angioplasty (PTCA) (abstr). *J Am Coll Cardiol* 9:1–7
54. Noboyushi M, Kimura T, Nosaka H, Mioka S, Ueno K, Yokoi H, Hamasaki N, Horiuchi H, Ohishi H (1990) Restenosis after successful percutaneous transluminal coronary angioplasty: serial angiographic follow-up of 229 patients. *J Am Coll Cardiol* 12: 616–623
55. Hjemdahl-Monsen C E, Ambrose J A, Borrico S, Cohen M, Sherman W, Alexopoulos D, Gorlin R, Fuster V (1990) Angiographic patterns of balloon inflation during percutaneous transluminal coronary angioplasty: role of pressure-diameter curves in studying distensibility and elasticity of the stenotic lesion and the mechanism of dilation. *J Am Coll Cardiol* 16: 569–575
56. Rensing B J, Hermans W R M, Beatt K J, Laarman G J, Suryapranata H, van den Brand M, de Feyter P J, Serruys P W (1990) Quantitative angiographic assessment of elastic recoil after percutaneous transluminal coronary angioplasty. *Am J Cardiol* 66:1039–44
57. Lehmann K G, Feuer J M, Kumamoto K S, Le Ha M (1990) Elastic recoil following coronary angioplasty: magnitude and contributory factors (abstr). *Circulation* 82:III-313
58. Rensing B J, Hermans W R, Strauss B H, Serruys P W (1991) Regional differences in elasic recoil after percutaneous transluminal coronary angioplasty. A quantitative angiographic study. *J Am Coll Cardiol* 17:343–383.
59. Isner J M, Rosenfield K, Mosseri M, Langevin R E, Palefski P, Losordo D W, Razvi S (1990) How reliable are images obtained by intravascular ultrasound for making decisions during percutaneous interventions? Experience with intravascular ultrasound employed in lieu of contrast angiography to guide peripheral balloon angioplasty in 16 patients (abstr). *Circulation* 82:III-440
60. Tobis J M, Mallery J A, Gessert J, Griffith J M, Mahon D, Bessen M, Moriuchi M, McLeay L, McRae M, Henry W L (1989) Intravascular ultrasound cross-sectional arterial imaging before and after balloon angioplasty in vitro. *Circulation* 80:873–882
61. Spears J R, Sandor T, Baim D S, Paulin S (1983) The minimum error in estimating coronary luminal cross-sectional area from cineangiographic diameter measurements. *Cathet Cardiovasc Diagn* 9:119–128
62. Jain A, Demer L L, Raizner A E, Hartley C J, Lewis J M, Roberts R (1987) In vivo assessment of vascular dilatation during percutaneous transluminal coronary angioplasty. *Am J Cardiol* 60:988–992
63. Losordo D W, Rosenfield K, Ramaswamy K, Harding M, Pieczek A, Isner J M (1990) How does angioplasty work? Intravascular ultrasound assessment of 30 consecutive patients demonstrating that angiographic evidence of luminal patency is the consistent result of plaque fractures and dissections (abstr). *Circulation* 82:III-338
64. Kahn J K, Rutherford B D, McConahay D R, Hartzler G O (1990) Inflation pressure requirements during coronary angioplasty. *Cathet Cardiovasc Diag* 21:144–147
65. Kleiman N S, Raizner A E, Roberts R (1990) Percutaneous transluminal coronary angioplasty: is what we see what we get? *J Am Coll Cardiol* 16:576–577
66. DeJesus S T, Rosenfield K R, Gal D et al (1989) Three-dimensional reconstruction of vascular lumen from images recorded during percutaneous two-dimensional intravascular ultrasound. *Clin Res* 37:838A
67. Kitney R I, Moura L, Straughan K (1989) 3-D visualization of arterial structures using ultrasound and Voxel modelling. *Int J Cardiac Imag* 4:177–185

148   *J.M. Isner et al*

68. Rosenfield K, Losordo D W, Ramaswamy K, Pastore J O, Langevin, R E, Razvi S, Kosowsky B D, Isner J M (1991) Three-dimensional reconstruction of human coronary and peripheral arteries from images recorded during two-dimensional intravascular ultrasound examination. *Circulation* 84:1938–1956
69. Rosenfield K, Losordo D W, Majzoubi D, Harding M, Pieczek A, Isner J M (1991) 3-Dimensional reconstruction of coronary and peripheral vessels from 2-D IVUS images: determination of optimal image acquisition rate during timed pullback (abstr). *J Am Coll Cardiol* 17:262A
70. Rosenfield K, Harding M, Pieczek A, Isner J M, Ramaswamy K, Losordo D W, Pastore J O, Kosowsky B D (1991) 3-Dimensional reconstruction of balloon dilated coronary, renal, and femoropopliteal arteries from 2-D intravascular ultrasound images: analysis of longitudinal sagittal versus cylindrical views. *J Am Coll Cardiol* 17:234A
71. Rosenfield K, Losordo D W, Palefski P, Langevin R E, Razvi S, Isner J M (1991) On-line 3-D reconstruction of 2-D intravascular ultrasound images during balloon angioplasty: clinical application in patients undergoing percutaneous balloon angioplasty. *J Am Coll Cardiol* 17:156A
72. Raya S P, Udupa J K, Barrett W A (1990) A PC-based 3D imaging system: algorithms, software, and hardware considerations. *Computerized Medical Imaging and Graphics* 14:353–370
73. Raya S P (1990) SOFVU – a software package for multidimensional medical image analysis. *Proc SPIE, Medical Imaging IV* 1232:152–156
74. Raya S P (1990) Low-level segmentation of 3D magnetic resonance brain images – a rule-based system. *IEEE Transactions on Medical Imaging* 9:327–337
75. Tobis J, Smolin M, Mallery J, Macleay L, Johnston W D, Connolly J E, Lewis G, Zuch B, Henry W, Bems M (1989) Laser-assisted thermal angioplasty in human peripheral artery occlusions: mechanism of recanalization. *J Am Coll Cardiol* 1989; 13:1547–1554
76. Isner J M, Donaldson R F, Funai J T, Deckelbaum L I, Pandian N G, Clarke R H, Bernstein J S (1985) Factors conibuting to perforations resulting from laser coronary angioplasty. Observations in an intact human post-mortem model of intra-operative laser coronary angioplasty. *Circulation* 72:II-191–199
77. Melchior J P, Meir B, Urban P, Finci L, Steffenino F, Noble J, Ratishouser W (1987) Percutaneous transluminal coronary angioplasty for chronic total arterial occlusion. *Am J Cardiol* 59:535–538
78. Chokshi S K, Hogan J, Desai V, Daod M, Cross F Parsonnet V, Isner J M (1990) Intravascular ultrasound assessment of implanted endovascular stents (abstr). *J Am Coll Cardiol* 15:29A
79. Siegel R J, Chae J S, Forrester J S, Ruiz C E (1990) Angiography, angioscopy, and ultrasound imaging before and after percutaneous balloon angioplasty. *Am Heart J* 120:1086–1090
80. Yock P G, Linker D T (1990) Intravascular ultrasound. Looking below the surface of vascular disease. *Circulation* 81:1715–1718

6. Evaluation of Restenosis Following New Coronary Interventions

RICHARD E. KUNTZ and DONALD S. BAIM

Introduction

Restenosis following conventional balloon coronary angioplasty is a well established phenomenon that has persisted despite growing operator experience and technical advancement [1, 2]. If significant restenosis is defined as late luminal narrowing greater than 50%, approximately 30–35% of patients will manifest such restenosis by 3 to 6 months following conventional balloon angioplasty [3–5]. Nearly two dozen "second generation" coronary interventional devices have been developed in an effort to improve immediate and long-term results, and widen the application of percutaneous techniques to include coronary lesions which are currently not optimal for conventional angioplasty [6–8]. Preliminary reports have suggested that *some* new devices may reduce restenosis [9], although the mechanism of that reduction remains unclear. Evaluation of restenosis by newer non-traditional approaches may allow insight into some of the geometric considerations responsible for this reduction, and for differences in restenosis based on multiple variables (e.g., vessel treated, patient demographics, etc.).

Restenosis appears to be due to local neo-intimal hypertrophy and hyperplasia, a process that occurs to some degree in virtually all patients after conventional angioplasty [10]. Incomplete initial dilatation is correlated with an increased likelihood of restenosis [11–13], but attempts to use oversized balloons (above a balloon:artery ratio of 1.1) to further improve the postangioplasty percent stenosis (typically 28–31% [3, 14], have been thwarted by an unacceptable increase in the rate of abrupt closure [14]. Thus, there is a limited "therapeutic window" in which conventional balloon angioplasty operates – usually providing a 30% residual stenosis immediately post-angioplasty that results in a >30% probability of restenosis. Moreover, no pharmacologic means of reducing the amount of intimal hyperplasia has yet been identified.

We have employed three new "second generation" devices: directional atherectomy, balloon-expandable stents, and laser balloon angioplasty, ob-

P.W. Serruys, B.H. Strauss and S.B. King III (eds), Restenosis after Intervention with New Mechanical Devices, 149–160.
© 1992 *Kluwer Academic Publishers. Printed in the Netherlands.*

taining immediate and 4 to 6 month follow-up angiographic data. Analysis of restenosis following these new devices may provide further insight into the mechanism of vessel re-narrowing since they provide different immediate results compared to conventional balloon angioplasty. This chapter evaluates several geometric indices relating to the treated coronary segment, and analyzes how these indices may relate to restenosis.

The Traditional View of Restenosis which Resulted in a Dichotomous Definition

Restenosis connotes the specific late-term failure of an acutely successful angioplasty, due to re-narrowing of a successfully dilated coronary segment that results in regional underperfused myocardium. A *clinical* definition of restenosis emerged to describe the 20–25% of patients who develop recurrent evidence of ischemia within six months following successful balloon angioplasty [15]. This definition was inherently dichotomous, since recurrent symptoms following angioplasty in patients with single vessel disease was the clinically important outcome of interest. As more patients with multivessel disease became candidates for PTCA, it became evident that recurrent symptoms were neither sensitive nor specific for angiographic restenosis of the previously dilated artery. Holmes et al reported that 44% of patients with definite or probable angina following PTCA did not have angiographic evidence of restenosis [16]. Since *clinical* restenosis depends on several variables (vessel size, collateralization, myocardial viability), "harder" *angiographic* definitions were subsequently developed to allow binary evaluation of restenosis in clinical trials [17]. Routine angiography performed from 4 to 6 months after balloon angioplasty shows a restenosis rate to 30–35% using such definitions.

With the increased interest in "angiographic restenosis," the outcome of PTCA was felt to be successful if the treated artery segment did not subsequently re-narrow beyond some prescribed threshold. The most common dichotomous definitions are: 1) loss of one-half the acute gain (National heart, Lung, and Blood Institute [NHLBI] IV [18], or 2) an absolute diameter stenosis >50% [19]. These definitions, however, have major limitations since many of the patients presenting with NHLBI IV restenosis have <50% stenosis and no demonstrable ischemia [3]. Moreover, this problem is exaggerated with new devices that produce less residual stenosis [3, 9], and the resulting restenosis rates depend strongly on the choice of an absolute stenosis cutoff [3]. The prevailing perspective remains, however, that restenosis is still a dichotomous event [3, 4, 17].

Beyond the disagreement among investigators as to which definition should be used in order to identify which coronary segments have restenosed at follow-up, there are issues regarding the methodology and reproducibility of angiographic measurements. When calculating restenosis, one generally has to determine the reference vessel size. Steil has shown that using of the diameter of the pre-stenotic segment to calculate percent stenosis is inaccurate, and generally causes underestimation of the severity of the index stenosis [20]. Beatt demonstrated progressive reduction in the reference diameter from immediately after intervention to 60 day follow-up, presumably due to balloon dilatation and subsequent fibrocellular proliferation of these adjacent segments [10]. Therefore, a reliable calculation of percent stenosis may be unachievable due to the compensatory dilatation of the diseased segment [21], and to covert diffuse atherosclerosis within the adjacent segment erroneously assumed to be an undiseased reference [22].

Further problems were brought to light regarding the limitations of angiographic measurements. Although quantitative coronary angiographic research has demonstrated the importance absolute measures of vessel dimensions for analysis of restenosis [23], repeat angiograms in the same vessel and the same gantry angle have inherent errors that reduce the reproducibility of exact measurements obtained. Reiber has suggested that a better angiographic criterion would be greater than 0.72 mm reduction in the absolute luminal diameter between post-procedure and late follow-up [24]. This value is based on twice the variation in duplicate angiographic determinations of luminal diameter by quantitative angiographic techniques, so that it detects intimal hyperplasia with 95% confidence. This method also avoids errors due to changes in reference segment size, that may otherwise influence calculations of "percent stenosis."

All current definitions of restenosis, however, rely on the simple hypothesis that restenosis is a dichotomous event, that is, it either does or does not occur. This is emphasized by Reiber's suggestion that a reduction of 0.72 mm in luminal diameter be utilized as a definition of restenosis, since this reduction reasonably assures a true change in luminal diameter. Indeed, implicit is the assumption that any "detectable" reduction in luminal diameter within a coronary segment following PTCA represents restenosis, while a "non-detectable" change in diameter should be considered as the absence of restenosis. Moreover, the extension of this angiographic definition to the underlying pathological process of restenosis suggests that intimal hyperplasia (the pathologic substrate of restenosis [25, 26]) might itself be a binary event.

Given the multiplicity of dichotomous definitions of restenosis at follow-up, comparison between PTCA and newer devices may be fraught with discrepancies in the determination of outcome. As demonstrated by Califf and coworkers [27], follow-up results based on absolute dimensions may result in different assessments (restenosis versus no restenosis) according to various definitions. Figure 1 demonstrates a similar disagreement among) three definitions of restenosis: the NHLBI IV (restenosis = late loss >1/2 the acute gain), the Reiber (restenosis = late loss >0.72 mm), and Emory (restenosis = 50% diameter stenosed) definitions, when these definitions are used to compare PTCA to stenting. Thus, the evaluation of newer devices such as stents (which may provide a −10% post-procedure percent stenosis),

Reference Diameter	Pre-procedure Diameter (% stenosis)		Post-procedure Diameter (% stenosis)

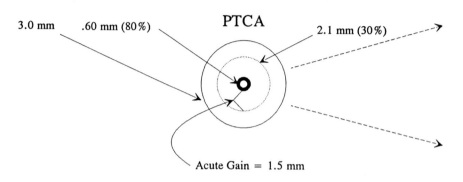

3.0 mm   .60 mm (80%)   PTCA   2.1 mm (30%)

Acute Gain = 1.5 mm

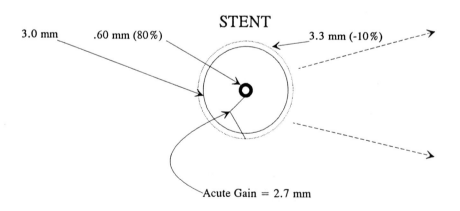

STENT

3.0 mm   .60 mm (80%)   3.3 mm (-10%)

Acute Gain = 2.7 mm

Figure 1. Left.

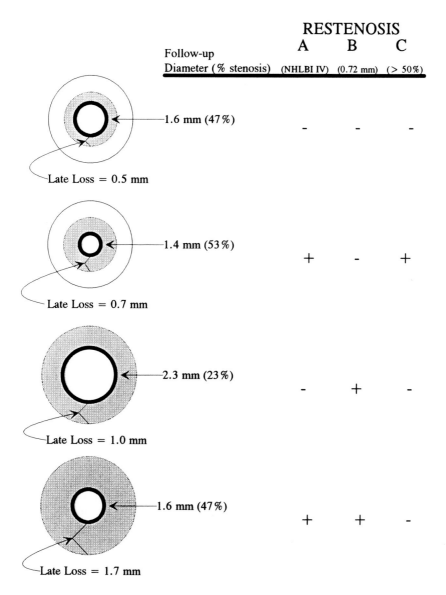

Figure 1. Effects of variable acute results in a 3.0 mm coronary artery on traditional definitions of restenosis. Illustrated in this figure, are typical acute and follow-up results that might result from conventional balloon angioplasty (PTCA) and stenting (STENT). Lumen diameters are analyzed in terms of differences in acute gain and late loss. Although the final luminal diameter in the first and fourth illustration are equivalent, differences in restenosis definitions cause discrepant categorizations of restenosis. The most consistent definition appears to be C. (Restenosis A = NHLBI IV – late loss >1/2 acute gain, B = Serruys – >0.72 mm, C = Emory – >50% reduction in reference luminal diameter).

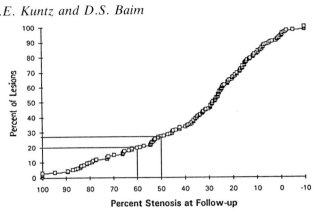

Figure 2. Distribution of percent stenosis among a hypothetical study group following a new intervention using a novel definition-independent restenosis graph. The lesions are ranked in descending order on the x-axis according to their percent stenosis at follow-up. The cumulative percent of lesions in the group that have a stenosis greater than the x-axis value is shown on the y-axis. Variations in dichotomous definitions of restenosis (shown are 50% and 60%) may be evaluated by this nomogram, as well as the overall distribution of percent stenosis.

may result in categorization of some angiographically excellent late results as "restenosis". Consequently, the late percent stenosis relative to the reference artery size (the Emory definition) may still be the most stable among devices that have consistently better acute results than conventional balloon angioplasty.

A Novel Graphical Technique of Percent Stenosis at Follow-up Provides a Definition-independent Display of Restenosis

To overcome the limitations of any such arbitrary definitional cut-offs, we have developed a method that depicts restenosis graphically, in a definition-independent rank fashion that allows comparison of follow-up results among interventions. By ranking the entire sample (subgrouped by various comparative strata such as device type or vessel size) a definition-independent comparison of percent stenosis may be made. This graphical technique allows the distribution of percent stenosis to be ordinally displayed, without application of any arbitrary threshold that dichotomizes angiographic restenosis.

The advantage of such a display is two-fold. First, the graph serves as a nomogram that allows any traditional dichotomous definition of restenosis to be applied to the study groups, in order to determine the percent of patients who qualify for restenosis (Fig. 2). Second, the graph is a standard non-parametric display of the percent stenoses (on the x-axis) against the cumulative distribution of patients (y-axis), that allows the use of routine statistical techniques to examine the distributions of percent stenoses in the individual study groups. That is, the distribution of percent stenoses within patient groups may be easily identified as parametric, uniform, bimodal, etc.,

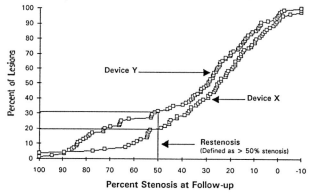

Figure 3. Comparison of restenosis between two hypothetical devices at follow-up using a definition-independent restenosis graph. In this scenario device X is clearly superior to device Y, as any dichotomous definition of restenosis will show a lower restenosis rate for device X. In this example, a 50% definition shows a restenosis rate of 19% for device X, and 31% for device Y.

based on examination of dispersion or clustering of data points along the x-axis. Furthermore, examination of multiple curves may allow insight into differences in restenosis when viewed as a continuous variable (Fig. 3). Such curves may demonstrate whether differences in restenosis are due to different distributions or to shifts in a similar distribution pattern.

Restenosis Is a Continuous Variable Rather Than a Discrete Event

In several serial angiographic studies, the variable luminal dimensions among vessels at restudy are summarized using parametric statistics (i.e., mean, standard deviation [4, 17], rather than by binary categories implying that the vessel is "patent" or "restenotic". It is evident that the vast majority of restudied segments following PTCA have at least *some* small reduction in luminal dimension [4, 17]. This concept is illustrated by Fig. 4. In this scheme, the "acute gain" provided by angioplasty is the increase in dimension from the pre-stenotic diameter to the post-procedure diameter. Following angioplasty, "late loss" is the subsequent reduction in luminal dimension from the post-procedure luminal diameter to 6 month following angioplasty – largely the result of local intimal hyperplasia. Both the acute gain and late loss may vary from procedure to procedure: acute gain ranges from 1.0 to 1.2 mm following conventional balloon angioplasty [4, 17], but may be as large as 2.7 mm following balloon expandable stenting [9]. Late loss appears to be ubiquitous, but the *amount* of late loss varies depending on the potential for the coronary segment to respond with intimal hyperplasia. Thus, the final diameter of the instrumented artery at follow-up is the result of both the opposing actions of the acute gain provided by the intervention, and the subsequent late loss due to intimal hyperplasia.

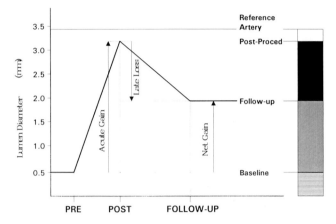

Figure 4. Diagram of luminal dimension with time following coronary intervention. The illustration depicts the separate indices of "acute gain" provided by the intervention, and the subsequent "late loss" that occurs over 4 to 6 months following the intervention. Consequently, the net gain at follow-up is a function of the magnitudes of the offsetting effects of acute gain and late loss. The bar graph shows the absolute coronary dimensions responsible for the calculation of the indices acute gain and late loss.

Among patients at our institution who were restudied following a newer intervention, late loss was found to be normally distributed [28] (Fig. 5). What determines the magnitude of this response is unknown presently, but it may be related to vessel size, coronary location, the type of vessel injury produced by the specific device, the amount of acute gain, or other demographic features such as smoking, cholesterol, etc. In particular, stenting, atherectomy and laser balloon angioplasty seem to have larger late losses [9,

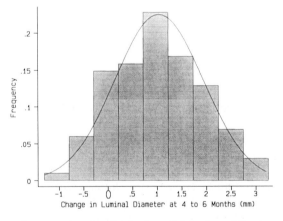

Figure 5. Histogram demonstrating the distribution of Late Loss following a new coronary intervention in patients at our institution (Kuntz et al [28]). Late Loss appears to be a ubiquitous and normally distributed phenomenon, rather than a dichotomous event.

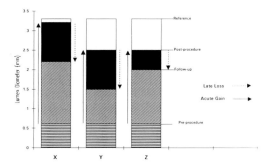

Figure 6. Bar graphs demonstrating hypothetical variations in follow-up dimensions in a 3.3 mm coronary artery based on differences in acute gain and late loss associated with 3 devices. Although the late loss is equivalent for X and Y, device X results in a larger lumen at follow-up compared to device Y because it produced a larger acute gain. Device Z, on the other hand, results in a larger lumen at follow-up (compared to device Y), because late loss is less even though the acute gains are equivalent.

29] (on average 1.0 mm) than that reported for conventional PTCA (on average 0.4 [4, 17].

This analysis of conventional balloon angioplasty and newer devices utilizing a more detailed breakdown of late luminal dimensions into its component indices (acute gain and late loss) may provide important additional insights (Fig. 4). It would be important to know how these two components contributed to the final luminal dimension at follow-up in a sample population. For example, if device X and Y are being compared because of lower restenosis rates with device X, analysis of acute gain and late loss may illuminate the mechanism of those superior results. Device X may be found to provide a greater acute gain compared to device Y, with a similar magnitude of late loss. In this case, the improved rate of restenosis would be due to the ability of device X to provide a very large immediate result (Fig. 6). On the other hand, device Z may be found to be superior to Y because the average of late loss following device Z is reduced even though the acute gains of the two devices were equivalent.

Linear and Logistic Modeling as Methods for Analysis of Restenosis

If indices such as acute gain and late losses have known (e.g., normal) distributions, linear regression might provide further insight into the mechanism of restenosis. By relating pre- or post-procedure luminal dimension to follow-up luminal dimension, a linear model could be fitted. The effects of other continuous variables, e.g. acute gain, cholesterol level, age, reference diameter, etc., could then be examined by linear regression techniques, while logistic regression could be used to examine important dichotomous variables (e.g., gender, vessel treated, etc). Furthermore, the effect of different pharmacologic and mechanical manipulations on these new indices of restenosis could be evaluated simultaneously in multivariable models. Restenosis may be detected with higher sensitivity and specificity when continuous, rather than dichotomous, outcomes are analyzed. Finally, the ultimate construction of a general model of restenosis that reflects the underlying biology of the coronary artery, may be constructed to allow incorporation of any device or other significant factor.

Conclusion

Conventional balloon angioplasty has consistently provided comparatively modest luminal improvements (30% post-procedure residual stenosis) and a relatively high restenosis rate (30–35%) over the past 15 years. Since the introduction of many newer coronary interventional devices, the acute results (and to some extent the subsequent restenosis rates) have improved. Evaluation of the mechanical effects of these newer interventions on the coronary artery, and their possible relationship to subsequent restenosis mandates a more sophisticated analysis than is currently utilized. By analyzing the mechanics of dilatation and vessel renarrowing in terms of absolute coronary dimensions and dissecting the component indices of "acute gain" and "late loss," further insight into the device-specific effect on the behavior of restenosis may be gained. Moreover, the observation that late loss which is ubiquitous and normally distributed, may allow inference about the biology of intimal hyperplasia. Finally, incorporation of regression techniques based on continuous variables may permit the identification of significant determinants of restenosis and allow the construction of a more general model of restenosis.

References

1. Gruentzig A R, King S B III, Schlumpf M, Siegenthaler W (1987) Long-term follow-up after perctuaneous transluminal coronary angioplasty. *N Engl J Med* 316:1127–32
2. Block P C (1990) Restenosis after percutaneous transluminal coronary angioplasty – anatomic and pathophysiological mechanisms. *Circulation* 81(suppl IV):IV-2–4
3. Beatt K J, Serruys P W, Hugenholtz P G (1990) Restenosis after coronary angioplasty: new standards for clinical studies. *J Am Coll Cardiol* 15(2):491
4. Nobuyoshi M et al (1988) Restenosis after successful percutaneous transluminal coronary angioplasty: serial angiographic follow-up of 220 patients. *J Am Coll Cardiol* 12:616
5. Guiteras Val P, Bourassa M G, David P R, Bonan R, Crepeau J, Dyrda I, Lesperance J (1987) Restenosis after successful percutaneous transluminal coronary angioplasty: the Montreal Heart Institute experience. *Am J Cardiol* 60:50–8
6. Baim D S, Detre K, Kent K (1989) Problems in the development of new devices for coronary intervention – possible role for a multicenter registry. *J Am Coll Cardiol* 14:1389
7. Waller B F (1989) "Crackers, breakers, stretchers, drillers, scrapers, shavers, burners,

welders and melters" – the future treatment of atherosclerotic coronary artery disease? A clinical-morphologic assessment. *J Am Coll Cardiol* 13:969–87

8. Litvack F (1989) Intravascular stenting for prevention of restenosis: in search of the magic bullet. *J Am Coll Cardiol* 13:1092–3

9. Levine M J, Leonard B M, Burke J A, Nash I D, Safian R D, Diver D J, Baim D S (1990) Clinical and angiographic results of balloon-expandable intracoronary stents in right coronary stenosis. *J Am Coll Cardiol* 16:332–9

10. Beatt K J, Luijten H E, de Feyter P J, van den Brand M, Reiber J H C, Serruys P W (1988) Change in diameter of coronary segments adjacent to stenosis after percutaneous transluminal coronary angioplasty: failure of percent diameter stenosis measurement to reflect morphologic changes induced by balloon dilation. *J Am Coll Cardiol* 12:315–23

11. Roubin G S, King S B III, Douglas J S Jr (1987) Restenosis after percutaneous coronary angioplasty – Emory University hospital experience. *Am J Cardiol* 60:39B–43B

12. Douglas J S Jr, King S B III, Roubin G S (1987) Influence of the methodology of percutaneous transluminal coronary angioplasty on restenosis. *Am J Cardiol* 60:29B–34B

13. Ellis S G, Roubin G S, King S B III, Douglas J S Jr, Cox W R (1989) Importance of stenosis morphology in the estimation of restenosis risk after elective percutaneous transluminal angioplasty. *Am J Cardiol* 63:30–4

14. Roubin G S, Douglas J S Jr, King S B III, Lin S, Hutchison N, Thomas R G, Gruentzig A R (1988) Influence of balloon size on initial success, acute complications, and restenosis after percutaneous transluminal coronary angioplasty. *Circulation* 78:557–65

15. Detre K et al (1989) One year follow-up results of the 1985–1986 National Heart, Lung, and Blood Institute's percutaneous transluminal coronary angioplasty registry. *Circulaton* 80:421

16. Holmes D R, Vliestra R E, Smith H C et al (1984) Restenosis after percutaneous transluminal coronary angioplasty (PTCA): a report from the PTCA Registry of the National Heart, Lung, and Blood Institute. *Am J Cardiol* 53:77C–81C

17. Serruys P W, Luijten H E, Beatt K J, Geuskens R, de Feyter P J, van den Brand M, Reiber J H C, ten Katen H J, van Es G A, Hugenholtz P G (1988) Incidence of restenosis after successful coronary angioplasty: a time-related phenomenon. *Circulation* 77:361–71

18. Holmes D R, Vliestra R E, Smith H C, Vetrovec G W, Kent K M, Cowley M J, Faxon D P, Gruentzig A R, Kelsey S F, Detre K M, van Raden M J, Mock M B (1984) Restenosis after percutaneous transluminal coronary angioplasty (PTCA): a report from the PTCA Registry of the National Heart, Lung, and Blood Institute. *Am J Cardiol* 53:77C

19. Leimgruber P P, Roubin G S, Hollman J, Cotsonis G A, Meier B, Douglas J S, King S B III, Greuntzig A R (1986) Restenosis after successful coronary angioplasty in patients with single vessel disease. *Circulation* 73:710

20. Stiel G M, Steil L S G, Schofer J, Donath K, Mathey D G (1989) Impact of compensatory enlargement of atherosclerotic coronary arteries on angiographic assessment of coronary artery disease. *Circulation* 80:1603

21. Glagov S, Weisenberd E, Zarins C K, Strakunavicius R, Kolettis G J (1987) Compensatory enlargement of human atherosclerotic coronary arteries. *N Engl J Med* 316:1371–5

22. McPherson D D, Hiratzka L F, Lamber W C et al (1987) Delineation of the extent of coronary atherosclerosis by high frequency echocardiography. *N Engl J Med* 316:394–9

23. Mancini G B J (1991) Quantitative coronary arteriographic methods in the interventional catheterization laboratory: an update and perspective. *J Am Coll Cardiol* 17:23B–33B

24. Reiber J H C, Serruys P W, van den Brand M et al (1985) Assessment of short-, medium- and long-term variations in arterial dimensions from computer-assisted quantitation of coronary cineangiograms. *Circulation* 71:280–8

25. Ueda M, Becker A E, Tsukada T, Numano F, Fujimoto T (1991) Fibrocellular tissue response after percutaneous transluminal coronary angioplasty. *Circulation* 83: 1327–1332

26. Nobuyoshi M, Kimura T, Ohishi H et al (1991) Restenosis after percutaneous transluminal coronary angioplasty: pathologic observations in 20 patients. *J Am Coll Cardiol* 17:433–439

27. Califf R M, Fortin D F, Frid DJ et al (1991) Restenosis after coronary angioplasty: An overview. *J Am Coll Cardiol* 17:2B–13B
28. Kuntz R E, Schmidt D A, Levine M J, Reis G J, Safian R D, Baim D S (1990) Importance of post-procedure luminal diameter on restenosis following new coronary interventions. *Circulation* 82(suppl III):III-314
29. Safian R D, Gelbfish J S, Erny R E, Schmidt S J, Schmidt D A, Baim D S (1990) Coronary atherectomy: clinical, angiographic, and histologic findings and observations regarding potential mechanisms. *Circulation* 82:69–79

PART THREE

Stents Restenosis and New Techniques

Introduction: Stenting for Restenosis?

ULRICH SIGWART

Introduction

Endoluminal support devices in blood vessels have been tried in animals long before angioplasty was born. While digging up appropriate literature, Dr Philip Urban, at that time a research fellow at the University Hospital of Lausanne in 1987, found an article published by Alexis Carrel from New York in September 1912 in the American monthly "Surgery, Gynaecology and Obstretrics" dealing with such ideas [1]. In this article Dr Carrel described the "results of the permanent intubation of the thoracic aorta" in 11 dog experiments; in 7 animals he placed short glass tubes, aluminium tubes in 3 dogs and in 1 animal a gold plated aluminium tube through a surgical incision inside the thoracic aorta. Thrombosis of the tube occurred in 5 cases between 5 and 97 days after the implantation. Two animals died from haemorrhage 8 and 11 days following the operation; in these cases no clot was found on the inner surface of the tube. Dr Carrel concluded that no thrombosis took place as long as no laceration of the vascular wall occurred and that improvement of the geometry and design of the glass or aluminium tube would prevent these problems. Unfortunately the author of this article had no materials available other than glass or aluminium. He suggested that the use of smooth edged gold tubes or tubes lined with a vein would probably yield better results.

Charles Dotter, who also felt the urge to support blood vessels from their luminal surface, made the same mistake when he used impervious plastic tube grafts which he positioned in normal dog femoral or popliteal arteries. He published his results in a Radiology journal in 1969, which showed that all stents thrombosed within the first 24 hours of implantation [2]. Dotter's results improved when he replaced the tubes with stainless steel coils [4]. He also altered his drug regimen to include administration of heparin for 4 days after implantation.

The goals behind these early experiments were similar. Both researchers tried to deal with degenerative arterial disease by providing a support device.

P.W. Serruys, B.H. Strauss and S.B. King III (eds), Restenosis after Intervention with New Mechanical Devices, 163–165.
© 1992 *Kluwer Academic Publishers. Printed in the Netherlands.*

Dr Carrel meant to insert tubes to treat aneurysms of the aorta and Dr Dotter hoped to be able to positively influence arteriosclerotic disease by stenting. A new incentive was brought about when coronary angioplasty became popular in the early eighties. Cardiologists were helpless when coronary arteries closed before their eyes when the dilating balloon was withdrawn. The only option was emergency surgery. With increasing numbers of percutaneous transluminal angioplasties performed, it also became obvious that restenosis occurred in just about one in three angioplasty cases. For these reasons several groups of researchers contemplated mechanisms of supporting arteries after angioplasty to prevent acute occlusion and chronic restenosis.

Restenosis occurs in 20 to 60% of patients who undergo coronary angioplasty; neither operator experience nor improvement in angioplasty equipment have changed these figures [3]. Although it is not clear whether restenosis is part of the disease process, it is often referred to as late complication of angioplasty. The knowledge about restenosis raises serious ethical and economic questions, especially when patients are known to produce myocardial ischaemia in the absence of angina.

All currently known drug trials have failed to substantially reduce restenosis. Removal of material that obstructs the artery has not been effective either in reducing restenosis, unless the removed plaque is very circumscript and eccentric [5]. A permanently implanted biocompatible and non thrombogenic support would therefore seem a logical way to reduce restenosis after angioplasty. Such a support device would not only prevent elastic recoil but also smooth the otherwise open wound with its uncontrolled fissures and flaps which may lead to an exaggerated healing process.

With the aim to reduce restenosis after coronary angioplasty, stents have been used in man since early 1986 [6]. Although the problem of acute closure can quite reproducibly be dealt with by stent implantation, the restenosis issue is far more complicated. So far all currently known stent models implanted in human coronary arteries have been associated with restenosis. Stent restenosis seems to vary between 10 and 60% according to preliminary data. Why is this so? – In contrast to the original lesion, namely atherosclerosis, restenosis is largely the result of exuberant healing. Even if elastic recoil can effectively be arrested by a scaffolding device, exuberant healing may still be an issue. If one looks at the early prototypes of stents one is not surprised that restenosis is still on the agenda. None of the existing stents provide a smooth laminar surface which most likely is the best insurance against exuberant healing. All stents exhibit large uncovered pores surrounded by thick metal struts. The struts measure between 60 to 150 micron in thickness; where these wires cross, the overall thickness is much greater. These struts create important turbulence and the remaining tissue islands, protruding into the arterial lumen, also add to the turbulence. Thus the fluid dynamics after stent implantation are far from being ideal despite the largely improved cross sectional area. Even in the absence of genuine tissue factors promoting exuberant smooth muscle cell proliferation, one would suspect the turbulence after stent implantation to play a major role as a stimulus for smooth muscle cell hyperplasia.

At least three conditions must be met before substantial reduction in restenosis rate by stenting can be expected:

(1) Laminar flow condition through modification of stent geometry.
(2) Non thrombogenic strut surfaces.
(3) Local drug modulation of uncontrolled healing.

New approaches are under way in order to control these three factors either individually or globally. The second and third generation of endoluminal support devices will use new delivery devices, new materials, different geometry and will function as drug delivery systems. They also may become biodegradable and vanish once the repair job is done.

References

1. Carrel A (1912) Results of the permanent intubation of the thoracic aorta. *Surgery, Gynaecology and Obstetrics* 3:245–8
2. Dotter C T (1969) Transluminally-placed coilspring endarterial tube grafts. *Invest Radiol* 4:329–32
3. Dotter C T, Buschmann R W, McKinney M K et al (1983) Transluminal expandable nitinol stent grafting: preliminary report. *Radiology* 147:259–60
4. Lambert M, Bonan R, Cote G et al (1988) Multiple coronary angioplasty: a model to discriminate systemic and procedural factors related to restenosis. *JACC* 12:310–14
5. Simpson J B, Bain D S, Hinohara T et al (1991) Restenosis of de novo lesions in native coronary arteries following directional atherectomy: multicentre experience. (abst). *J Am Coll Cardiol* 17:346A
6. Sigwart U, Puel J, Mirkovitch V et al (1987) Intravascular stents to prevent occlusion and restenosis after transluminal angioplasty. *N Engl J Med* 316:701–6

7. The Wallstent Experience: 1986–1990

PATRICK W. SERRUYS and BRADLEY H. STRAUSS*

On behalf of Michel E. Bertrand, Jacques Puel, Bernhard Meier, Urs Kaufmann, Jean-Christopher Stauffer, Anthony F. Rickards, Lucas Kappenberger and Ulrich Sigwart

Introduction

In 1986, the first coronary Wallstent implantation ushered in a new era in interventional cardiology with the purpose of circumventing the two major limitations of coronary angioplasty, early acute occlusion and late restenosis [1]. As with all new procedures, operators of the device had to struggle with their own learning curves at the same time that anticoagulation regimens and clinical indications and contraindications evolved from their clinical experience. Since March 1986, the coronary Wallstent[R] has been the most intensively studied endovascular prosthesis in Europe. As a result of cooperation among the six participating European centers, a central core laboratory was set up in Rotterdam to objectively assess the follow up of stents with quantitative coronary angiography.

In a previous publication from our group, the late angiographic and clinical follow-up of the inital 105 patients implanted between 1986–1988 was reported [2]. In the period from January 1989 until March 1990, a further 160 patients underwent stent implantation in the coronary circulation.

In this chapter, we compare the late quantitative angiographic and clinical follow-up of this second group of patients with the initial group, and, to further characterize the factors associated with angiographic restenosis within the stented segment, we retrospectively studied the predictive ability of several angiographic variables.

Methods

Study Patients. Two hundred and sixty-five patients (308 lesions) were enrolled after obtaining informed consent between March 1986 and March 1990 at the participating centers.

*Dr. Strauss is a Research Fellow of the Heart and Stroke Foundation of Canada.

P. W. Serruys, B. H. Strauss and S. B. King III (eds), Restenosis after Intervention with New Mechanical Devices, 167–189.
© 1992 Kluwer Academic Publishers. Printed in the Netherlands.

Table 1. Stent implantations according to date of implantation.

	Group 1 (March 1986–Dec 1988)		Group 2 (Jan 1989–March 1990)	
Vessels	107		175	
Bypass	18%		60%	
Native	82%		40%	
LAD		54%		15%
CX		7%		5%
RCA		21%		20%
Stent/Lesions	117/114		266/194	

The study patients were grouped according to the date of implantation (prior to or after January 1, 1988; Groups 1 and 2 respectively) and the vessel type stented (native vessel versus bypass graft) (Tables 1, 2).

In Group 1, 117 stents were implanted in 114 lesions, of which 82% were in native vessels (and in particular the left anterior descending artery). In group 2, 266 stents were implanted in 194 lesions, predominantly in bypass grafts (60% of cases). In this group, the right coronary artery was the most common vessel stented in the native circulation.

The indications for stenting also differed between the two vessel types (Fig. 1). Native vessels were primarily stented to prevent a second restenosis or as a bail-out procedure for angioplasties complicated by abrupt closure or large dissections that interrupted anterograde flow and were associated with clinical and electrocardiographic signs of ischemia. However, in bypass grafts, the principle indication was for primary lesions in bypass grafts that had not been previously treated with angioplasty.

In the overall group, angiographic follow up was obtained in 216 patients (82%). However, in-hospital occlusions occurred in 40 patients (41 lesions).

Follow-up angiograms were quantitatively analyzed in 176 patients (78%) of the 225 patients who were discharged from hospital without known occlusion (Fig. 2 and 3).

They had a total of 259 stents implanted in 214 lesions. The mean length of angiographic follow-up in the study group was 6.6 ± 4.8 months.

The anticoagulation for the first period of implantation has previously

Table 2. Stent implantations according to vessel type.

	Natives	Bypass Grafts
Patients	166	101
Vessels	171	110
Stent/Lesion	193/173	192/135
LAD	55%	
CX	10%	
RCA	35%	

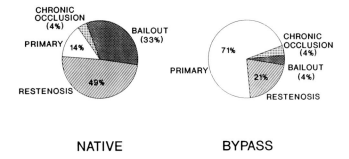

NATIVE   BYPASS

Figure 1. The indications for stenting in native arteries and bypass grafts. (Primary = Primary atherosclerotic lesion that has not been previously treated by PTCA or stenting.)

been described [2]. Based on this initial clinical experience, a uniform anti-coagulation schedule was followed at the centers. Acetylsalicylic acid 1 gram orally was started 1 day before the procedure. At the beginning of the procedure, patients received heparin 10,000 international units intravenously and in some cases, dextran infusions (500 mg/ 4 hours) were also given. Additional heparin (10,000 international units) and urokinase 100,000 units

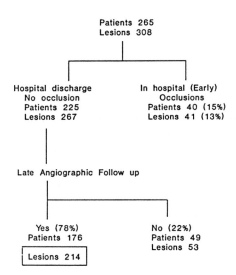

Figure 2. Flow diagram showing the angiographic follow-up in 265 stented lesions. In hospital (early) occlusions occurred in 40 patients (15%). In the remaining 225 patients that were discharged from hospital without known stent occlusion, 176 patients (78%) with 214 stented lesions had quantitative angiographic follow-up.

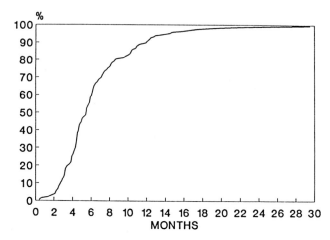

Figure 3. Timing of late angiographic follow-up after stent implantation. In this cumulative curve, the interval (in months) between date of implantation and final angiographic follow-up is shown for the study group.

intracoronary were administered during the procedure. Following the procedure, the heparin infusion was adjusted according tho the activated partial thromboplastin time (APTT 80–120 seconds) in addition to initiating oral Vitamin K antagonist therapy. Heparin was discontinued after the therapeutic oral anticoagulation level was stabilized (International Normalized Ratio of 2.3 or more). Acetylsalicylic acid 100 mg daily, dipyridamole (300 to 450 mg/day) and in some patients sulfinpyrazone 400 mg daily were also administered.

In this trial, the endovascular prosthesis, Wallstent[R], was provided by Medinvent SA, Lausanne. The method of implantation and description of this stent has previously been reported [1, 2]. This stent is a self-expandable stainless steel woven mesh prosthesis that can be positioned in the coronary artery using standard over-the-wire technique through a 8F or 9F guiding catheter. The device is constructed of 16 wire filaments, each 0.08 mm wide. It is constrained in an elongated configuration on a 1.57 mm diameter delivery catheter with the distal end covered by a removable plastic sleeve. As the sleeve is withdrawn, the constrained device returns to its original unconstrained larger diameter and becomes anchored against the vessel wall. Unconstrained stent diameter ranged from 2.5–6 mm and was selected to be 0.50 mm larger than the stented vessel based on a visual estimate of the pre stent angiogram by the investigator. In an effort to alleviate the problem of acute thrombosis, the stent design was changed in April 1989 with the introduction of a polymer coated stent (Biogold[R]) for certain stent sizes. By August 1989, all manufactured stents contained this particular polymer coating.

Quantitative Coronary Arteriography

All cineangiograms were analyzed at the core laboratory in Rotterdam using the computer assisted cardiovascular angiography analysis system (CAAS) which has previously been discussed in detail [3, 4]. The important steps will be briefly described. Selected areas of the cineframe encompassing the desired arterial segment (from side branch to side branch) are optically magnified, displayed in a video format and then digitally converted. Vessel contour is determined automatically based on the weighted sum of the first and second derivative functions applied to the digitized brightness information. A computer-derived estimation of the original arterial dimension at the site of the obstruction is used to define interpolated reference diameter and area. The absolute diameter of the stenosis as well as the reference diameter are measured by the computer which uses the known guiding catheter diameter as a calibration factor, after correction for pincushion distortion. The percentage diameter of the narrowed segment is derived by comparing the observed stenosis dimensions to the reference values. *The length* of the lesion (mm) is determined from the diameter function on the basis of a curvature analysis. Using the reconstructed borders of the vessel, the computer can calculate a symmetry coefficient for the stenosis. Differences in distance between the actual and reconstructed vessel contours on both sides of the lesion are measured. *Symmetry* is determined by the ratio of these two differences with the largest distance between actual and reconstructed contours becoming the denominator. Values for symmetry range from 0 for extreme eccentricity to 1 for maximal symmetry (that is, equal distance on both sides between reconstructed and actual contours). The angiographic analysis was done pre and post angioplasty, immediately post stent implantation and at long term follow-up in all patients using the average of multiple matched views with orthogonal projections wherever possible.

Restenosis

Two different set of criteria were applied to determine the restenosis rate. We have found a change in minimal luminal diameter (MLD) of 0.72 mm or more to be a reliable indicator of angiographic progression of vessel narrowing and by no means implies functional or clinical significance [3, 4]. This value takes into account the limitations of coronary angiographic measurements and represents two times the long term variability (ie. the 95% confidence intervals) for repeat measurements of a coronary obstruction using CAAS. The other criterion for restenosis chosen was an increase of the diameter stenosis from less than 50% after stent implantation to greater than or equal to 50% at follow-up. This criterion was selected since common clinical practice continues to assess lesion severity by a percentage stenosis.

Table 3. Angiographic follow-up.

Implantations (Lesions/Pts)	308/265	
Early Occlusions	41/40	
Late Follow Up	214/176	
Total	255/216	(82%)
No Angiographic Follow-up	53/49	(18%)
Death	10	(4%)
Early CABG	11	(4%)
Refusal	25	(9%)
Technical	3	(1%)
Time to Angiographic Follow Up		
Excluding Early Occlusions	6.6 ± 4.8	
Including Early Occlusions	5.7 ± 5.0	

The two criteria were assessed within the stent and in the segment immediately adjacent (proximal and distal) to the stent.

Late (i.e., documented after the initial discharge from hospital) occlusion (n = 10 patients, 16 lesions) were regarded as restenoses.

Angiographic Variables

Based on the quantitative angiographic data, multiple variables were identified and recorded for each lesion. These variables, either discrete (two or three distinct responses) or continuous (a range of responses), were grouped according to lesion, stent or procedural factors (Tables 3, 4). These particular variables were of a priori clinical interest on the basis of previously published PTCA and stent reports [5–11].

Statistical Methods

The data obtained by quantitative angiographic analysis are given as mean ± SD. The mean of each angiographic variable pre PTCA, post stent and at follow-up were compared using analysis of variance. If significance differences were found, two tailed T-tests were applied to pairs of data. The occlusion and restenosis rates were compared using a chi square test. A statistical probability of less than 0.05 was considered significant.

A relative risk analysis was performed for the aforementioned discrete

Table 4. Angiographic results: early occlusions.

	Total	Group 1	Group 2	Native Vessels	Bypass Grafts
Lesions/Pts	308/265	114/105	194/160	173/166	135/101
Early Occlusions	41(13%)/40(15%)	21(18%)/21(20%)	20(10%)/19(12%)	32(18%)/32(19%)	9(7%)/8(8%)

and continuous variables [12]. The continuous variables were dichotomized for the risk ratio analysis. To avoid arbitrary subdivision of data in continuous variables, cutpoints were derived by dividing the data into two groups, each containing roughly 50% of the total population. This method of subdivision has the advantage of being consistent for all variables and thus avoids any bias in selection of subgroups which might be undertaken to emphasize a particular point. The incidence of restenosis in the two groups was compared using a relative risk analysis. A relative risk of 1 for a particular variable implies that the presence of that variable poses no additional risk for restenosis; relative risks greater than 1 or less than 1 imply additional or a reduction in risk, respectively. For example a relative risk of 2 for a particular parameter implies that the presence of that factor increases the likelihood of restenosis by a factor of two. The 95% confidence intervals were calculated to describe the statistical certainty. Statistical significance was defined as $p < 0.05$. and was determined using the Pearson Chi square (BMDP statistical software, University of California, Berkeley, California, 1990).

The late clinical follow-up was determined according to a life table format using the Kaplan-Meier method [13].

The following events were considered clinical endpoints: death, myocardial infarction, bypass surgery or nonsurgical revascularization (PTCA or atherectomy). The life table was constructed according to the initial clinical event.

Results

A. *Occlusion and Restenosis Rate*

The angiographic follow-up for the entire study population was 82% (Table 3). This includes patients with documented early occlusions during hospital admission ($n = 40$) in addition to patients who had late (after the initial hospital discharge) angiographic controls. The reasons why follow-up angiography could not be performed are listed in Table 3. The time to angiographic follow-up was 6.6 ± 4.8 months if early occlusions are excluded and 5.7 ± 5.0 months with the early occlusions.

The angiographic data for individual lesions in bypass grafts and native vessels are presented in Figs 4 A and B. In native vessels, there was a mean increase in minimal luminal diameter from $1.17 \pm .52$ mm to $2.53 \pm .53$ mm immediately post stenting but a late deterioration to $1.99 \pm .81$ mm if early occlusions are excluded and 1.59 ± 1.08 mm with the inclusion of the early occlusions ($p < 0.0001$) (Fig. 5). Similarly, the minimal luminal diameter increased in bypass lesions from $1.39 \pm .64$ mm to $2.81 \pm .69$ mm post stenting with a late reduction to 2.21 ± 1.16 mm and 2.03 ± 1.27 mm with the exclusion and inclusion of early occlusions, respectively ($p < 0.0001$). Diameter stenosis was reduced from immediately post stenting in bypass grafts

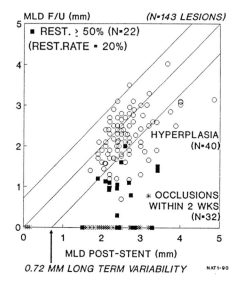

a   *0.72 MM LONG TERM VARIABILITY*   NAT1-90

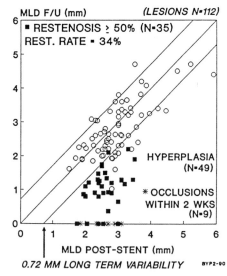

b   *0.72 MM LONG TERM VARIABILITY*   BYP2-90

Figure 4. Change in the minimal luminal diameter (MLD) for individual lesions in native vessels (Fig. 4A) and in bypass grafts (Fig. 4B) between stent implantation and angiographic follow-up (F/U). The diameter of each segment immediately after implantation is plotted against the diameter at follow-up. The lines on each side of the identity line (diagonal) represent the limits of long-term variability of repeat measurements (a change of ≥0.72 mm [arrow]). All symbols below the right-hand line represent stents with involvement of angiographic detectable hyperplasia. The filled squares represents lesions with follow-up diameter stenosis ≥50%. Occlusions are located along the x-axis and those lesions that occurred within the first two weeks are marked by an asterisk.

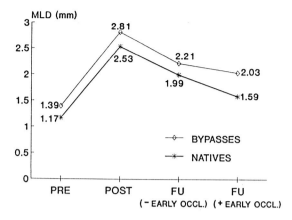

Figure 5. Minimal luminal diameter (MLD) of native vessels and bypass grafts pre procedure, post stenting, and at follow-up. The mean values at follow-up have been calculated with and without the inclusion of the early in-hospital occlusions.

from $60 \pm 14\%$ to $23 \pm 10\%$ but increased at late follow-up to $43 \pm 31\%$ and to $38 \pm 27\%$ with and without the early occlusions respectively ($p < 0.0001$). Similar changes were observed in native vessels (data not shown).

In the overall group, the incidence of early in-hospital occlusion was 15% by patient and 13% by lesion (Table 4). In bypass grafts, early occlusions were documented in 7% of lesions (8% of patients) versus 18% of lesions (19% of patients) in native vessels (by lesion $p = 0.005$; by patient $p = 0.016$). Three of these native vessel occlusions occurred during the procedure and could not be recanalized. The remaining occlusions presented clinically as acute ischemic syndromes following a successful stenting procedure. Early occlusions were less frequent in Group 2 patients (12%) than in Group 1 (20%) but not statistically significant. Detectable angiographic narrowing (0.72 mm loss in MLD) in the overall group was 42% by lesion and 43% by

Table 5. Late angiographic follow-up: Restenosis within and immediately adjacent to the Stent.

	Total	Group 1	Group 2	Native vessels	Bypass grafts
Lesions/Patients	214/176	85/75	129/101	111/104	103/74
0.72 mm Criterion					
Within Stent	75/61	25/21	50/40	34/30	40/31
Adjacent to Stent	14/14	5/5	9/9	5/5	9/9
Total	89/75	30/26	59/49	40/35	49/40
	(42%/43%)	(37%/35%)	(46%/49%)	(36%/34%)	(48%/54%)
50% DS Criterion					
Within Stent	51/42	17/15	34/27	21/18	30/24
Adjacent to Stent	6/6	1/1	5/5	1/1	5/5
Total	57/48	18/16	39/32	22/19	35/29
	(27%/27%)	(22%/21%)	(30%/32%)	(20%/18%)	(34%/39%)

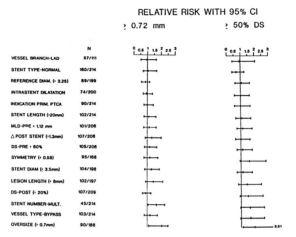

Figure 6. Relative risk ratios (with 95% confidence intervals) for the angiographic variables using the two restenosis criteria (≥0.72 mm loss in minimal luminal diameter from immediately post stenting to follow-up and diameter stenosis ≥50% at follow-up). The relative risk is indicated by the thick vertical line in the center and the outside vertical line represent the 95% confidence limits. The hatched vertical line signifies a relative risk of 1 (no additional risk for restenosis). Variables with values greater than or less than 1 imply additional or a reduction in risk respectively (see text for details). The variables are listed in the left hand column. N represents the number of lesions analyzed for each particular variable. Although 214 lesions were analyzed in total, some lesions could not be analyzed for certain variables. The denominator for vessel branch (111) represents the total number of lesions that were stented in native vessels. (CI, confidence interval; DS, diameter stenosis; LAD, left anterior descending artery; DIAM., diameter; PRIM., primary; PTCA, percutaneous transluminal coronary angioplasty; MLD, minimal luminal diameter; Δ, absolute change; MULT., multiple)

patient (Table 5). Using the 50% diameter stenosis criterion, restenosis occurred in 27% of lesions (27% of patients).

Restenosis according to either definition was significantly higher in bypass grafts (MLD criterion:54% by patient; DS criterion:39% by patient) than in native vessels (34% and 18% respectively) (MLD: p = 0.016; DS: p = 0.001). Group 2 patients (MLD criterion:49% by patient; DS criterion: 32% by patient) did not have significantly greater restenosis than Group 1 patients (MLD criterion:35%; DS criterion:21%).

B. *Relative Risk Analysis*

The relative risk and 95% confidence intervals for each variable using either of the two criterion for restenosis are shown in Fig. 6. The variables with statistically significant associations with restenosis using the 0.72 mm criterion were multiple stents and oversizing the stent (unconstrained diameter) with respect to the reference diameter by more than 0.70 mm which had relative risk ratios (RR) (and 95% confidence intervals (CI)) of 1.56 (1.08–2.25) and

Table 6. Restenosis rates according to Criterion 1.
(≥0.72 mm Loss in Minimal Luminal Diameter)

		n	Restenosis Rate
Stent Number	Multiple	22/44	50%
	Single	53/165	32%
Stent Oversize	>0.7 mm	40/90	44%
	≤0.7 mm	26/96	27%

1.64 (1.10–2.45) respectively. The second criterion, ≥50% diameter stenosis at follow up, was associated with oversizing by >0.70 mm (RR 1.93, 95% CI 1.13–3.31), bypass grafts (RR 1.62, 95% CI 0.98–2.66), multiple stents/lesion (RR 1.61, 95% CI 0.97–2.67) and residual diameter stenosis >20% post stenting (RR 1.51, 95% CI 0.91–2.50). The actual restenosis rates for these variables are included in Tables 6 and 7.

C. *Long Term Follow-up*

The overall mortality during the study period was 8.9% for bypass grafts and 6.6% for native vessels (7.9% and 6% at 1 year respectively). In the bypass group, four of the nine deaths occurred during the initial hospitalization. Two of these deaths resulted from intracerebral hematomas related to the anticoagulation and two were from myocardial infarctions due to stent occlusion. Two of the 5 late deaths were sudden (at 2 and 18 months), two were clearly unrelated to the stent (chronic congestive heart failure, chronic renal failure) and the other death occurred after bypass surgery. In the group with native vessels, 7 of the 11 deaths were in-hospital. These were all due to myocardial infarctions resulting from stent occlusion with the exception of one intracerebral bleed and one patient who was stented 24 hours after an extensive myocardial infarction with cardiogenic shock. Two of the four

Table 7. Restenosis rates according to Criterion 2.
(>50% Diameter Stenosis at Follow-Up)

Parameter		n	Restenosis Rate
Vessel Type	Bypass	30/103	30%
	Native	20/111	19%
Stent Oversize	>0.7 mm	29/90	32%
	≤0.7 mm	16/96	17%
Diameter Stenosis Post Stent	>20%	30/107	28%
	≤20%	19/102	19%

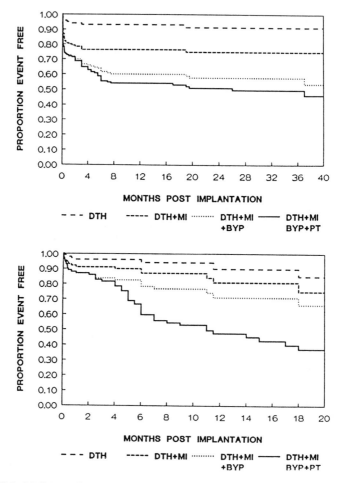

Figure 7. Clinical follow-up in native vessels up to 40 months (Fig. 7A) and bypass grafts up to 20 months (Fig. 7B). Death, myocardial infarction, bypass surgery, and PTCA or atherectomy were considered clinical end points.

late deaths were sudden (at 1.5 and 19 months), one was noncardiac (pneumonia) and the other resulted from complications post bypass surgery.

The actuarial event-free survival (freedom from death, myocardial infarction, bypass surgery or PTCA) for native artery patients was 46% at 40 months and for bypass graft patients was 37% at 20 months (Fig. 7).

Discussion

Despite progress in techniques and equipment, the rate of late angiographic narrowing following PTCA, a process popularly termed "restenosis," has not been altered since its clinical introduction 13 years ago. This failure has provided the impetus for the development of newer alternative forms of coronary revascularization such as stenting, atherectomy and laser. However the effectiveness of all forms of nonoperative coronary interventions remains limited by the restenosis process(es).

A. *Early Occlusion, Late Restenosis*

The coronary Wallstent was initially introduced as an endovascular device to prevent the late restenosis process that limits percutaneous transluminal coronary angioplasty. The indications for and management of patients implanted with this particular prosthesis have evolved as experience and knowledge have increased. In this study, an attempt has been made to separate two important factors in the late outcome of patients with stent implantations. The first division, according to date of implantation, provides the clearest picture of the changes in stent applications based on the early experience. Investigators originally believed that the stent could be safely implanted in native vessels and that the benefit of stents would be most apparent in lesions that had already restenosed on at least one occasion. However, a high in-hospital occlusion rate was noted, particularly in patients with unstable syndromes, evolving myocardial infarction or angiographic evidence of thrombus. These occlusions, often with disastrous clinical sequelae, convinced most of the investigators that native vessels in general and particularly in the left anterior descending artery (due to the large territory at risk), should only be stented in bail-out situations. Group 2 mainly consisted of patients with bypass grafts who were stented for primary lesions and native vessels who were stented as part of a bail-out strategy following complicated balloon angioplasty. Bypass grafts in particular were selected for stent implantations due to an extremely high rate of restenosis after PTCA alone and the larger diameter of these grafts seemed less likely to thrombose than smaller calibre native arterial vessels [14–17].

Bypass lesions, which were the majority of lesions stented in Group 2, were more complex in general than Group 1 lesions due to the advanced age and diffuse nature of the disease in the bypass grafts. As a result, more stents per lesion (1.4 versus 1.1 in native vessels) were required to cover these lesions. Therefore, the significantly lower rate of in-hospital occlusion in bypass graft patients versus patients with native vessels (8% versus 19%) and trend in Group 2 versus Group 1 (12% versus 20%) is indicative of several possible factors including improvements in anticoagulation regimens, operator experience and/or larger calibre vessels despite more complex case selection.

Recently, the initial clinical experience with the Palmaz-Schatz stent has been reported [18]. Using a similar anticoagulation schedule in 174 patients, a 0.6% in hospital occlusion rate was demonstrated. The discrepancy between a substantially higher occlusion rate in our series with the Wallstent and the Schatz study can not be entirely explained. The stent itself does not appear to be more thrombogenic. In a model of stents placed inside a polytetrafluo-ethylene graft in exteriorized arteriovenous shunts in baboons, no difference in acute platelet deposition and thrombus formation was noted between the two types of stents [19]. Differences in study design such as patient selection (collateralized vessels, predominantly right coronary arteries and exclusion of patients with recent myocardial infarction and abrupt closure following PTCA in the Schatz study) may account for some of the differences.

Higher restenosis rates by both criteria were demonstrated in bypass grafts compared with native vessels and in Group 2 than in Group 1. There are two possible explanations for this increase. First, bypass grafts, which are overrepresented in Group 2, are known to have higher restenosis rates than native vessels [14–16]. Secondly, higher restenosis rates may be the "price" for lower occlusion rates. Organization of thrombus at the site of intimal damage may be an important cause of late restenosis after stenting. Although it is often difficult to histologically differentiate thrombus organization from intimal hyperplasia, we have observed an extremely disorganized pattern of intimal thickening in the stented segments of several bypass grafts that have been surgically retrieved or obtained by atherectomy 1–5 months following stent implantation [20]. By diminishing the formation of early occlusive thrombus with more effective anticoagulation, the residual non occlusive thrombus could form the substrate for late restenosis. Although the second group had a higher proportion of bail-out cases, we did not identify increased relative risk for restenosis from bail-out cases in comparison to stent implantations performed in primary or restenosed lesions [21].

B. *Relative Risk Analysis*

Restenosis is a complex process that is only partially understood. Pathological studies of patients who have died more than 1 month following angioplasty have demonstrated the presence of intimal hyperplasia, presumably due to proliferation and migration of medial smooth muscle cells into the intima, and associated production of extracellular matrix collagen and proteoglycans [22, 23]. It has been suggested by Liu et al that the two major factors that determine the absolute amount of intimal hyperplasia are (1) the depth of injury and (2) the regional flow characteristics (which are determined by the geometry of the dilated lumen of the lesion and blood flow velocity patterns across that lumen) [24]. Two separate PTCA follow-up reports support the concept that the greater the diameter change post PTCA (implying a greater degree of disruption to the vessel wall), the more extensive is the absolute amount of reactive hyperplasia [25, 26]. On the basis of several angiographic studies from the Thoraxcenter, immediate results following stent implantation are superior to angioplasty alone (mean minimal luminal diameter of

2.5 mm versus 2.0–2.1 mm) and thus favor a more aggressive proliferative response post procedure [2, 4, 27]. The second factor is illustrated by the inverse relationship between the level of wall shear stress and subsequent intimal thickening. In the presence of a significant residual stenosis, the post stenotic region is a site of flow separation and low wall shear stress. This may retard endothelial recovery and prolong the period of smooth muscle cell proliferation which is partially dependent on restoration of regenerated endothelial barrier [28]. Stenting appears to diminish the effect of post stenotic wall shear stress by significantly improving the hemodynamic effects of the stenosis (based on the calculated reductions in Poisseuille and turbulent contributions to flow resistance) [29].

It is extremely difficult if not impossible to predict restenosis in the individual patient following PTCA (30). This problem can be partially understood when one considers that the two factors (ie. depth of injury and regional flow characteristics) affecting the extent of intimal proliferation act in opposition to the other and thus make it hazardous to predict outcome of this interaction in a particular patient. In large population of patients, relative risk analyses following PTCA have identified several patient, lesion, and procedural variables that predict late restenosis. However, the situation following stenting may be different where the mean loss of minimal luminal diameter at late follow-up is twice that of PTCA alone (0.62 mm versus 0.31 mm) [2, 27]. Therefore, this study was designed to identify factors that were associated with an increased risk of restenosis following stenting.

Lesion Factors

Stented bypass grafts had a greater risk of restenosis than native vessels (30% versus 19%) but this finding was restricted to the DS criterion. The increased susceptibility of bypass grafts to the restenosis process has previously been documented following PTCA [9, 31–35]. Although left anterior descending (LAD) lesions have been shown to be a risk factor in several PTCA studies [5], this was not evident in our study. The reference diameter of the vessel also had no relationship to restenosis. Forty-three percent of the vessels had reference diameter between 3–4 mm and 43% were 3 mm or less. Lesion length and the severity of the lesion, in absolute minimal luminal diameter or diameter stenosis, prior to the procedure have been cited by several authors as important risk factors for restenosis following angioplasty although our data did not show this association [5–7]. Lesion length is probably not an important factor for restenosis if lesions can be covered by a single stent (see below). We believe that this is due to a more uniform and optimal dilatation with stenting. Long lesions treated with angioplasty are frequently less successfully dilated along the entire length of the lesion and the ragged irregular surface of the vessel may predispose to rheological factors critically involved in restenosis. Total occlusions have been reported as an important predictor of restenosis in angioplasty studies. However, this accounted for only 4.5% of the lesions in our study which was too few for this analysis. Although there was a trend for higher restenosis in more eccentric lesions, this was not statistically significant.

Stent Factors

Multiple stents (RR: MLD 1.56 (1.08–2.25); DS 1.61 (0.9–2.67)) and unconstrained stent diameter exceeding reference diameter by > 0.7 mm (RR: MLD 1.64 (1.10–2.45); DS 1.93 (1.13–3.31)) significantly predicted restenosis with both criteria. Preliminary reports from four separate groups working with the Palmaz-Schatz stent have shown a similar relationship between multiple stents/lesion and restenosis [36–39]. In our study, multiple stents placed in tandem were overlapped at the extremities (so called "telescoping") which may be the reason for the observed increase in restenosis rates. The segment of the vessel that was covered by the overlapping stents was subjected to the dilating force of two separate stents as well as an increased density of metal. We have observed that restenosis commonly occurred at these sites of overlapping between extremities of stents. Since the length of the lesion and the absolute length of the stent required to cover a lesion were not significant predictors, it seems prudent to implant longer stents rather than two or more shorter stents in tandem.

Selecting an oversized stent (unconstrained diameter >0.7 mm larger than the reference diameter) was a particularly important stimulus for hyperplasia with the self-expanding Wallstent. Schwartz et al have described an aggressive proliferative response in a porcine model as a result of severe stent oversizing (0.5 to 1.5 mm) [40]. This effect, which they attributed to penetration of the internal elastic lamina by the stent wires and subsequent deep medial injury, was much less pronounced when the stent diameter was matched more closely to the vessel diameter. Furthermore, due to its self expanding property, the Wallstent (and particularly when it is oversized) continues to expand the vessel wall for at least 24 hours post implantation [41]. The vessel is subjected to increasingly higher wall stress than after implantation of a balloon expandable stent (which is maximally expanded at the time of implantation), a factor which may adversely stimulate the proliferative process. It may seem paradoxical that oversizing the stent by >0.7 mm would result in a higher restenosis rate with the 50% DS criterion. However, the diameter stenosis post stent was not different in the two groups despite the oversizing. The main effect of oversizing then was not particularly a superior immediate result but rather a more aggressive "hyperplastic" reaction and a smaller MLD at follow-up than if less oversized stents were implanted. The absolute value of the unconstrained stent diameter and the addition of the polymer coating (Biogold[R]) had no significant relationship to late restenosis.

Procedural Factors

No significant relative risk could be attributed to a particular indication for the procedure. Restenosis rates for primary cases were not significantly different than for bail-out or restenosis cases (MLD Criterion:37%, 42%, 33%; DS Criterion: 24%, 27%, 24%) although an increased rate of restenosis has been described with the Palmaz-Schatz stent in patients with previous restenosis [39]. The absolute change in diameter from the pre to the post stent result and dilatation within the stent after implantation (the so-called "Swiss Kiss") did not appear to affect the late restenosis. This post stent dilatation was performed to dissipate clot within the stent and to accelerate early expansion of the stent. A post stent diameter stenosis >20% tended to be predictive of a follow-up diameter stenosis >50% (RR 1.51, 95% CI 0.91–2.50) although not for the MLD criteria. The larger the residual stenosis following stenting (ie. less optimal result), the less hyperplasia is required to reach a reach a particular diameter stenosis at follow-up such as the 50% diameter stenosis criterion.

Limitations of Study

Several important limitations of this study must be mentioned. Although this study suggest several factors that may be predictive of restenosis following stenting, it does not address the actual mechanisms of restenosis in the stented vessel. By comparing the predictors of restenosis following stenting to angioplasty, we have assumed that the underlying mechanism(s) responsible for late angiographic narrowing are similar (i.e. primarily intimal hyperplasia). Although almost every stenting procedure was accompanied by balloon dilatation at some particular time during the procedure, several other mechanisms may be important. Elastic recoil, which in the first few days following the procedure may be a significant factor in causing renarrowing, may be less important in stented vessels than angioplasty alone due to the scaffolding function of the stent. Although organization of thrombus at the site of intimal damage following PTCA has been recognized as a cause for late restenosis, it has not been particularly regarded as an important factor based on late pathological studies following PTCA. However, this may be an extremely important cause of late restenosis after stenting. Although it is difficult to histologically discriminate thrombus organization from intimal hyperplasia, we have observed a disorganized layer of intimal thickening directly above the stent wire associated with remnants of thrombus in segments of several bypass grafts that have been surgically retrieved up to 10 months following stent implantation [20, 42] (Fig. 8). Therefore we consider organization of residual thrombus to be a potentially important cause of late angiographic narrowing in addition to the major occlusion problems early after stenting. This may partially explain why commonly regarded determi-

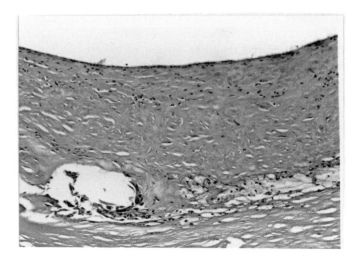

Figure 8. Light micrograph of stented bypass graft removed 10 months after stent implantation. The void (*) represents a 70 micron diameter stent wire. Immediately adjacent to the stent wire are cellular debris and foam cells (arrowhead). Directly above the stent wire is a layer of disorganized fibrointimal hyperplasia. Courtesy of HMM van Beusekom.

nants of restenosis following PTCA (eg. lesion length, Left Anterior Descending Artery) do not appear to be significant in this analysis since a different pathological processes may predominate. This also has important clinical implications since therapy to limit smooth muscle proliferation may be quite different than therapy to minimize thrombus formation.

There are two statistical limitations to this study. Due to the relatively small sample size, we can not rule out a significant beta error. Secondly, in performing multiple statistical comparisons, there is a risk that some of them may be significant by chance alone. Therefore, this data requires confirmation by other studies.

In conclusion, the European coronary Wallstent experience has demonstrated that restenosis following stenting is increased in bypass grafts and in the presence of multiple stents and excessive oversizing of the stent (>0.7 mm) and less optimal results immediately post stenting (>20% diameter stenosis). Since some of these factors can be modified, we recommend against the use of multiple stents and excessive oversizing to reduce the probability of late restenosis.

C. *Short and Long Term Follow-up: Clinical Events*

The problems of prolonged anticoagulation are an additional consideration. Increased morbidity (increased femoral hematomas, gastrointestinal and genito-urinary tract bleeding) and mortality (3 patients died from intracerebral hemorrhage) are directly attributable to the intensive anticoagulation regimen. The duration of hospitalization is also lengthened to ensure therapeutic levels of anticoagulation.

The high incidence of late adverse clinical events in stented patients is a cause for concern. A mortality rate of 8.9% in bypass grafts and 6.6% in native vessels is higher than in reported PTCA studies [43, 44, 45]. However, it must be stressed that a large number of stents in native vessels were implanted for abrupt closure following PTCA which dramatically increases the risk of the procedure [45]. Actuarial event free survival (freedom from death, myocardial infarction, bypass surgery or repeat PTCA or atherectomy) was 37% at 20 months in bypass patients and 46% at 40 months in native vessels. In the bypass group, about 30% of the adverse events were unrelated to the stented lesion and were due to worsening of a different lesion or to development of new lesions. In the native vessel group, 12% of the adverse events were unrelated to the stented lesion. In addition, 9 of the 30 bypass operations in stented native vessel patients were performed as part of a protocol for patients stented for the bail-out indication [46]. Although there are no comparable series of native vessel patients in the literature because of the unique set of indications in our study, three recent reports have been published of late clinical follow-up (Kaplan-Meier analysis) after PTCA in bypass grafts. The Thoraxcenter reported that only 41% of patients were alive and event-free (myocardial infarction, repeat CABG, repeat PTCA) at a median follow-up of 2.1 years [47]. A review of the overall Dutch experience also showed limited late beneficial results with a two year and five year event free survival of 52% and 26% respectively in 454 bypass patients [48]. Webb et al have described a 71% freedom from death, infarction and surgery at 5 years in bypass patients who underwent PTCA at their institution but did not include the 27% incidence of second angioplasty procedures also required in their patient group [14]. However, it must be stressed that our study was not a randomized trial designed to compare stenting with PTCA but rather an observational study with a first generation coronary stent. Nevertheless, all of these late follow-up studies of nonoperative coronary revascularization clearly show that these are palliative procedures and not long-term solutions to the underlying problems of progression of underlying coronary disease and iatrogenically induced restenosis.

Several important points emerge from this study. Although in hospital occlusion rates improved in the later experience, Wallstent^R coronary thrombosis continues to limit its use. Restenosis rates with the 50% DS criterion do not seem to be significantly improved when compared with historical post angioplasty results, although definitive statements must await randomized trials. Bypass grafts in particular have a high incidence of late restenosis rate although early occlusion occurred less significantly than in patients with native vessels. Based on our experience, there is insufficient evidence at this time to suggest implantation of this particular stent outside of a randomized trial with the following exceptions: (1) bail-out for abrupt occlusion, (2) suboptimal (inadequate dilalatation) results following PTCA, and (3) bypass grafts at high risk for distal embolization with PTCA (friable lesions that may benefit from the scaffolding property of the Wallstent[R]).

Appendix

Participating Centers and Collaborators: Catheterization Laboratory for Clinical and Experimental Image Processing, Thoraxcenter, Rotterdam, The Netherlands: B. H. Strauss, MD, K. J. Beatt, MB BS, M. v.d. Brand, MD, P. J. de Feyter, MD, H. Suryapranata, MD, I. K. de Scheerder, MD, J. R. T. C. Roelandt, MD, P. W. Serruys, MD; Department of Cardiology, Hôpital Cardiologique, Lille, France: M. E. Bertrand; Department of Invasive Cardiology, The Royal Bromptom and National Heart Institute, London, United Kingdom: A. F. Rickards, MD, U. Sigwart, MD; Department of Clinical and Experimental Cardiology, CHRU Rangeuil, Toulouse, France: J. P. Bounhoure, MD, A. Courtault, MD, F. Joffre, MD, J. Puel, MD, H. Rousseau, MD; Division of Cardiology, Department of Medicine, CHUV, Lausanne, Switzerland: J. -J. Goy, MD, J. -C. Stauffer, MD, U. Kaufmann, MD, L. Kappenberger, MD, P. Urban, MD; Cardiology Center, University Hospital, Geneva, Switzerland: B. Meier, MD, P. Urban, MD.

Acknowledgements

We gratefully acknowledge the assistance of Hanneke Roerade in preparation of the manuscript and Dr. Edward Murphy (Portland, Oregon) for critical comments. We appreciated the technical assistance of Marie-Angèle Morel and Eline Montauban van Swijndregt.

This study was supported in part by grants from the Dutch Ministry of Science and Education, Den Haag, The Netherlands (87159) and the Swiss National Fund (3,835,083).

References

1. Sigwart U, Puel J, Mirkovitch V, Joffre F, Kappenberger L (1987) Intravascular stents to prevent occlusion and restenosis after transluminal angioplasty. *N Engl J Med* 316:701–6
2. Serruys P W, Strauss B H, Beatt K J, Bertrand M E, Puel J, Rickards A F, Meier B, Kappenberger L, Goy J J, Vogt P, Sigwart U (1991) Quantitative follow-up after placement of a self-expanding coronary stent. *New Engl J Med* 324:13–17
3. Reiber J H C, Serruys P W, Kooijman C J, Wijns W, Slager C J, Gerbrands J J, Schuurbiers J C H, den Boer A, Hugenholtz P G (1985) Assessment of short-, medium-, and long-term variations in arterial dimensions from computer-assisted quantitation of coronary cineangiograms. *Circulation* 71:280–288
4. Serruys P W, Luijten H E, Beatt K J, Geuskens R, de Feyter P J, van den Brand M, Reiber J H C, ten Katen H J, Es G A van, Hugenholtz P G (1988) Incidence of restenosis after succesful angioplasty: a time related phenomenon. *Circulation* 77:361–371
5. Leimgruber P P, Roubin G S, Hollman J, Cotsonis G A, Meier B, Douglas J S Jr, King S B III, Gruentzig A R (1986) Restenosis after succesful coronary angioplasty in patients with single-vessel disease. *Circulation* 73:710–717

6. Myler R K, Topol E J, Shaw R E, Stertzer S H, Clark D A, Fishman J, Murphy M C (1987) Multiple vessel coronary angioplasty: classification, results, and patterns of restenosis in 494 consecutive patients. *Cathet Cardiovasc Diagn* 13:1–15

7. Vandormael M G, Deligonul U, Kern M J et al (1987) Multilesion coronary angioplasty: clinical and angiographic follow-up. *J Am Coll Cardiol* 10:246–252

8. Mata L A, Bosch X, David P R et al (1985) Clinical and angiographic assessment 6 months after double vessel percutaneous coroanry angioplasty. *J Am Coll Cardiol* 6:1239–1244

9. Holmes D R Jr, Vliestra R E, Smith H C et al (1984) Restenosis after percutaneous transluminal coronary angioplasty (PTCA): a report from the PTCA registry of the National Heart, Lung, and Blood Institute. *Am J Cardiol* 53:77C–81C

10. Levine S, Ewels C J, Rosing D R, Kent K M (1985) Coronary angioplasty: clinical and angiographic follow-up. *Am J Cardiol* 55:673–676

11. Disciascio G, Cowley M J, Vetrovec G W (1986) Angiographic patterns of restenosis after angioplasty of multiple coronary arteries. *Am J Cardiol* 58:922–925

12. Gardner M J, Altman D G (1989) Statistics with confidence. *British Medical Journal*, London

13. Kaplan E L, Meier P (1958) Nonparametric estimation from incomplete observations. *J Am Stat Assoc* 53:457–481

14. Webb J G, Myler R K, Shaw R E, Anwar A, Mayo J R, Murphy M C, Cumberland D C, Stertzer S H (1990) Coronary angioplasty after coronary bypass surgery: initial results and late outcome in 422 patients. *J Am Coll Cardiol* 16:812–820

15. Douglas JS, Gruentzig AR, King III SB, Hollman J, Ischinger T, Meier B, Craver JM, Jones EL, Waller JL, Bone DK, Guyton R (1983) Percutaneous transluminal coronary angioplasty in patients with prior coronary bypass surgery. *J Am Coll Cardiol* 2:745–754

16. Block P C, Cowley M J, Kaltenbach M, Kent K M, Simpson J (1984) Percutaneous angioplasty of stenoses of bypass grafts or of bypass graft anastomosis sites. *Am J Cardiol* 53:666–668

17. Bucx J J J, de Scheerder I, Beatt K, van den Brand M, Suryapranata H, de Feyter P, Serruys P W (1991) The importance of adequate anticoagulation to prevent early thrombosis following stenting of stenosed venous bypass grafts. *Am Heart J* 121:1389–1396

18. Schatz R A, Baim D S, Leon M et al (1991) Clinical experience with the Palmaz-Schatz coronary stent. Initial results of a multicenter study. *Circulation* 83:148–161

19. Krupski W C, Bass A, Kelly A B, Marzec U M, Hanson S R, Harker L A (1990) Heparin-resistant thrombus formation by endovascular stents in baboons: interruption by a synthetic antithrombin. *Circulation* 82:570–577

20. Serruys P W, Strauss B H, van Beusekom H M, van der Giessen W J (1991) Stenting of coronary arteries. Has a modern Pandora's Box been opened? *J Am Coll Cardiol* 17:143B–154B

21. Strauss B H, Serruys P W, de Scheerder I K et al (1990) A relative risk analysis of the angiographic predictors of restenosis in the coronary Wallstent[R] (abstract). *Circulation* 82(III):540

22. Austin G E, Ratliff N B, Hollman J, Tabei S, Phillips D F (1985) Intimal proliferation of smooth muscle cells as an explanation for recurrent coronary artery stenosis after percutaneous transluminal coronary angioplasty. *J Am Coll Cardiol* 6:369–375

23. Waller B F, Gorfinkel H J, Rogers F J, Kent K M, Roberts W C (1984) Early and late morphologic changes in major epicardial coronary arteries after percutaneous transluminal coronary angioplasty. *Am J Cardiol* 53:42C–47C

24. Liu M W, Roubin G S, King S B III (1989) Restenosis after coronary angioplasty: potential biologic determinants and role of intimal hyperplasia. *Circulation* 79:1374–1387

25. Beatt K J, Luijten H E, Suryapranata H, de Feyter P J, Serruys P W (1989) Suboptimal post angioplasty result, the principle risk factor for "restenosis" (abstract). *Circulation* 80:II–257

26. Liu M W, Roubin G S, King S B III (1989) Does an optimal luminal result after PTCA reduce restenosis? (abstract) *Circulation* 80:II–63

27. Serruys P W, Rutsch W, Heyndrickx G, Danchin N, Mast G, Wijns W, Rensing B J (1991) Effect of long term thromboxane A2 receptor blockade on angiographic restenosis and clinical events after coronary angioplasty. The CARPORT study (abstract). *J Am Coll Cardiol* 17:2:283A

28. Haudenschild C C, Schwartz S M (1979) Endothelial regeneration. Restitution of endothelial continuity. *Lab Invest* 41:407–418

29. Serruys P W, Juilliere Y, Bertrand M E, Puel J, Rickards A F, Sigwart U (1988) Additional improvement of stenosis geometry in human coronary arteries by stenting after balloon dilatation. *Am J Cardiol* 61:71G–76G

30. Renkin J, Melin J, Robert A, Richelle F, Bachy J-L, Col J, Detry J-M, Wijns W (1990) Detection of restenosis after successful coronary angioplasty: improved clinical decision making with the use of a logistic model combining procedural and follow-up variables. *J Am Coll Cardiol* 16:1333–1340

31. Douglas J S, Gruentzig A R, King III S B, Hollman J, Ischinger T, Meier B, Craver J M, Jones E L, Waller J L, Bone D K, Guyton R (1983) Percutaneous transluminal coronary angioplasty in patients with prior coronary bypass surgery. *J Am Coll Cardiol* 2:745–754

32. Block P C, Cowley M J, Kaltenbach M, Kent K M, Simpson J (1984) Percutaneous angioplasty of stenoses of bypass grafts or of bypass graft anastomosis sites. *Am J Cardiol* 53:666–668

33. Corbell J, Franco I, Hollman J, Simpfendorfer C, Galan K (1985) Percutaneous transluminal coronary angioplasty after previous coronary artery bypass surgery. *Am J Cardiol* 56:398–403

34. Pinkerton C A, Slack J D, Orr C M (1988) Percutaneous transluminal angioplasty in patients with prior myocardial revascularization surgery. *Am J Cardiol* 61:15G–22G

35. Webb J G, Myler R K, Shaw R E, Anwar A, Mayo J R, Murphy M C, Cumberland D C, Stertzer S H (1990) Coronary angioplasty after coronary bypass surgery: initial results and late outcome in 422 patients. *J Am Coll Cardiol* 16:812–820

36. Ellis S G, Savage M, Baim D, Hirschfeld J, Cleman M, Teirstein P, Topol E (1990) Intracoronary stenting to prevent restenosis. Preliminary results of a multicenter study using the Palmaz-Schatz stent suggest benefit in selected high risk patients (abstract). *J Am Coll Cardiol* 15:18A

37. Levine M J, Leonard B M, Burke J A, Nash I D, Safian R D, Diver D J, Baim D S (1990) Clinical and angiographic results of balloon-expandable intracoronary stents in right coronary artery stenoses. *J Am Coll Cardiol* 16:332–339

38. Schatz R A, Goldberg S, Leon M B, Fish R D, Hirshfield J W, Walker C M (1990) Coronary stenting following "suboptimal" coronary angioplasty results (abstract). *Circulation* 82:III–540

39. Teirstein P S, Cleman M W, Hirshfeld J W, Buchbinder M, Walker C (1990) Influence of prior restenosis on subsequent restenosis after intracoronary stenting (abstract). *Circulation* 82:III–657

40. Schwartz R S, Murphy J G, Edwards W D, Camrud A R, Vliestra R E, Holmes D R (1990) Restenosis after balloon angioplasty. A practical proliferative model in porcine coronary arteries. *Circulation* 82:2190–2200

41. Beatt K J, Bertrand M, Puel J, Rickards A F, Serruys P W, Sigwart U (1989) Additional improvement in vessel lumen in the first 24 hours after stent implantation due to radial dilating force (abstract). *J Am Coll Cardiol* 13:224A

42. van Beusekom H M M, Serruys P W, van der Giessen W J, Strauss B H, de Feyter P J, van Loon H, van Suylen R J, Suryapranata H, van der Brand M J (1991) Histological features 3 to 320 days after stenting of human saphenous vein bypass grafts (abstract). *J Am Coll Cardiol* 17:53A

43. Kent K M, Bentivoglio L G, Block P C et al (1984) Long-term efficacy of percutaneous transluminal coronary angioplasty (PTCA): Report from the National Heart, Lung, and Blood Institute PTCA Registry. *Am J Cardiol* 53:27C–31C

44. Gruentzig A R, King S B III, Schlumpf M, Siegenthaler W (1987) Long-term follow-up

after percutaneous transluminal coronary angioplasty. The early Zurich experience. *New Engl J Med* 316:1127–1132

45. Detre K, Holubkov R, Kelsey S et al (1989) One-year follow-up results of the 1985–1986 National Heart, Lung, and Blood Institute's percutaneous transluminal coronary angioplasty registry. *Circulation* 80:421–428

46. de Feyter P J, de Scheerder I, van den Brand M, Laarman G, Suryapranata H, Serruys P W (1990) Emergency stenting for refractory acute coronary artery occlusion during coronary angioplasty. *Am J Cardiol* 66:1147–1150

47. Meester B J, Samson M, Suryapranata H, Bonsel G, van den Brand M, de Feyter P J, Serruys P W (1991) Long-term follow-up after attempted angioplasty of saphenous vein grafts: the Thoraxcenter experience 1981–1988. *Eur Heart J* (in press)

48. Plokker H W T, Meester B H, Serruys P W (1991) The Dutch experience in percutaneous transluminal angioplasty of narrowed saphenous veins used for aortocoronary arterial by-pass. *Am J Cardiol* 67:361–366

8. Restenosis after Palmaz-Schatz™ Stent Implantation

DAVID L. FISCHMAN, MICHAEL P. SAVAGE, STEPHEN G. ELLIS, RICHARD A. SCHATZ, MARTIN B. LEON, DONALD BAIM and SHELDON GOLDBERG

Introduction

Efforts currently directed at reducing restenosis in coronary arteries after transcatheter interventions have met with little success. A variety of pharmacologic [1–6] and mechanical interventions [7–11] have been tested but without proven benefit. This failure to prevent restenosis should not be surprising given our limited understanding of the complexity of the biologic response to arterial injury. This response to injury phenomenon occurs independent of the specific type of intervention and is a result of plaque disruption and subintimal injury, endothelial denudation, platelet activation and release of growth factors which lead to intimal smooth muscle cell proliferation. This response has been described as an example of "wound healing" [12]. It would be simplistic to expect that any currently available device would abolish the problem of coronary restenosis. The best that any mechanical intervention could do would be to provide a larger smoother initial lumen compared with standard balloon angioplasty. This enhanced acute gain in lumen diameter would accommodate a greater degree of intimal hyperplasia before hemodynamically significant luminal compromise would occur. Coronary stents are permanent implants which provide this greater "growing room" for smooth muscle cells and may potentially reduce the rate of restenosis by this mechanical effect. The purpose of this chapter is to review the results of the angiographic follow-up studies with one type of intravascular scaffold, the balloon expandable Palmaz-Schatz™stent.

Stent Design

The original stent design developed by Palmaz for use in the peripheral vasculature consisted of a single rigid slotted stainless steel tube. The design was subsequently modified by Schatz for use in the coronary arteries

P. W. Serruys, B. H. Strauss and S. B. King III (eds), Restenosis after Intervention with New Mechanical Devices, 191–205.
© 1992 Kluwer Academic Publishers. Printed in the Netherlands.

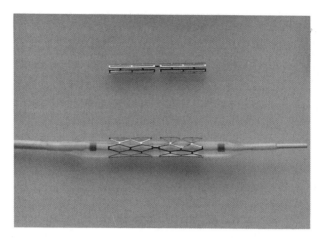

Figure 1. The Palmaz-Schatz™ stent.

(Fig. 1). The currently used device consists of two 7.0 mm tubes connected by a central bridging 1 mm strut. The stent fits over an angioplasty balloon. It is 15 mm in length and 1.6 mm in diameter in its unexpanded state; with balloon inflation, the struts of the stent take on a diamond configuration with a high free space to metal ratio, a factor which in part accounts for the relatively low thrombogenicity of this device [13]. The articulation point of the stent imparts longitudinal flexibility which enhances passage through tortuous segments of preformed catheters and the coronary vasculature. In early trials the stent was hand crimped on a standard balloon and delivered bare to the target lesion; later because of problems with stent embolization, a subselective sheath system was used for stent delivery.

In Vivo Laboratory Studies

Schatz studied the biologic response to stent implantation in non-diseased coronary arteries in the canine model [14]. Stents were implanted in the coronary arteries of animals pretreated with aspirin and dypyrimadole and for 3 months after the procedure. Heparin and low molecular weight Dextran 40 were administered during the procedure. Coronary angiography was performed at 1, 3, 6, and 12 months after stent implantation. Gross pathology and electron microscopic studies were performed on sacrificed animals. Angiography revealed patency in all stented coronary segments without evidence of spasm, thrombosis, perforation or migration. Histology showed that the stents were initially covered by a thin layer of fibrin and thrombus with immature endothelial cells covering the thrombus. After 3 weeks myofibroblastic cells had replaced the thrombus; the peak of the fibrocellular response was noted at 8 weeks which resulted in a neointimal thickness of 300

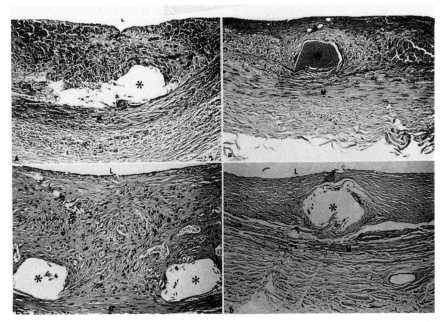

Figure 2. Time course of proliferative response following stent implantation in the canine model
(From Schatz et al, *Circulation* 76:450. *Reprinted with permission*).

microns. This response regressed by 32 weeks; at which time mature endothelial cells were noted to cover a sclerotic ground substance. The time
course of this response is noted in Fig. 2.

Encouraged by these preliminary experimental results, a multicenter
group of investigators was organized to assess the safety and efficacy of
coronary stenting using this device in patients. A major endpoint of the
group was to determine the effects of stenting on restenosis rates. The
principal investigators and their institutional affiliation are noted in the ap-
pendix. A core angiographic laboratory was established at Thomas Jefferson
University Hospital, where qualitative and quantitative coronary analyses
were performed.

Patient Studies

Inclusion criteria: Patients were selected for stenting if they met the following
criteria:
· objective evidence of myocardial ischemia
· critical coronary stenosis ≥ 70% by visual estimate
· preserved left ventricular function
· suitability for coronary artery bypass surgery
Patients were excluded for the following reasons:

· recent acute myocardial infarction
· diffuse disease
· ostial stenosis
· large diseased side branches
· preexistent coronary thrombi
· unprotected left main coronary stenosis
· extreme vessel tortuosity

It should be noted that initially patients with long lesions (>15 mm) requiring placement of multiple overlapping stents were included into the study. However, based on the suboptimal results of follow-up angiography for multiple stents, we are currently performing stenting only if lesions can be spanned by a single stent.

Medication Protocol

Because of the potential for subacute thrombosis a rigorous anticoagulation regimen is followed. The current approach includes the following:
Before stent placement
· ASA 325 mg daily
· Dipyrimadole 75 mg tid
· calcium channel antagonist
· low molecular Dextran 40
Intraoperatively
· Heparin 10,000 units with continuous infusion and intermittent boluses to maintain activated clotting time > 300 seconds
· low molecular Dextran 40
After stent placement
· heparin   (until PT > 16 seconds)
· warfarin   (1–3 months)
· aspirin   (indefinitely)
· dipyrimadole   (3 months)
· calcium antagonist   (3 months)

Angiographic Analysis at the Core Laboratory

In all patients enrolled in the stent trial, coronary angiography was performed before angioplasty, after conventional angioplasty, and after stent implantation. In addition, as part of the protocol, followup angiography was performed at 4 to 6 months following stent implantation. Detailed morphologic analysis of the cineangiograms was performed at the core angiographic laboratory by a panel of three experienced angiographers. Qualitatively, lesions were assessed for eccentricity, calcification, thrombus, plaque ulceration, diffuse disease and tortuosity.

Quantitative analysis of selected coronary segments was performed using a computer based coronary angiography analysis system [15, 16]. Paired cine frames, in orthogonal views whenever possible, were selected from the pre-angioplasty, post-angioplasty, post-stent, and followup angiograms. These frames were projected on a cine 35 mm viewer (General Electric, CAPS 35, King of Prussia, PA.) optically coupled to a video camera. The video signal was digitized at $512 \times 512 \times 8$ bit resolution onto a digital angiographic computer (ADAC laboratories, Model DPS-4100, Milpedas, CA.) Images were magnified 4 fold using bilinear interpolation. The lesion of interest was determined by the operator through placement of variable size circles. The vessel lumen was then determined by the computer using an automatic edge detection algorithm that has previously been validated. Quantitative measurements of stenosis length and diameter (in mm) were determined using the guiding catheter as a scaling reference. Proximal and distal segments, considered to be without coronary disease and outside the stented segment were selected and averaged; this average value was considered the normal reference diameter used to calculate the percentage diameter stenosis. Validation of this quantitative technique at our laboratory has been made using phantom models and patient studies. A series of 12 precision drilled plexiglass stenosis models along with a contrast-filled 7 French coronary catheter were filmed at 30 frames/second over the left hemithorax. Correlation between quantitative angiography and actual measurements were 0.98 for luminal diameter and 0.96 for percent diameter stenosis. For repeated measurements of patient cineangiograms made on separate days the intraobserver variability at the core laboratory is 0.16 mm for absolute diameter and less that 5% for percent diameter stenosis.

Restenosis in Patients Undergoing Palmaz-Schatz^{TM} Stent Placement

In the first phase of our trial a total of 226 patients underwent attempted placement of the Palmaz-Schatz^{TM} stent [13]. Successful implantation was achieved in 213 patients (94%). Subacute thrombosis occurred in 8 patients (3.8%). Therefore, 205 patients remained eligible for follow-up angiography which was performed 5.5 ± 1.7 months (mean ± s.d.) in 165 patients for an angiographic followup rate of 80%. The demographic characteristics of these patients and associated lesions characteristics are listed in Tables 1–3.

Overall Restenosis Rate

Various definitions has been used to define restenosis in the major restenosis studies. Among these definitions are: 1) loss of at least 50% of the initial gain achieved at angioplasty [2], 2) Deterioration of 0.72 mm in minimal luminal diameter or greater from immediately postangioplasty to follow-up

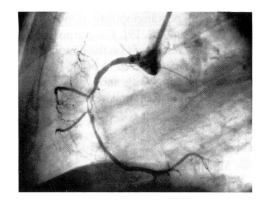

a

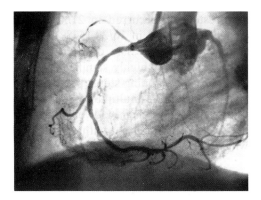

b

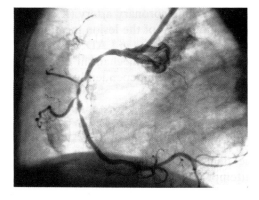

c

Figure 3. Severe restenosis despite excellent angiographic result: A) Baseline angiogram revealing a critical stenosis in the mid-right coronary artery is shown. B) The post stent result. C) Follow-up angiography which shows severe restenosis.

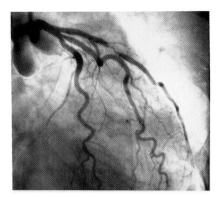

a

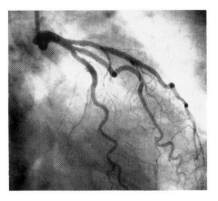

b

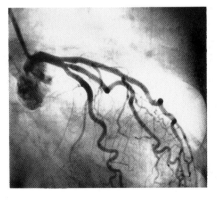

c

Figure 4. Excellent long term followup after stenting. A) Baseline angiogram which shows a critical lesion in the proximal left anterior descending coronary artery. B) Post-stent result. C) 6 month follow-up angiogram revealing a widely patent stented segment.

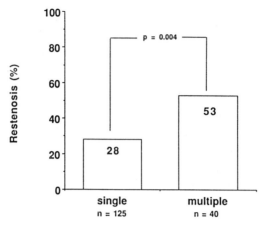

Figure 5. Restenosis as a function of single versus multiple stents.

Influence of Vessel Diameter

We analyzed the effect of vessel diameter on future development of restenosis. The mean reference vessel diameter of all patients stented was
3.2 mm. Forty-three percent of patients had a normal reference diameter
> 3.2 mm; the restenosis rate in this group was 21%. By contrast, the
restenosis rate was 37% in those patients with smaller vessels ≤3.2 mm in
diameter as shown in Fig. 7. Although, there appeared to be a trend towards
a lower restenosis rate in larger diameter vessels, these results did not reach
statistical significance ($X^2 = 3.0$, p = 0.09).

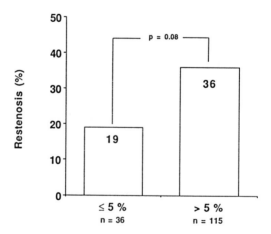

Figure 6. Restenosis as a function of the initial angiographic result.

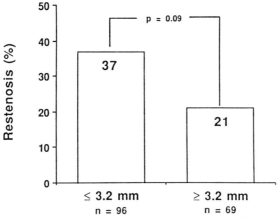

Figure 7. Restenosis as a function of reference vessel diameter.

Effect of Prior PTCA Procedures

We compared those patients who underwent stenting of de novo lesions with those in whom the stent was placed in lesions that had previously undergone balloon angioplasty. Of the initial 226 patients, 157 (69%) patients had previous coronary angioplasty with clinical and angiographic restenosis of the lesion to be stented. Of the 165 patients who underwent angiographic follow-up, 65% had previous coronary angioplasty. Overall no significant difference was noted in the restenosis rate for de novo lesions versus lesions that had undergone previous balloon dilatation (25% versus 36%, p = 0.07). However, for patients with de novo lesions who received a single stent the restenosis rate was 13% in contrast to 36% for patients with previous restenosis (X^2 = 6.8, p = 0.009). These results are shown in Fig. 8.

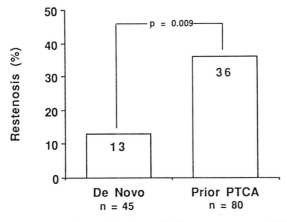

Figure 8. Restenosis as a function of DeNovo versus repeat PTCA.

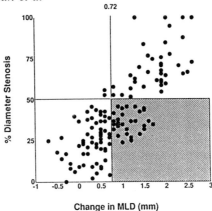

Figure 9. Restenosis as a function of the change in minimal luminal diameter afforded by stent implantation.

Mechanism of Potential Stent Benefit

The mechanism of stent benefit in reducing restenosis could be related to either an enhanced acute gain or a decrease in intimal hyperplasia. Accordingly, we analyzed the change in minimal luminal diameter as a function of the percent stenosis at follow-up as depicted in Fig. 9. A significant change in minimal luminal diameter (>0.72mm) was observed in 50% of lesions, in contrast to significant restenosis ($\geq$50% diameter stenosis) which was present in 34%. As shown in the right lower quadrant of Fig. 9, 42% of lesions which demonstrated a change of >0.72 mm were not categorized as restenosis. Thus while the majority of patients developed significant intimal hyperplasia, this was not always sufficient to compromise the lumen by $\geq$50%, the arbitrary definition of restenosis. Therefore, the degree of acute gain which the stent achieves compared with standard balloon angioplasty appears to be responsible for the reduction in restenosis rate.

Long Term Follow-up

Finally, we sought to determine whether the permanent metallic implant affects the time course over which restenosis occurs [21]. Follow-up coronary angiography was performed in a cohort of 37 patients (39 lesions) who reached their one year anniversary from the date of stent implantation. Comparison of the 6 and 12 month angiograms revealed no difference in minimum luminal diameter (1.92 ± 0.57 versus 1.93 ± 0.56) or % stenosis (36 ± 17 versus 35 ± 17). The overall restenosis rate for the 39 lesions was 23% at 6 months and 21% at 12 months. Therefore, stent implantation does not appear to prolong the temporal course of the restenosis process.

Clinical Implications and Future Goals

We have demonstrated that coronary stenting with the Palmaz-Schatz^{TM} device *may* limit restenosis in certain subgroups: These include patients in whom a single stent is placed in a relatively large vessel. Furthermore, the effect on reducing restenosis is most pronounced in patients with de novo lesions. The mechanism of stent benefit in reducing restenosis is due to the enhanced acute gain achieved by stenting as compared to standard balloon angioplasty. The degree of luminal loss due to intimal hyperplasia seems similar to other transcatheter interventions. It should be pointed out that the conclusions drawn concerning reduction in restenosis rates need to be formally tested by means of a prospective randomized trial comparing stenting to standard balloon angioplasty. We are currently involved in such a trial which will enroll approximately 400 patients with de novo lesions which could be treated with placement of a single stent. The primary endpoint of the trial will be restenosis (defined by $\geq 50\%$ narrowing) on the 6 month angiogram. Importantly, periprocedural complication rates including the incidence of vessel closure, myocardial infarction, death, emergent surgery, and major bleeding will be analyzed for the two groups.

A major lesson learned from our experience with stenting is that for any new intervention to significantly reduce restenosis, a major effort will need to be expended on interfering with the steps in the pathway which result in the intense proliferative response to intracoronary trauma caused by these devices. Efforts are currently underway to coat stents with antiproliferative compounds such as heparin which might achieve this goal. Other novel approaches include seeding of stents with genetically engineered endothelial cells which could secrete antithrombotic and antiproliferative molecules [22]. Clearly the devices being used today in clinical trials need to undergo further evaluation and development before elimination of restenosis as a major clinical problem is achieved.

Appendix

Johnson and Johnson Interventional Systems Intracoronary Stent Study Group.

Clinical Sites and Investigators

Scripps Clinic & Research Foundation – LaJolla, CA
  Richard A Schatz, M.D.
  Paul Teirstein, M.D.
Washington Hospital Center – Washington, D.C.
  Martin B. Leon, M.D.
Beth Israel Hospital – Boston, MA
  Donald S. Baim, M.D.

University of Michigan Medical Center – Ann Arbor, MI
    Stephen G. Ellis, M.D.
    Eric J. Topol, M.D.
Thomas Jefferson University Hospital – Philadelphia, PA
    Sheldon Goldberg, M.D.
    Michael P. Savage, M.D.
Yale University Medical School – New Haven, CT
    Michael W. Cleman, M.D.
    Henry S. Cabin, M.D.
Cardiovascular Institute of the South – Houma, LA
    Craig M. Walker, M.D.
    Jody Stagg, M.D.
University of California – San Diego, CA
    Maurice Buchbinder, M.D.
Hospital of the University of Pennsylvania – Philadelphia, PA
    John W. Hirshfeld, M.D.
Arizona Heart Institute – Phoenix, AZ
    Richard Heuser, M.D.
The University of Texas Health Science Center at San Antonio – San Antonio, TX
    Julio A. Perez, M.D.
    Steven Bailey, M.D.
Florida Hospital – Orlando, Fl
    R. Charles Curry, M.D.
    Hall B. Whitworth, M.D.

Core Angiographic Laboratory

Thomas Jefferson University Hospital
    David L. Fischman, M.D.
    Glenn Morales, R.C.P.T
    Michael Savage, M.D.
    Sheldon Goldberg, M.D.

References

1. Schwartz L, Bourassa M G, Lesperance J, Aldridge H E, Kazim F, Salvator V A, Henderson M, Bonan R, David P (1988) Aspirin and dipyrimadole in the prevention of restenosis after percutaneous transluminal coronary angioplasty. *N Engl J Med* 318:1714
2. Thorton M A, Gruentzig A R, Hollman J, King S B, Douglas J S (1984) Coumadin and aspirin in prevention of recurrence after transluminal coronary angioplasty: a randomized study. *Circulation* 69:721
3. Corcos T, David P R, Val P G, Renkin J, Dangoisse V, Rapold H G, Bourassa M G (1985) Failure of diltiazem to prevent restenosis after percutaneous transluminal coronary angioplasty. *Am Heart J* 109:926
4. Whiteworth H B, Roubin G S, Hollman J, Meier B, Leimgruber P P, Douglas J S Jr, King S B, Gruentzig A R (1986) Effect of nifedipine on recurrent stenosis after percutaneous transluminal coronary angioplasty. *J Am Coll Cardiol* 8:1271
5. Pepine C J, Hirshfeld J W, Macdonald R G, Henderson M A, Bass T A, Goldberg S, Savage M P, Vetrovec G, Cowley M, Taussig A S, Margolis J R, Hill J A, Bove A A,

Jugo R (1990) A controlled trial of corticosteroids to prevent restenosis after coronary angioplasty. *Circulation* 81:1

6. Ohman E M, Califf R M, Leek L, Fortin D F, Frid D J, Bengtson J R (1990) Restenosis after angioplasty: overview of clinical trials using aspirin and omega-3 fatty acids (abstr). *J Am Coll Cardiol* 15 (Suppl A):88A

7. Simpson J, Rowe M, Robertson G, Selmon M, Vetter J, Braden L, Hinohara T (1990) Directional coronary atherectomy: success and complication rates and outcome predictors (abstr). *J Am Coll Cardiol* 15:196A

8. Hinohara T, Rowe M, Sipperly M E, Johnson D, Robertson G, Selmon M, Leggett J, Simpson J (1990) Restenosis following directional coronary atherectomy of native coronary arteries (abstr). *J Am Coll Cardiol* 15:196A

9. Rogers P J, Garratt K N, Kaufman U P, Vlietstra R E, Bailey K R, Holmes D R (1990) Restenosis after atherectomy versus PTCA (abstr). *J Am Coll Cardio* 15:197A

10. Haase K K, Mauser M, Baumbach A, Voelker W, Karsch K R (1990) Restenosis after excimer laser coronary atherectomy (abstr). *Circulation* 82 (Suppl III): III–672

11. Sanborn T A, Bittl J A, Hershman R A, Siegal R M (1991) Percutaneous coronary excimer laser-assisted angioplasty: initial multicenter experience in 141 patients. *J Am Coll Cardiol* 17 (Suppl B):169B

12. Forrester J S, Fishbein M, Helfant R, Fagin J (1991) A paradigm for restenosis based on cell biology: clues for the development of new preventive therapies *J Am Coll Cardiol* 17:758

13. Schatz R A, Baim D S, Leon M, Ellis S G, Goldberg S, Hirshfeld J W, Cleman M W, Cabin H S, Walker C, Stagg J, Buchbinder M, Teirstein P S, Topol E J, Savage M, Perez J A, Curry R C, Whitworth H, Sousa J E, Tio F, Almagor Y, Ponder R, Penn I M, Leonard B, Levine S L, Fish R D, Palmaz J C (1991) Clinical experience with the Palmaz-Schatz coronary stent: initial results of a multicenter study. *Circulation* 83:148

14. Schatz R A, Palmaz J C, Tio F O, Garcia F, Garcia O, Reuter S R (1987) Balloon expandable intracoronary stents in the adult dog. *Circulation* 76:450

15. LeFree M T, Simon S B, Mancini G B J, Vogel R A (1986) Digital radiographic assessment of coronary arterial geometric diameter and videodensitometric cross-sectional area. *SPIE* 626:334

16. Mancini G B J, Simon S B, McGillem M J, LeFree M T, Friedman H Z, Vogel R A (1978) Automated quantitative coronary arteriography: morphologic and physiologic validation in vivo of a rapid digital angiographic method. *Circulation* 75:452

17. Serruys P W, Luijten H E, Beat K J, Geuskens G A, DeFeyter P J, VanDerBrand M, Reiber J H C, Katen H J, Es G A, Hugenholtz P G (1988) Incidence of restenosis after successful angioplasty: a time-related phenomenon. *Circulation* 77:361

18. Leimgruber P P, Roubin G S, Hollman J, Cotsonis G A, Meier B, Douglas J S, King S B, Gruentzig A R (1986) Restenosis after successful coronary angioplasty in patients with single vessel disease. *Circulation* 73:710

19. Holmes D R Jr, Vliestra R E, Smith H C, Vetrovec G W, Kent K M, Cowley M J, Faxon D P, Gruentzig A R, Kelsey S F, Detre K M, VanRaden M J, Mouk M B (1984) Restenosis after percutaneous transluminal coronary angioplasty: a report from the PTCA Registry of the National Heart, Lung, and Blood Institute. *Am J Cardiol* 53:77C

20. Hirshfeld J W, Schwartz J S, Jugo R, Macdonald R G, Goldberg S, Savage M P, ass T A, Vetrovec G, Cowley M, Taussig A S, Whitworth H B, Margolis J R, Hill J A, Pepine C (in press) Restenosis after coronary angioplasty: a multivariate statistical model to relate lesion and procedure variable to restenosis.

21. Savage M, Fischman D, Ellis S, Leon M, Cleman M, Teirstein P, Walker C, Hirshfeld, Schatz R, Goldberg S (1990) Does late progression of restenosis occur beyond 6 months following coronary artery stenting? (abstr). *Circulation* 82:III–540

22. Dichek D A, Neville R F, Zwiebel J A, Freeman S M, Leon M B, Anderson W F (1989) Seeding of Intravascular stents with genetically engineered endothelial cells. *Circulation* 80:1347

9. Restenosis after Gianturco-Roubin Stent Placement for Acute Closure

JAMES A. HEARN, SPENCER B. KING III, JOHN S. DOUGLAS and GARY S. ROUBIN

Introduction

Acute closure of a dilated coronary artery after PTCA results in an increase in morbidity and mortality in patients in whom it occurs [1–5]. Periprocedural occlusions occurred in 6.8% of patients in the 1985–1986 NHLBI Registry and was associated with a five-fold increase in the incidence of death (5% compared to 1%) and an increase in myocardial infarction incidence from a few percent in those without acute closure to 27% in those who closed and were reopened with repeat PTCA alone and to 56% in those requiring emergency coronary artery bypass grafting (CABG) [4]. In addition to suffering an increased early mortality, this acute closure group also tended to have further increases in mortality during the next 18 months of follow-up. It has been shown that one of the most potent predictors of acute closure after PTCA is the occurrence of an intimal tear or coronary artery dissection with an odds ratio of 5.2 [5–7]. Risk factors associated with increased mortality after acute closure include collateral vessels originating from the dilated artery, female gender, and multivessel disease [8]. When multiple repeat inflations, as well as prolonged inflations, fail to resolve an acute closure, patients have traditionally undergone emergency coronary bypass surgery. However, our own experience demonstrates that in-hospital death (1.2%) and new, non-fatal, Q-wave myocardial infarction (21.2%) are not eliminated in the group of patients having emergency CABG after a failed PTCA [9]. Strategies for acute closure have included prolonged inflations, bailout catheters, or perfusion catheters. While these are successful to varying degrees, our stented patients had failed one or more of these strategies before receiving a stent. The goals of stent placement are to avert the imminent ischemic complications of myocardial infarction and death. In so doing coronary artery stenting has created a new subgroup of patients whose long term outcome is unknown. Over the last four years we have stented patients with threatened or actual acute closure and have begun to accumulate the long term follow-up.

P.W. Serruys, B.H. Strauss and S.B. King III (eds), Restenosis after Intervention with New Mechanical Devices, 207–214.
© 1992 *Kluwer Academic Publishers. Printed in the Netherlands.*

Benefits of Coronary Artery Stenting

Coronary artery stents offer the hypothetical advantages of scaffolding intimal/medial flaps away from the center of the artery and maintaining radial support to offset elastic recoil and collapse of plaque material and flaps into the lumen of the artery. This provides greater volumetric blood flow which may serve to carry away coagulation factors which are activated or undergoing activation. It has long been held by our pathology colleagues that increased flow itself is anti-thrombotic in nature. Stents may also retard the tendency of freshly dilated arteries to passively, or actively, recoil following the procedure. This leaves a larger overall lumen than balloon angioplasty and may better *accomodate* the *obligatory* intimal hyperplasia following any arterial injury. A recently published pathology report lends support to the idea that the degree of injury (e.g., rupture through intima, media, and adventitia) has a significant influence on the amount of resultant neointimal formation [10]. With greater injury more intimal hyperplasia forms and there is a greater risk of restenosis. For example, in a reference (native) artery segment of 3,000 μm (3.0 mm) a residual lumen after PTCA might be 2,000 μm (2 mm), giving a 30% residual stenosis, which is not uncommon. If intimal hyperplasia grows to an additional thickness of 250 μm then restenosis, by definition, is present (1–((250 μm+250 μm+1,000 μm residual stenosis) $\div$ 3,000 μm) $\times$ 100% = 50%). Stents may provide a better initial lumen dimension (e.g., 15% or 450 μm narrowing) so that the same amount of intimal hyperplasia regrowth now fails to qualify as restenosis (1–(250 μm + 250 μm + 550 μm) $\div$ 3,000 μm) $\times$ 100% = 35%). If intimal hyperplasia is a process that is "transient" and followed by scarring, as suggested by recent post-PTCA autopsy data [10], then stents may allow the opportunity to wait through this process until the hyperplasia subsides.

Use of Other Stents for Acute Closure

It is important to consider that stenting for acute closure selects arteries that are maximally damaged and may have a greater potential for restenosis. Investigations using the Medinvent stent have served to point out the risk of subsequent thrombotic stent closure in the days to weeks following placement. Twenty-seven stents out of 117 (24%) were totally occluded at follow-up catheterization, including 21 occlusions that occurred within the first 14 days after implantation [11]. However, only 14 of 105 patients received a stent for acute closure after PTCA. A separate study [12] details the outcome of emergency stenting for acute closure, but most of these patients underwent semi-elective CABG because of early studies showing a potential for thrombus formation [11, 13]. This thrombotic complication was felt to be due to the metallic foreign body stimulus of the stent perhaps in the face of less than optimal anticoagulation. However, it is unclear how important the metal content or composition of the stent is in comparison with the unknown natural history of a closure-prone, acutely damaged artery. It is instructive to recall that the 1–year myocardial infarction rate in the new NHLBI Registry of single vessel disease patients was 1.9%, a rate that is infrequent but not rare [3]. These were patients undergoing a first PTCA in a non-infarct setting, a situation clearly different from the acutely closed, or closing, artery. The metal content (amount, type and configuration) may be important during the short term follow-up after placement. Also, mural/stent thrombus formation may also be important in the process of restenosis over the ensuing six months. Thrombus may potentiate the formation of intimal hyperplasia through provision of growth promoting biomolecules like platelet-derived growth factor, thrombin, fibrin and fibrinogen, and serotonin.

Use of The Gianturco-Roubin Stent for Acute Closure

We have recently described some of our initial results with the Gianturco-Roubin stent, a balloon-expandable, stainless steel stent in the treatment of acute and threatened acute closure after PTCA. This stent had been tested at the Andreas Gruentzig Cardiovascular Center of Emory University in dog coronary arteries and rabbit iliac arteries and was found to be well tolerated. Clinical evaluation began on September 3, 1987, when the Phase 1 study started in which patients proceeded to coronary artery bypass grafting routinely after stent placement [14, 15]. Following this favorable experience a second phase began in which emergency CABG was not mandated. Under this protocol, between September 20, 1988 and December 31, 1990, one hundred stents were placed into ninety-three patients for imminent or actual acute closure after PTCA. A portion of this data has been previously reported [16].

The entry criteria included coronary dissections combined with arteriographic or hemodynamic evidence of closure, imminent closure, or threatened closure following repeated balloon inflations which failed to improve the artery satisfactorily. It was intended that stents be placed in large arteries or vein grafts supplying critical areas of myocardium only if a good collateral system existed. If not, and it was judged that closure of the stented artery would pose a prohibitive risk, then early surgery was planned. This criterion would be obviated if the vascular distribution of the stented artery was small or moderate in size. Examples of such segments would be a right coronary or left circumflex artery in a co-dominant system, large branches of a dominant right coronary or left circumflex artery, large diagonal branches of the left anterior descending artery, and left anterior descending artery at or beyond its mid portion, or after the take-off of large branches supplying the septal and diagonal territories. Exclusions from stent placement were vessels that were diffusely diseased, the presence of triple vessel disease or multiple stenoses in a single vessel, moderate or severely impaired left ventricular function (ejection fraction <35%), an akinetic wall segment or Q waves in the distribution of the artery to be stented, a vessel diameter of <2.5 mm, distal segments beyond severe bends or branch points (precluding stent placement), the presence of a bleeding diathesis or other disorder (e.g., peptic ulceration or recent cerebrovascular accident) limiting the use of anti-platelet and anti-coagulant therapy, and the presence of an angiographically evident thrombus in the proposed stent site.

Stent Procedure

Stenting was considered once a standard PTCA procedure had been completed and all conventional efforts to maintain adequate vessel patency had failed. In addition to the standard pre-procedural 10,000 IU of intravenous heparin, 325 mg aspirin and 60 mg diltiazem, patients received 75 mg oral dipyridamole and intravenous dextran 40 at a rate of 100 ml/hour. Intracoronary nitroglycerin was also given prior to stenting. Stent sizes selected were slightly larger than the estimated diameter of the artery to be stented. Additional heparin was given as deemed necessary. Intracoronary urokinase was given if an intraluminal filling defect was seen. Repeat coronary angiography was performed prior to, and after, balloon PTCA and stent placement. Femoral artery sheaths were removed when the activated clotting time (ACT) declined to 1.5 times normal. After hemostasis was achieved patients were restarted on heparin (intravenous bolus of 2,000 to 5,000 IU and a constant infusion of 1,000 IU/hour). Partial thromboplastin times were monitored frequently with a target of 60 to 90 seconds. Aspirin, 80 mg p.o. Q.D., dipyridamole, 75 mg p.o. T.I.D., diltiazem 60 mg p.o. Q.I.D., and a trans-dermal nitroglycerin patch were continued. Daily coumadin was administered in order to raise the prothrombin time to 1.5 to 2 times control. Creatine kinase isoenzymes and electrocardiograms were obtained serially. Telemetry was continued and the patient was typically discharged on the fifth to seventh day post-stent. Patients underwent telephone follow-up and repeat coronary angiography of the stented segment 6 months after implantation.

Acute Results and Follow-up Angiographic Study

Placement of 109 stents was attempted after 104 PTCA procedures in 102 patients with actual, or imminent, acute closure. Five patients received 2 stents at a single procedure and two patients received 2 stents at two separate procedures. Stents could not be deployed in nine patients (91% successful deployment rate) for various reasons (e.g., unable to pass the stent through the guiding catheter or the stenosis) and were removed. This left 93 patients who received 100 stents during 95 procedures. Three stent deployments were

Table 1. Deaths in stented patients.

Number	Date	Circumstances
24	10/7/89	Severe COPD, esophagitis, nausea, vomiting, aspiration, asystolic cardiac arrest, unable to resuscitate, stent patent and thrombus-free at autopsy
37	9/20/89	Semi-urgent CABG, post-op peptic ulcer and perforation, abdominal surgery, COPD, ventilator dependence, expired two months later without evidence of ischemia
41	9/26/89	CABG for RCA with two stents because of evidence of severe hypotension with occlusion prior to the stents; post-op RVMI after protamine heparin reversal, leading to refractory shock
5	1/18/90	LMCA acute closure during diagnostic cath; prolonged CPR prior to PTCA; successful stent placement but paucity of distal reflow
91	11/10/90	Rapidly fatal stroke several days after stenting while on heparin; presummed intracranial hemorrhage

angiographically unsuccessful (% diameter stenosis remained ≥ 50), but are part of this analysis. Eighty-five procedures were carried out in native arteries and 10 procedures (11 stents) in saphenous vein grafts. The average age of these patients was 57 ± 11 years; 79% were males. Unstable angina was present in patients who underwent 75 of 95 procedures (79%) with 69 of the 95 (73%) being classified as class 3 and 4 angina. One patient with an acute MI received a stent following reclosure after primary balloon PTCA for his evolving infarction. Thirty-two of 93 patients had a remote myocardial infarction. Multi-vessel CAD was present in 43% of the patients. The average ejection fraction was $56 \pm 13\%$. Forty-two stented sites (44%) had previously been dilated. In addition to balloon angioplasty, the pre-stenting procedure included atherectomy in 2 patients, excimer laser in 6 patients, and laser balloon angioplasty in 7 patients. Prior to stenting, angina was recorded in 58 procedures with ST elevation in 57 and an average TIMI flow of 2.0 ± 1.2. The pre-angioplasty percent stenosis was $80 \pm 14\%$. The post-balloon percent stenosis was $59 \pm 27\%$, which increased to $67 \pm 25\%$ just before stent placement. After stent placement angina was relieved in 51/58 (88%), and ST elevation resolved in 46/57 (81%). The post-stent percent stenosis was $16 \pm 15\%$. The in-hospital complications, by procedure, included death in five (5.4%) (Table 1), urgent or emergent CABG in 18/95 (18.9%), Q-wave MI in 5/95 (5.2%), subacute closure in 7/95 (7.3%) and repeat PTCA in 5/95 (5.2%). More than one of these complications occurred in several patients. Sixty-seven patients (74%) had none of these complications. Other complications included femoral artery hematoma in 33%, pseudoaneurysm repair in 8%, and cerebral contusion after fall in one patient. With a median follow-up of 14 months the events included two deaths (one from acute respiratory failure and one following CABG), CABG in 11, Q-MI in 2, and repeat PTCA in 15.

Angiographic Follow-up

Angiographic follow-up post-discharge was obtained in 50 patients at the time symptoms developed or when they became eligible for 6 month cath (82% of those alive and without early CABG). Patients who had in-hospital urgent/emergent bypass with grafting beyond the stented segment were not analyzed for late stent patency due to the likely effect on the stented segment. In those patients with a follow-up angiogram restenosis ($\geq$50% diameter reduction) was present in 25 (50%). Restenosis rates were higher in the left circumflex artery (79% vs 42% in LAD and 39% in RCA), in SVBGs (100% vs 44%), and in patients with prior CABG (77% vs 40%) and tended to be higher in those with diabetes mellitus (79% vs 44%). The difference in restenosis rates between the left circumflex artery and the others was thought not due to differences in size, since the average native artery diameters were not different. There were more diabetic patients in the left circumflex artery group and perhaps this accounts for their excess restenosis.

Effort at Controlling Restenosis Post Stent Placement

In addition to the antiplatelet and anti-thrombotic regimens previously described, an attempt at controlling restenosis with anti-inflammatory and anti-mitotic agents was also tried in a subset of these stented patients. Hydrocortisone followed by tapering doses of prednisone over 2 weeks was combined with colchicine for six months in some of the patients. Among this group, 15 have undergone late restudy to evaluate symptoms or to perform the 6 month restudy. Although the overall restenosis rate was not reduced by this strategy, a curious phenomenon of aneurysm formation was seen in the dilated and stented segments. We have not seen this in stented patients without such therapy and feel that in the setting of a dissected and subsequently stented artery, the addition of such drugs may impede the normal healing process thereby allowing formation of aneurysms.

   Although this is not a desired outcome, it demonstrated an effect of an intervention in altering a proliferative response in patients. This knowledge will influence our thinking about antiproliferative strategies in the future. The goal will be to control the healing process but not to eliminate it. Notably, 3 of the 6 artery segments with aneurysms also exhibited areas of restenosis.

Repeat Angioplasty in Restenotic Stented Arteries

Fifteen patients who developed restenosis within the stent have undergone a repeat PTCA procedure. All were successfully redilated without major complications. There was one non-obstructive coronary dissection and one small intimal tear. These procedures were notable for the fact that following balloon angioplasty, the lumen diameter stenosis was similar to that seen in the post stenting group (15.7% residual stenosis vs. 16%). In other words, there was no elastic recoil suggesting that the stent, which is now buried within the wall of the artery, produces a rigid media which does not allow for elastic recoil or spasm. Although the acute results of redilating stent restenosis are excellent, the long-term results are unknown. Five patients have been restudied at an average of 3.2 months after repeat PTCA of the stented segment and one remains open without restenosis.

Conclusion

Acute dissection and threatened closure of the artery at the time of angioplasty remain significant problems. When other therapies fail to solve the problem, intracoronary prostheses have the ability to open most of the vessels. The threat of post-stent thrombosis remains the major limitation of the procedure and mandates a vigorous anticoagulation program. This in itself produces certain hemorrhagic complications and prolongs hospitalization significantly. Development of non-thrombogenic and perhaps antithrombotic stents is sorely needed. If such stents can be developed and proved effective locally without the necessity for systemic anticoagulation, then the use of stents for suboptimal PTCA results could be greatly expanded. Until that day, however, the enthusiasm for stenting such patients must be moderated by the rather cumbersome post-stent management and potential thrombotic and hemorrhagic complications. Restenosis in arteries with such significant damage will probably differ markedly from restenosis seen with elective stent placement.

References

1. Detre K, Holubkov R, Kelsey S, et al (1988) Percutaneous transluminal coronary angioplasty in 1985–1986 and 1977–1981. The National Heart, Lung, and Blood Institute Registry. *N Engl J Med* 318:265–270.
2. Holmes D R, Holubkov R, Vlietstra R E, et al (1988) Comparison of complications during percutaneous transluminal coronary angioplasty from 1977 to 1981 and from 1985 to 1986: The National Heart, Lung, and Blood Institute Percutaneous Transluminal Angioplasty Registry. *J Am Coll Cardiol* 12:1149–1155.
3. Detre K, Holubkov R, Kelsey S, et al (1989) One-year follow-up results of the 1985–1986 National Heart, Lung, and Blood Institute's Percutaneous Transluminal Coronary Angioplasty Registry. *Circulation* 80:421–428.
4. Detre K M, Holmes D R, Holubkov R, et al (1990) Incidence and consequences of periprocedural occlusion. The 1985–1986 National Heart, Lung, and Blood Institute Percutaneous Transluminal Coronary Angioplasty Registry. *Circulation* 82:739–750.
5. Bredlau C E, Roubin G S, Leimgruber P P, Douglas Jr J S, King III S B, Gruentzig A R

(1985) In-hospital morbidity and mortality in patients undergoing elective coronary angioplasty. *Circulation* 72:1044–1052.

6. Black A J R, Namay D L, Niederman A L, Lembo N J, Roubin G S, Douglas Jr J S, King III S B (1989) Tear or dissection after coronary angioplasty. Morphologic correlates of an ischemic complication. *Circulation* 791035–1042.

7. Ellis S G, Roubin G S, King III S B, Douglas Jr J S, Weintraub W S, Thomas R G, Cox W R (1988) Angiographic and clinical predictors of acute closure after native vessel coronary angioplasty. *Circulation* 77:372.

8. Ellis S G, Roubin G S, King III S B, Douglas Jr. J S, Shaw R E, Stertzer S H, Myler R K (1988) In-hospital cardiac mortality after acute closure after coronary angioplasty: analysis of risk factors from 8,207 procedures. *J Am Coll Cardiol* 11:211–6.

9. Talley J D, Weintraub W S, Roubin G S, Douglas Jr J S, Anderson H V, Jones E L, Morris D C, Liberman H A, Craver J M, Guyton R A, King III S B (1990) Failed elective percutaneous transluminal coronary angioplasty requiring coronary artery bypass surgery – in-hospital and late clinical outcome at 5 years. *Circulation* 82:1203–1213.

10. Nobuyoshi M, Kimura J, Ohishi H, Horiuchi H, Nosaka H, Hamasaki N, Yokoi H, Kim K (1991) Restenosis after percutaneous transluminal coronary angioplasty: pathologic observations in 20 patients. *J Am Coll Cardiol* 17:433–439.

11. Serruys P W, Strauss B H, Beatt K J, Bertrand M E, Puel J, Rickards A F, Meier B, Goy J-J, Vogt P, Kappenberger L, Sigwart U (1991) Angiographic follow-up after placement of a self-expanding coronary artery stent. *N Engl J Med* 324:13–17.

12. de Feyter P J, de Scheerder I, van den Brand M, Laarman G, Suryapranata H, Serruys P W (1990) Emergency stenting for refractory acute coronary artery occlusion during coronary angioplasty. *Am J Cardiol* 66:1147–1150.

13. Sigwart U, Urban P, Golf S, Kaufmann U, Imbert C, Fischer A, Kappenberger L (1988) Emergency stenting for acute occlusion after coronary balloon angioplasty. *Circulation* 78:1121–1127.

14. Roubin G S, Douglas Jr. J S, Lembo N J, Black A J, King III S B (1988) Intracoronary stenting for acute closure following percutaneous transluminal coronary angioplasty (PTCA). *Circulation* 78(suppl II):II–407.

15. Roubin G S, King III S B, Douglas Jr. J S, Lembo N J, Robinson K A (1990) Intracoronary stenting during percutaneous transluminal coronary angioplasty. *Circulation* 81(suppl IV):IV–92–IV–100.

16. Roubin G S, Hearn J A, Carlin S F, Lembo N J, Douglas Jr J S, King III S B (1990) Angiographic and clinical follow-up in patients receiving a balloon expandable, stainless steel, stent (Cook, Inc.) for prevention or treatment of acute closure after PTCA. *Circulation* 82(suppl III):III–191

17. Rab S T, King S B III, Roubin G S, Carlin S, Hern J A, Douglas J S Jr. (1991) Coronary aneurisms after stent placement: a suggestion of altered vessel wall healing in the presence of anti-inflammatory agents. *J Am Coll Cardiol* 18:1524–1528.

10.   Immediate and Long-term Morphologic
      Changes in Stenosis Geometry after Wiktor™
      Stent Implantation in Native Coronary Arteries
      for Recurrent Stenosis Following Balloon
      Angioplasty. Report on the First Fifty
      Consecutive Patients

PETER DE JAEGERE, PATRICK W. SERRUYS, WILLEM
VAN DER GIESSEN and PIM DE FEYTER

On behalf of the Wiktor Study Group: Michel Bertrand, Volker
Wiegand, Gisbert Kober, Jean-François Marquis, Bernard Valeix,
Rainer Uebis, Jan Piessens

Introduction

Percutaneous Transluminal Coronary Angioplasty (PTCA) has established
its role as a nonsurgical revascularization procedure in selected patients with
obstructive coronary artery disease. In most western countries, the number
of PTCA's equals or even exceeds the number of coronary artery bypass
operations [1]. Although most stenoses can now be traversed and dilated by
balloon angioplasty with a high initial success rate and a low complication
rate, the unpredictable problems of abrupt closure and late restenosis continue to compromise the overall results. Restenosis is a time-related phenomenon with an occurrence of 20–40% [2–5]. Recurrence of stenosis following
balloon angioplasty may increase the risk of future restenosis [6, 7]. Despite
improvements in catheter technology and gained operator experience, the
problem of restenosis has not yet been solved. Intracoronary stents are
one of the new technologies that (along with pharmacological interventions,
atherectomy and laser techniques) have entered clinical testing with the goal
of providing a practical and predictable solution to this problem. Different
prostheses have been developed, tested in animal experiments and implanted
in humans [8–12]. Although the exact pathophysiological mechanism(s) responsible for restenosis are largely unknown, stent implantation may lead to
a reduced restenosis rate. There is a large body of evidence indicating that
suboptimal angiographic result after balloon angioplasty contributes to restenosis. The stent optimizes the dilatation process by preventing recoil and
containing the irregular surface of the atherosclerotic plaque created by the
disruptive action of the ballon, resulting in a larger cross-sectional area and
a smoother vessel surface [8]. Thereby, the hemodynamic disturbances are
minimized and flow across the dilated segment is normalized [13, 14]. As a
result, the response of the vessel to balloon-induced trauma is mitigated and
presumably the healing process modified.

P.W. Serruys, B.H. Strauss and S.B. King III (eds), Restenosis after Intervention with New Mechanical
Devices, 215–234.
© 1992 *Kluwer Academic Publishers. Printed in the Netherlands.*

The stent used in this study is the Medtronic Wiktor stent which, in contrast to the Wallstent (Schneider, Zürich, Switzerland) and Palmaz-Schatz stent (Johnson & Johnson, Warren, USA), is not a mesh made of stainless steel, but a radiopaque single loose interdigitating tantalum wire. As a result of this loose configuration, it has been hypothesized that the Wiktor[TM] stent design conforms more adequately to the natural bending of the coronary artery in contrast to the stents with a more rigid and stiff mesh architecture such as the Palmaz-Schatz stent. The Wiktor[TM] stent, like the Palmaz-Schatz stent, is a balloon expandable endoluminal prosthesis and does not exert an active radial force on the vascular wall after deployment as occurs with the Wallstent [12]. However, the loose configuration of the Wiktor[TM] stent may have less scaffolding properties compared to the other two intravascular prostheses.

In this study the immediate and the long-term changes in stenosis geometry after Wiktor[TM] stent implantation in the first fifty consecutive patients were evaluated by quantitative coronary angiography using automated edge detection. The hemodynamic changes were assessed by the calculation of the theoretical pressure drop across the dilated and stented stenosis and by calculation of the Poiseuille and turbulent resistances assuming a coronary blood flow of either 0.5, 1 or 3 ml/s.

Methods

Patients. Between January 1990 and October 1990, a single Wiktor[TM] stent implantation was attempted in 50 patients (44 male, age [mean ±SD] 55 ± 9 years). The patients were treated in the following centers: the Catheterization Laboratory, Thoraxcenter, Rotterdam, The Netherlands; Department of Cardiology, Hôpital Cardiologique, Lille, France; Department of Cardiology, Georg August Universität Göttingen, Germany; Department of Cardiology, Klinikum der J. W. Goethe Universität Frankfurt, Germany; Department of Cardiology University of Ottawa Heart Institute, Canada; Departement of Cardiology, Clinique la Casamance, Marseille, France; Department of Cardiology Medical Clinic I RWTH Aachen, Germany; Department of Cardiology, University Hospital Gasthuisberg, Leuven, Belgium. All patients gave informed consent. The study protocol was approved by the ethics committee of the individual hospitals. Stent implantation was attempted because of recurrence of stenosis in a native coronary artery lesion following balloon angioplasty: a first restenosis in 33 patients, a second restenosis in 13 patients and a third restenosis in 4 patients. In all patients objective evidence of ischemia was documented. The implantation success rate was 98% (49/50 patients): In one patient, a tortuous proximal segment of the right coronary artery prevented stent delivery at the target site.

The dilated and stented coronary artery of the remaining 49 patients was the left anterior descending artery in 26 patients (53%), the circumflex artery

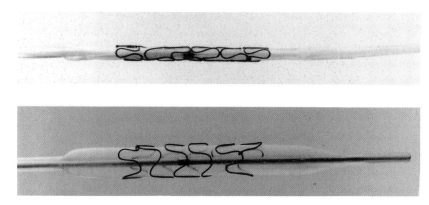

Figure 1. Wiktor stent mounted on a conventional balloon catheter when de- and inflated.

in 7 patients (14%) and the right coronary artery in 16 patients (33%). The nominal size of the balloon on which the stent was mounted was 3.0 mm in 23 patients (47%), 3.5 mm in 19 patients (39%) and 4.0 mm in 7 patients (14%). The nominal diameter of the balloon for the total study group (mean ±SD) was 3.34 ± 0.36 mm.

In hospital angiographically documented (sub)acute stent occlusion occurred in 5 patients (10%): day 0 = 1 patient, day 1 = 1 patient, day 4 = 1 patient and on day 5 in 2 patients. Successful recanalisation was achieved in 4 patients (rePTCA in 3 patients and rePTCA in combination with thrombolysis in another patient). All 4 patients had follow-up angiography at 5 to 6 months. The remaining patient sustained a thrombotic occlusion of the stent the fifth day after implantation and underwent emergency bypass surgery. No attempt was made to use thrombolytic therapy or to redilate the occlusion.

Angiographic follow-up was completed in 47 of 49 patients (94%) at a mean (±SD) period of 5.3 ± 1.5 months. Control angiography could not be performed in the patient referred for bypass surgery because of subacute thrombotic occlusion and in a patient who died 3 months post stenting following prostate surgery (not stent-related death).

Description of the Stent. The endoprosthesis used in this study is a balloon-expandable stent (Wiktor^{TM}, Medtronic Inc., Minneapolis, USA) constructed of a single loose interdigitating radiopaque tantalum wire (0.125 mm in diameter) which is formed into a sinusoidal wave and wrapped into a helical coil structure. This prosthesis is crimped onto the deflated polyethylene balloon of a standard angioplasty catheter (Fig. 1). The features of this prosthesis design are such that by inflating the balloon the diameter of the stent increases without any alteration in length (14–16 mm, Fig. 1).

The crimped stent profile is approximately 1.5 mm. The maximal diameter of the balloon during inflation determines the ultimate size of the prosthesis on implantation. One inflation at 6–8 atmospheres is sufficient to deploy the stent. The surface of the vascular endothelium covered by a fully expanded stent amounts to 6.7, 7.7 and 8.4% for a 4.0, 3.5 and 3.0 mm stent, with an open space of 93.3, 92.3 and 91.6%, respectively. After implantation, the tantalum wire undergoes oxidation, resulting in a stable and corrosion resistant oxide (TaO_5). Potentially, the smaller amount of endothelial surface covered by the stent in conjunction with the electrochemical characteristics of this stent should protect against thrombus formation.

Stent Implantation. One day prior to stent implantation acetylsalicylic acid 300 mg/day was started. Dextran (100cc/hour) was administered 2 hours before the implant and continued throughout the procedure. A minimum of 500 cc was infused. A total of 20,000 units of heparin was injected intravenously. Full heparinization was maintained until therapeutic levels of coumadin therapy were achieved. Conventional balloon angioplasty was performed until the desired angiographic result was obtained. After control coronary angiography for subsequent quantitative analysis, the balloon/stent system was advanced towards the target lesion over a 0.014 inch steerable guidewire under fluoroscopic control. The balloon was then inflated until full expansion of the stent was achieved. Subsequently the balloon was deflated and the catheter was removed under negative pressure while leaving the stent in place. In case of incomplete expansion of the stent, a repeat balloon dilatation within the stent was performed. The post-procedure drug therapy consisted of coumadin for a minimum of 3 months and acetylsalicylic acid (300 mg/day) for six months.

Quantitative Coronary Angiography. The coronary cineangiograms were analyzed at the core laboratory in Rotterdam by means of a computer-assisted Cardiovascular Angiography Analysis System (CAAS), described in detail elsewhere [15, 16]. Briefly, this system allows an objective and reproducible quantification of a coronary artery stenosis. A 35 mm cineframe was selected and digitized with a CCD-camera at very high resolution (1330×1770 pixels) and electronically a region of interest (512×512 pixels) encompassing the arterial segment to be analyzed was selected for subsequent analysis by the computer.

Contours of the arterial segment were detected automatically on the basis of the first and second derivative functions of the brightness profile, and corrected for pincushion distortion from the image intensifiers. A calibration factor was derived from a computer processed segment of the angio-catheter.

From the arterial contour data, a diameter function was computed. The minimal luminal diameter and a reference diameter, computer-estimated by the interpolated diameter technique, were expressed in millimeters. On the basis of the proximal and distal centerline segments and the computed reference diameter function, the reference contours over the obstructed region were reconstructed. The extent of the obstruction was determined from the diameter function on the basis of curvature analysis and expressed in millimeters. The curvature is computed as the average value of all the individual curvature values along the centerline of the coronary segment, with the curvature defined as the first derivative of the tangent as it moves along the centerline which for a circle is equal to the reciprocal of the radius. The difference in area between the reference and the detected contours over the lesions ("plaque area", in mm^2) is a measure for the atherosclerotic plaque [17]. The inflow angle is the average slope of the diameter function between the position of the minimal obstruction diameter and the position of the proximal boundary of the stenotic lesion. The outflow angle is the average slope of the diameter function of the minimal obstruction diameter and the position of the distal boundary of the stenotic segment.

The severity of the stenosis can also be expressed as a percentage area stenosis, assuming a circular cross-section at the obstruction and reference position, corresponding luminal areas (mm^2) were calculated by comparing the minimal area value at the obstruction with the reference value obtained following the interpolated diameter technique. An illustration of such a quantitative analysis of a coronary artery is shown in Fig. 2. Elastic recoil was calculated as the difference between the mean diameter of the balloon when fully inflated and the mean diameter of the stented segment filmed in the same angiographic view immediately after stent delivery and withdrawal of the balloon.

Hemodynamic Assessment. To assess the physiological significance of the obstruction and its changes after angioplasty and stenting, the theoretical pressure drop was calculated using the arteriogram and digital computation, according to the formulae described in the literature: Pgrad = Q. (Rp + Rt) where Pgrad is the theoretic transtenotic pressure decrease (mmHg) over the stenosis, Q the mean coronary blood flow (ml/s), Rp the Poiseuille resistance and Rt the turbulent resistance [18, 19].

These resistances have been defined as follows:

Rp = C1 · (length obstruction)/(minimal cross-sectional area)^2
where C1 = 8 · π · (blood viscosity) with blood viscosity = 0.03 g/cm · s.
Rt = C2 · (1/minimal cross-sectional area − 1/normal distal area)^2
where C2 = (blood density)/0.266 with blood density = 1.0 g/cm^3.

The theoretic transtenotic pressure drop was calculated for theoretic coronary blood flow of 0.5, 1 and 3 ml/s. The Poiseuille and turbulent contributions to the flow resistance were determined from stenosis geometry assessed by quantitative coronary angiography.

Restenosis. Two different sets of criteria were applied to determine the rate of restenosis. A reduction of 0.72 mm or more in the minimal luminal diameter has been found to be a reliable indicator of angiographic progression of vessel narrowing [2, 16, 20]. This value takes into account the limitations of coronary angiographic measurements and represents twice the long-term

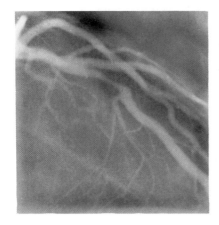
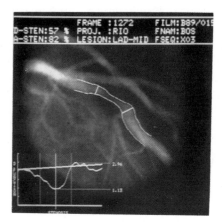

Pre
PTCA

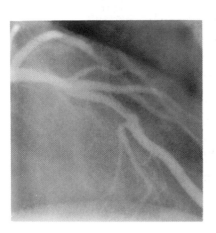
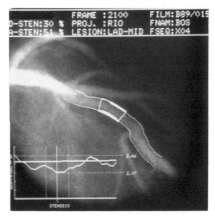

Post
PTCA

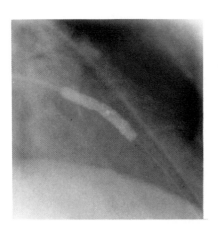
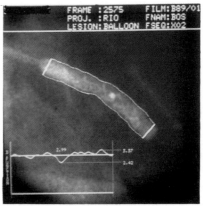

Balloon full
inflated wit
stent

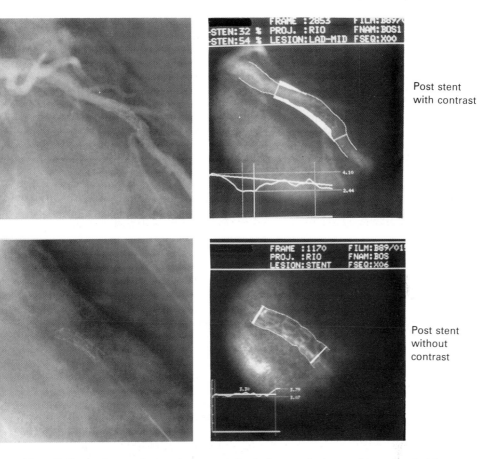

Post stent
with contrast

Post stent
without
contrast

Figure 2. Single plane angiograms before and after balloon angioplasty and immediately following stent implantation with superimposition of the contours computed by the CAAS system. Below each angiogram is shown the diameter function of the detected contours of the artery. The minimal luminal diameter (vertical line) and the interpolated diameter function (horizontal line) from which the reference diameter is derived are shown. For further explanation, see text.

variability of repeat measurements of a coronary artery obstruction with the Cardiovascular Angiographic Analysis System. The other criterion for restenosis is an increase in the percentage of stenosis from less than 50 percent after stent implantation to 50 percent or more at follow-up evaluation. This criterion was selected since common clinical practice has continued to express lesion severity as a percentage of stenosis.

Statistical Analysis. Values obtained by quantitative angiographic analysis are expressed as means $\pm$ SD. The means for each angiographic variable before PTCA, after PTCA, immediately after stent implantation and at follow-up were compared by analysis of variance. If significant differences were found, two-tailed t-tests were applied to paired data. A statistical probability of less than 0.05 was considered to indicate significance.

Results

1. Immediate Changes in Stenosis Geometry

The morphologic changes in stenosis geometry observed immediately after stent implantation and the associated hemodynamic changes (mean ±SD) are presented in Tables 1, 2 and 3. Stent implantation after balloon angioplasty resulted in an additional increase in minimal luminal cross-sectional area and minimal luminal diameter with a concommitant decrease in percentage area and percentage diameter stenosis compared with the postangioplasty state. (Table 1) Moreover, there was a significant decrease in plaque area, in- and outflow angle while the curvature of the lesion was respected. (Table 2) This morphologic improvement was associated with a drastic decrease in both the calculated turbulent and Poiseuille resistance, resulting in the virtual disappearance of the theoretical transtenotic pressure drop for a theoretical flow of 0.5, 1 and 3 ml/s. (Table 3)

In most patients the measured diameter of the fully inflated balloon was higher than the measured diameter of the stent (Fig. 3). During maximum inflation the mean diameter of the balloon for the total study group was 3.02 ± 0.38 mm, the mean diameter of the stented segment immediately following implantation was 2.92 ± 0.37 mm (Table 4). This implies a recoil of 0.11 ± 0.30 mm ($p < 0.05$)

2. Long-term Changes in Stenosis Geometry

The immediate and long-term changes in stenosis geometry following stent implantation are shown in Tables 1–3. Figure 4 displays the cumulative distribution of the minimal luminal diameter and its changes immediately after balloon angioplasty and stent implantation and at follow-up. The additional improvement in the minimal luminal diameter immediately after stent implantation is lost at follow-up. The incidence of restenosis depended on the definition used. When a change of ≥ 0.72 mm in minimal luminal diameter was used as a criterion, restenosis was observed within the stent in 22 patients (46%, Fig. 5), and in the distal segment adjacent to the stent in another patient (2%). Therefore, the total restenosis rate was 48 percent. At follow-up the percentage of stenosis had increased to ≥ 50 percent within the stent in 13 patients (27%, Figure 5), in the segment distal to the stent in 1 patient (2%), resulting in a total rate of 29 percent.

Table 1. Immediate and long-term morphologic changes following Wiktor stent implantation.

	Pre-PTCA	Post-PTCA	Post-Stent	Follow-up	P_1	P_2	P_3	P_4
Extent obstruction (mm)	7.18 ± 2.46	6.75 ± 2.59	5.31 ± 1.84	7.15 ± 2.77	NS	0.0004	0.0003	NS
Reference diameter (mm)	2.81 ± 0.48	2.80 ± 0.48	2.98 ± 0.42	2.90 ± 0.55	NS	NS	0.03	0.03
MLD (mm)	1.09 ± 0.26	1.80 ± 0.32	2.45 ± 0.35	1.71 ± 0.68	0.0001	0.001	0.0001	NS
Diameter stenosis (%)	60.57 ± 9.26	34.15 ± 10.58	17.53 ± 6.97	40.17 ± 21.65	0.0001	0.001	0.0001	NS
Reference area (mm2)	6.38 ± 2.17	6.26 ± 2.21	7.15 ± 2.04	6.86 ± 2.63	NS	0.0001	NS	0.02
MLCA (mm^2)	1.00 ± 0.44	2.65 ± 0.91	4.83 ± 1.40	2.61 ± 1.72	0.0001	0.0001	0.0001	NS
Area stenosis (%)	83.47 ± 7.66	55.52 ± 13.71	31.38 ± 11.30	60.92 ± 23.11	0.0001	0.0001	0.0001	NS

MLCA: minimal luminal cross-sectional area, MLD: minimal luminal diameter. All parameters are expressed in mean ± SD.

Table 2. Immediate and long-term morphologic changes following Wiktor stent implantation.

	Pre-PTCA	Post-PTCA	Post-Stent	Follow-up	P_1	P_2	P_3
Curvature	23.22 ± 11.87	22.33 ± 9.71	21.39 ± 10.67	24.59 ± 20.71	NS	NS	NS
Plaque area (mm)	8.57 ± 4.37	5.20 ± 3.47	3.31 ± 2.32	5.97 ± 4.13	0.0001	0.0002	0.0001
Inflow angle	23.13 ± 6.27	14.68 ± 5.16	6.17 ± 14.54	10.66 ± 7.98	0.0001	0.001	NS
Outflowangle	22.05 ± 9.85	15.83 ± 13.91	4.46 ± 14.05	7.41 ± 7.44	0.02	0.0001	NS

All parameters are expressed in mean ± SD.

Table 3. Immediate and long-term hemodynamic changes following Wiktor stent implantation.

	Pre-PTCA	Post-PTCA	Post-Stent	Follow-up	P_1	P_2	P_3
Rpois	18.66 ± 39.26	1.24 ± 1.73	0.46 ± 0.25	5.60 ± 12.59	0.003	0.002	0.008
Rturb	11.37 ± 29.47	0.31 ± 0.72	0.02 ± 0.02	1.86 ± 5.26	0.01	0.006	0.02
Pgrad (0.5 ml/s)	30.03 ± 68.36	1.52 ± 2.44	0.48 ± 0.27	7.83 ± 17.93	0.005	0.004	0.008
Pgrad (1 ml/s)	48.68 ± 66.90	3.67 ± 6.30	0.98 ± 0.56	19.41 ± 46.30	0.0001	0.004	0.01
Pgrad (3 ml/s)	92.13 ± 129.07	6.45 ± 11.61	1.49 ± 0.92	34.70 ± 85.17	0.0001	0.004	0.01

Rpois: Poiseuille resistance, Rturb: turbulent resistance, Pgrad: pressure drop. All parameters are expressed in mean ±SD.

Table 4. Nominal diameter of the balloon, measured diameter of balloon at maximal inflation pressure and of stented segment by edge detection.

Nominal diameter balloon	Measured diameter balloon	Measured diameter stented segment	P1	P2
3.34 ± 0.36 mm	3.02 ± 0.38 mm	2.92 ± 0.37 mm	0.0001	0.01

All parameters are expressed in mean ±SD.

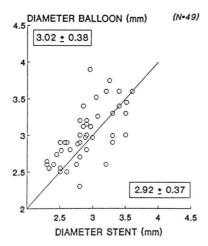

Figure 3. Recoil assessed by comparing the mean diameter of the fully expanded balloon on which the stent is mounted and the mean diameter of the stented segment immediately following stent delivery.

Discussion

1. *Quantitative Method Used*

Coronary artery stenting has been introduced as an adjunct to PTCA in obstructive coronary artery disease [8–10, 21–23]. The implantation of vascular endoprostheses may provide a useful approach to prevent occlusion and restenosis [21]. As for every therapeutic procedure, an objective and reproducible technique evaluating efficacy is needed. Computer based automated edge detection angiographic analysis systems have reduced the variability

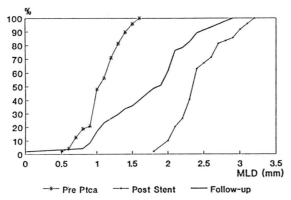

Figure 4. Cumulative distribution of the minimal luminal diameter before and immediately after stent implantation and at follow-up.

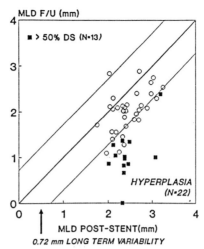

Figure 5. Change in the minimal luminal diameter between stent implantation and angiographic follow-up. The diameter of each segment immediately following stent implantation is plotted against the diameter at follow-up. The lines on each side of the diagonal (line of identity) represent the limits of long-term variability of repeat measurements (≥0.72 mm or twice the standard deviation of a duplicate measurement).

resulting from visual and caliper-determined contour detection of coronary cineangiograms [24–26].

The optimal method to quantitatively analyze the immediate angiographic results of coronary stenting in native coronary arteries is still a matter of debate. At present, two techniques are available; automated edge detection and videodensitometry. The technique of automated edge detection is limited in eccentric lesions and in particular following balloon angioplasty when acute tears and dissections distort the anatomy. Videodensitometric measurements of cross-sectional areas are independent of geometric assumptions regarding the shape of the stenosis and should in theory be more reliable than edge detection, especially after the disruptive action of balloon angioplasty which is known to cause asymmetric enlargement of the lumen [27, 28]. However, a recent study has shown that edge detection and videodensitometry are equally acceptable methods of analysis after coronary stenting with the non radiopaque Wallstent [29]. This may be explained by the more regular and smooth vessel contours after stenting, with tacking back of the intimal flaps by the scaffolding property of the stent in some cases and by the remodelling of the stented segment into a more circular geometry. However, it has been shown that videodensitometry overestimates the minimal luminal cross-sectional area after Wiktor[TM] stent implantation, particularly in smaller vessels [30]. This is presumably due to the radiographic characteristics of the stent itself. X-ray energy dispersion spectrometry studies from our laboratory has shown that the Wiktor[TM] stent is made of only one element, tantalum, which has a higher atomic number than the elements contained in the Palmaz-Schatz stent and Wallstent. Consequently more X-ray energy is absorbed by the Wiktor^TM stent wire. Furthermore, the Wiktor^TM stent has a greater wire cross-sectional area than the other two stents. The cross-sectional wire area of a stent is dependent on the number and thickness of the wire(s) at any particular point along the stent. Due to the asymmetric and helical design and the orientation of the loops of the Wiktor stent, the cross-sectional area of this stent is not uniform at any segment over its length. It is estimated that at any one segment, a cross-section contains 4 to 8 cut wires with a average of 6 wires. This corresponds to a cross-sectional area of the stent ranging from 0.0005 to 0.001 cm^2 with an average value of 0.00075 cm^2. The total cross-sectional area of the Wall-stent and Palmaz-Schatz stent, which are easier to calculate due to the more uniform stent design, are 0.00062 cm^2 and 0.00039 cm^2 respectively. These physical characteristics result in a higher radiopacity of the Wiktor stent in comparison with the stainless steel stents. As a result, the intraluminal bright-ness profile generated by the Wiktor^TM stent makes automated edge detec-tion the more appropriate technique for quantification of the stented seg-ment. Conversely, when edge detection is not able to distinguish between the radiopaque stent embedded in the vessel wall and the actual luminal boundaries in case of restenosis (e.g. due to incomplete contrast mixing resulting in poor film quality), videodensitometry may be the technique of choice to assess restenosis.

2. Immediate Angiographic Results

The initial increase in minimal luminal diameter after predilatation with the balloon in this study (1.09 ± 0.26 mm to 1.80 ± 0.32 mm), is what has been observed after conventional balloon angioplasty in other series [2, 31, 32]. The additional improvement after implantation of the Wiktor^TM stent is comparable to what has been observed with either self expanding or balloon expandable stents [8, 14, 33]. The same holds for the minimal luminal cross-sectional area. There is a five fold increase in the minimal luminal cross-sectional area after stenting (1.00 ± 0.44 mm^2 to 4.83 ± 1.40 mm^2). As pre-viously demonstrated, a normalization of the coronary flow reserve may be expected with such an increase in the minimal luminal cross-sectional area [30]. As indirect confirmation of the above findings, the theoretical pressure drop across the stenosis remains virtually zero even with a theoretical flow of 3 ml/s and a normalization of the calculated resistances. In addition to the increase in the minimal luminal cross-sectional area, there is a significant change in plaque area, in the in- and outflow angles and in the extent of obstruction, while the natural curvature of the artery is respected.

However, the smaller mean diameter of the stented segment (2.92 ± 0.37 mm) in comparison with the measured diameter of the fully expanded balloon (3.02 ± 0.38 mm) suggests some recoil of the stented segment. This minimal recoil appears to be a true phenomenon since the accuracy and the precision of the CAAS system is -30 u and 90 u respectively [13, 15, 16]. Furthermore, the recoil phenomenon has also been observed, even to a larger extent, after Wiktor[TM] stent implantation in Yorkshire pigs [12]. The more pronounced recoil (10%) observed in the animal model compared to recoil (3%) observed in this study may be explained by the fact that in the former animal study the stent was implanted in normal coronary arteries. All these angiographic data indicate that in contrast to balloon angioplasty, where recoil amounting to 50% has been documented [35], the Wiktor[TM] stent appropriately scaffolds the vessel. The measured diameter of the inflated balloon at an average inflation pressure of 6–8 atmospheres (3.02 ± 0.38 mm) did not achieve the nominal size of the balloon (3.34 ± 0.36 mm) as specified by the manufacturer. The inflation pressure needed to obtain the nominal size of the balloon has been tested in air. It is conceivable that a higher inflation pressure is needed to overcome the opposing forces exerted by the arterial wall and possibly by the stent itself to achieve full expansion of the balloon.

3. Long-term Angiographic Results/restenosis

A. Criteria for Restenosis Used

Essentially, angiographic definitions of restenosis either are based on an increase in narrowing with respect to the immediate post-angioplasty angiographic appearance or are defined as a loss of the gain achieved by the successful angioplasty. Definitions based on percent diameter stenosis may fail to identify lesions undergoing significant deterioration. These criteria are chosen to reflect the change in minimal luminal diameter in relation to the so-called normal diameter of the vessel in the immediate vicinity of the obstruction. It also assumes that this normal diameter (or reference diameter) does not change either as a result of the angioplasty or during the immediate follow-up period when restenosis of the dilated lesion is a well recognized phenomenon. Quantitative angiographic studies have shown this premise to be false [5, 20]. This observation has led to the concept of the decrease in the minimal luminal diameter as a parameter for restenosis [2, 16, 20, 36].

To define restenosis a cutoff point dividing the restenosis group from the nonrestenosis group can be selected. In such a categorical approach, the cutoff point can be derived by determining the variability of measurement (1 SD of the difference in means) of the same lesion taken from separate catheter sessions. Twice the variability (95% confidence intervals) defines with reasonable certainty those lesions that have undergone significant deterioration from those that have not. This value has been found to be 0.72 mm on the basis of angiograms taken 90 days apart [16]. Another example of a more commonly used categorical approach is the increase in diameter stenosis from less than 50% after angioplasty to greater than 50% at follow-up. As discussed earlier, one should realize that the so called normal diameter or reference diameter may change [20].

In studies evaluating the biology of restenosis, a continuous measure of the degree of luminal obstruction is preferable since any progression of the stenosis reflects the process of interest whether or not an arbitrarily defined threshold is reached. Keeping in mind that an angiographic restenosis study assesses only the anatomical component of the restenosis problem, there is no threshold above which a loss of luminal diameter would have clinically significant functional or symptomatic consequences. Why then should one bother to try to define a threshold above which there would be "significant" quantitatively determined angiographic restenosis? In the present study, the results have been presented according to the three methodological approaches (50% diameter stenosis criterion, change in minimal luminal diameter of ≥ 0.72 mm and cumulative distribution of the minimal luminal diameter and its changes). Future randomised trials will certainly favor the continuous approach since statistically, the quantitative outcome determined from direct measurements of continuous variables can be evaluated with only one third of the number of the patients required for the categorical outcome. This is indeed logical because the categorical end points does not take full advantage of the available information [32].

B. *Long-term Angiographic Results*

The exact incidence of recurrent restenosis after repeat balloon angioplasty is not known. Data from previous studies suggest that this incidence increases with the number of repeat interventions (Table 5). This table shows the angiographic documented recurrent restenosis rate relative to the number of patients in whom a second, third or fourth angioplasty was successful. It is clear that the reported incidence is an underestimation of the actual incidence due to the incomplete angiographic follow-up. Control angiography is mandatory in all patients, even in patients free of angina at follow-up since approximately 25% of the patients with restenosis are asymptomatic [37]. The recurrent restenosis rate after Wiktor stent implantation in this study amounts to 27% using the 50% diameter stenosis criterion and 46% using the 0.72 mm criterion. The lower restenosis rate using the former criterion is consistent with the concept of stent implantation. As shown in this study, stent implantation results in a further increase in minimal luminal diameter and effectively prevents elastic recoil. Consequently, with the same degree of intimal proliferation, the lumen can remain widely patent after stent implantation, while a significant residual stenosis would be present when a lesser increase in minimal luminal diameter would be achieved at the end of the procedure.

There are some encouraging reports that coronary stenting may reduce the overall restenosis rate to 23–27 percent and even less then 20 percent [8, 38–44, 46]. These data are stemming from non-randomized (preliminary)

Table 5. Angiographic documented recurrent restenosis rate after repeat balloon angioplasty.

Author	Reference	n	angiographic FU	Time interval procedure angiographic FU (months, mean)	Definition restenosis	2° restenosis	3° restenosis	4° restenosis
Williams	1984 (47)	173*	62 (36%)	73	≥30% increase or ≥50% loss	21 (34%)	–	–
Meier	1984 (48)	92*	56 (61%)	?	≥50% loss	23 (25%)	–	–
Black	1988 (49)	384*	151 (39%)	recommended 6 mths earlier if indicated	>50% DS	47 (31%)	–	–
Teirstein	1989 (50)	69**	36 (52%)	18 (7–49)	>50% DS of previously dilated lesion to <40%	–	27(39%)	–
Teirstein	1989 (50)	15***	8 (53%)	16 (7–38)		–	–	6(40%)

n = number of patients who underwent successful second PTCA (*), third PTCA (**) or fourth PTCA (***). Only the incidence of the angiographic documented restenosis relative to the number of patients with successful repeat angioplasty is shown.

reports in which single and multiple stent implantation has been performed in both native coronary arteries and venous bypass grafts in patients with either acute ischemic syndromes or stable angina for a variety of indications (primary stent implantation, restenosis, bail out). Furthermore, different criteria to define restenosis are being used, the angiographic follow-up differs in time and is incomplete. Another factor to be considered when defining restenosis following stent implantation, is that neointimal hyperplasia within the stent may progress beyond 6 months after implantation. Only one brief report indicates that this is not the case [51].

There is evidence that the restenosis rate is lower after stenting a primary lesion with one single Palmaz-Schatz stent [39, 42]. This is contradicted by a recent study from our group, in which the Wallstent was used, showing no difference in the restenosis rate between primary or secondary stenting [45]. It may be a fallacy to compare the incidence of restenosis between different stents. Stents currently available differ not only in their geometry (mesh, coil) and thickness of filaments and composition but also in their composition (metal, plastic), mechanical behavior (active or passive expansion), electrostatic properties, biocompatibility and coatings. These different physico-chemical properties may result in a different restenosis rate.

In conclusion, changing the stenosis geometry by stent implantation does not eliminate the late neointimal hyperplasia. However, the further increase in minimal luminal diameter and cross-sectional area after stent implantation compensates to some degree for the restenosis process. To assess the proper role of intracoronary stenting in the prevention of (recurrent) restenosis, further studies with randomised comparisons are needed.

Acknowledgement

We are greatly indebted to Marie-Angèle Morel for performing the quantitative coronary angiography.

References

1. Sigwart U (1990) Percutaneous transluminal coronary angioplasty: what next? *Br Heart J* 63:321–322
2. Serruys P W, Luijten H E, Beatt K J, Geuskens R, de Feyter P J, van den Brand M, Reiber J H C, ten Katen H J, van Es G A, Hugenholtz P G (1988) Incidence of restenosis after successful coronary angioplasty: a time-related phenomenon. *Circulation* 77:361–371
3. Leimgruber P P, Roubin G S, Hollman J, Cotsonis G A, Meier B, Douglas J S, King S B III, Gruentzig A R (1986) Restenosis after successful coronary angioplasty in patients with single-vessel disease. *Circulation* 73:710–717
4. Levine S, Ewel C J, Rosing D R, Kent K M (1985) Coronary angioplasty: clinical and angiogarphic follow-up. *Am J Cardiol* 55:673–676
5. Nobuyoshi M, Kimura T, Nosaka H, Mioka S, Ueno K, Yokoi H, Hamasaki N, Horiuchi H,

Ohishi H (1988) Restenosis after successful percutaneous transluminal coronary angioplasty: serial angiographic follow-up of 229 patients. *J Am Coll Cardiol* 12:616–623

6. Teirstein P S, Hoover C A, Lignon R W, Giorgi L V, Rutherford B D, McConahay D R, Johnson W L, Hartzler G O (1989) Repeat coronary angioplasty: efficacy of a third angioplasty for a second restenosis. *J Am Coll Cardiol* 13:291–296

7. Black A, Anderson H, Roubin G, Powelson S, Douglas J, King III S (1988) Repeat coronary angioplasty: correlates of a second restenosis. *J Am Coll Cardiol* 11:714–718

8. Serruys P W, Strauss B H, Beatt K J, Bertrand M E, Puel J, Rickards A F, Meier B, Kappenberger L, Goy J J, Sigwart U (1991) Quantitative angiographic follow-up of the coronary Wallstent in the initial 105 patients. *N Engl J Med* 324:13–17

9. Schatz R A (1989) A view of vascular stents. *Circulation* 79:445–457

10. Roubin G S, King III S B, Douglas J S, Lembo N J, Robinson K A (1990) Intracoronary stenting during percutaneous transluminal coronary angioplasty. *Circulation* 81(suppl IV):IV–92–IV–100

11. Burger W, Hartmann A, Kandyba J, Keul H G, Sievert H, Niemöller E, Schneider M, Kober G (1990) Angiographic and histologic course after implantation of balloon expandable intravascular stents in miniswine coronary arteries: short- and mid-term observations. *J Interven Cardiol* 3:87–98

12. van der Giessen W J, Serruys P W, van Beusekom H M M, van Woerkens L J, van Loon H, Loe Kie Soei, Strauss B H, Beatt K J, Verdouw P (1991) Coronary stenting with a new, radiopaque, balloon-expandable endoprosthesis in pigs. *Circulation* 83:1788–98

13. Serruys P W, Julliere Y, Bertrand M E, Puel J, Rickards A F, Sigwart U (1988) Additional improvement of stenosis geometry in human coronary arteries by stenting after balloon dilatation. *Am J Cardiol* 61:71G–76G

14. Puel J, Julliere Y, Bertrand M, Rickards A, Sigwart U, Serruys P W (1988) Early and late assessment of stenosis geometry after coronary arterial stenting. *Am J Cardiol* 61:546–553

15. Reiber J H C, Serruys P W, Slager C J (1986) *Quantitative Coronary and Left Ventricular Cineangiography*. Martinus Nijhoff Publishers

16. Reiber J H C, Serruys P W, Kooijman C J (1985) Assessment of short-, medium, and long-term variations in arterial dimensions from computer-assisted quantitation of coronary cineangiograms. *Circulation* 71:280–288

17. Crawford D W, Brooks S H, Selzer R H, Brandt R, Beckenbach E S, Blankenhorn D H (1977) Computer densitometry for angiographic assessment of arterial cholesterol contents and gross pathology in human atherosclerosis. *J Lab Clin Med* 89:378–392

18. Gould K L, Kelley K O, Bolson E L (1982) Experimental validation of the quantitative coronary arteriography for determining pressure-flow characteristics of coronary stenosis. *Circulation* 66:930–937

19. Wijns W, Serruys P W, Reiber J, van den Brand M, Simoons M, Kooijman C, Balakumaran K, Hugenholtz P (1985) Quantitative angiography of the left anterior descending coronary artery: correlations with pressure gradient and results of exercise thallium scintigraphy. *Circulation* 71:273–279

20. Beatt K J, Luijten H E, de Feyter P J, van den Brand M, Reiber J H C, Serruys P W (1988) Change in diameter of coronary artery segments adjacent to stenosis after percutaneous transluminal coronary angioplasty: failure of percent diameter stenosis measurement to reflect morphologic changes induced by balloon dilatation. *J Am Coll Cardiol* 12:315–323

21. Sigwart U, Puel J, Mirkovitch V, Joffre F, Kappenberger L (1987) Intravascular stent to prevent occlusion and restenosis after transluminal angioplasty. *N Engl J Med* 316:701–706

22. Serruys P W, Beatt K J, van der Giessen W J (1989) Stenting of coronary arteries. Are we the sorcerer's apprentice? *Eur Heart J* 10:774–782

23. Levine M J, Leonard B M, Burke J A, Nash I D, Safian R D, Diver D J, Baim D S (1990) Clinical and angiographic results of balloon-expandable intracoronary stents in right coronary artery stenoses. *J Am Coll Cardiol* 16:332–329

24. De Rouen T A, Murray J A, Owen W (1977) Variability in the analysis of coronary arteriograms. *Circulation* 55:324–328

25. Trask N, Califf R M, Conley M J, Kong Y, Peter R, Lee K L, Hackel D B, Wagner D B,

Wagner G S (1984) Accuracy and interobserver variability of coronary cineangiography: a comparison with postmortem evaluation. *J Am Coll Cardiol* 3:1145–1154

26. Holder D A, Johnson A L, Stolberg H O, Campell M, Gustensen J, Joyal M, Roberts R, Biagioni E M, Vaughan W, Romeo M (1985) Inability of caliper measurements to enhance observer agreement in the interpretation of coronary cineangiograms. *Can J Cardiol* 1:24–29

27. Serruys P W, Reiber J H C, Wijns W, van den Brand M, Kooijman C J, ten Katen H J, Hugenholtz P G (1984) Assessment of percutaneous transluminal coronary angioplasty by quantitative coronary angiography: diameter versus densitometric area measurements. *Am J Cardiol* 54:482–488

28. Smalling R (1987) Can the immediate efficacy of coronary angioplasty be adequately assessed? *J Am Coll Cardiol* 10:261–263

29. Strauss B H, Julliere Y, Rensing B J, Reiber J H C, Serruys P W (1991) Edge detection versus densitometry for assessing coronary stenting quantitatively. *Am J Cardiol* 67:484–490

30. Strauss B H, Rensing B J, Reiber J H C, den Boer A, van der Giessen W J (1990) Do stents interfere with the videodensitometric assessment of a lesion? An in-vitro model. *Circulation* 82:2610(A)

31. Hermans W, Rensing B J, Strauss B H, Serruys P W (1991) Methodological problems related to the quantitative assessment of strech, elastic recoil and balloon-artery ratio. Submitted for publication

32. Serruys P W, Rutsch W, Heyndrickx G R, Danchin N, Mast G, Wijns W, Rensing B, Vos J, Stibbe J (1991) Prevention of restenosis after percutaneous transluminal coronary angioplasty with thromboxane A2 receptor blockade. A randomized, double-blind, aspirin-placebo controlled trial. *Circulation* 84: 1568–1580.

33. Erbel R, Höpp H W, Haude M, Dietz U, Franzen D, Straub U, Rupprecht H J, Schatz R, Hilger H H, Meyer J (1990) Success, complication and restenosis rate of intracoronary placing of balloon expandable stents. *Eur Heart J* 11:1413(A)

34. Zijlstra F, van Ommeren J, Reiber J H C, Serruys P W (1987) Does quantitative assessment of coronary artery dimensions predict the physiological significance of a coronary stenosis? *Circulation* 75:1154–1161

35. Rensing B J, Hermans R M, Beatt K J, Laarman G J, Suryapranata H, van den Brand M, de Feyter P J, Serruys P W (1990) Quantitative angiographic assessment of elastic recoil after percutaneous transluminal coronary angioplasty. *Am J Cardiol* 66:1039–1044

36. Beatt K J, Serruys P W, Hugenholtz P G (1990) Restenosis after coronary angioplasty: New standards for clinical studies. *J Am Coll Cardiol* 15:491–498

37. Holmes D, Schwartz R, Webster M (1991) Coronary restenosis: what have we learned from angiography? *J Am Coll Cardiol* 17:14B–22B

38. Marco J, Fajadet J, Cassagneau B G, Laurent J P, Robert G P (1990) Balloon expandable intracoronary stents: immediate and mean term results in a series of 122 consecutive patients. *Eur Heart J* 11:2034(A)

39. Ellis S, Fischman D, Hirsfeld J, Savage M, Goldberg S, Erbel R, Cleman M, Teirstein P, Schatz R (1990) Mechanism of stent benefit to limit restenosis following coronary angioplasty: regrowth versus larger initial lumen? *Circulation* 82:2143A

40. Teirstein P, Cleman M, Hirshfeld J, Buchbinder M, Walker C (1990) Influence of prior restenosis on subsequent restenosis after intracoronary stenting. *Circulation* 82:2612A

41. Levine M, Cleman M, Schatz R, Buchbinder M, Erbel R, Baim D (1990) Management of restenosis following Palmaz-Schatz intracoronary stenting: multicenter results. *Circulation* 82:2611A

42. Schatz R, Goldberg S, Leon M, Fish D, Hirshfeld J, Walker C (1990) Coronary stenting following "suboptimal" coronary angioplasty results. *Circulation* 82:2145A

43. Shaknovich A, Teirstein P S, Stratienko A A, Walker C M, Cleman M W, Schatz R A (1991) Restenosis in single Palmaz-Schatz coronary stents: effects of prior PTCA and interval to prior PTCA. *J Am Coll Cardiol* 17:269A

44. Fajadet J, Marco J, Cassagneau B G, Robert G P, Vandormael M, Jordan C G, Flores M

Y, Laurent J P (1991) Restenosis following successful Palmaz-Schatz intracoronary stent implantation. *J Am Coll Cardiol* 17:346A

45. Strauss B, Serruys P W, de Scheerder I, Tijssen J, Bertrand M, Puel J, Meier B, Kaufmann U, Stauffer J C, Rickards A, Sigwart U (1991) A relative risk analysis of the angiographic predictors of restenosis within the coronary Wallstent. *Circulation* 84: 1636–1643

46. Strauss B, Serruys P W, Bertrand M, Puel J, Meier B, Goy J J, Kappenberger L, Rickards A, Sigwart U (1992) Quantitative angiographic follow-up of the coronary Wallstent in native and bypass grafts: the evolving European experience from March 1986– March 1990. *Am J Cardiol* 69: 475–481

47. Williams D, Gruentzig A, Kent K, Detre K, Kelsey S, To T (1984) Efficacy of repeat percutaneous transluminal coronary angioplasty for restenosis. *Am J Cardiol* 53:32C–35C

48. Meier B, King III S, Gruentzig A, Douglas J, Hollman J, Ischinger T, Galan K, Tankersley (1984) Repeat coronary angioplasty. *J Am Coll Cardiol* 4:463–466

49. Black A, Anderson V, Roubin G, Powelson S, Douglas J, King III S (1988) Repeat coronary angioplasty: correlates of a second restenosis. *J Am Coll Cardiol* 11:714–718

50. Teirstein P, Hoover C, Ligon R, Giorgi L, Rutherford B, McConahay D, Johnson W, Hartzler G (1989) Repeat coronary angioplasty: efficacy of a third angioplasty for a second restenosis. *J Am Coll Cardiol* 13:291–296

51. Savage M, Fischman D, Ellis S, Leon M, Cleman M, Teirstein P, Walker C, Hirshfeld J, Schatz R, Goldberg S (1990) Does late progression of restenosis occur beyond six months following coronary artery stenting? *Circulation* 82:(Suppl III) 2144A

PART FOUR

Atherectomy

Atherectomy Introduction

JOHN SIMPSON

The concept of atherectomy, the removal of atheroma, was introduced to overcome some of the limitations of percutaneous transluminal coronary angioplasty (PTCA) [1]. Dilatation of stenoses by balloons frequently causes splitting of the atheroma or normal vessel wall while creating a larger lumen. In contrast, atherectomy was designed to create a larger lumen by removing obstructive tissue [2, 3]. The concept of atherectomy is based on the hypothesis that removal of tissue will (1) create a smoother surface than PTCA without dissection and, (2) result in a larger intravascular lumen. If atherectomy truly achieves the above-described conditions, it may improve the acute outcome compared to PTCA by preventing dissections or elastic recoil and possibly reducing restenosis.

Potential mechanisms of reducing restenosis following atherectomy are as follows: (1) less stimulation of smooth muscle cell proliferation; (2) wider space for the tissue to grow, and; (3) prevention of elastic recoil. A smooth residual surface without dissection may be less thrombogenic or less of a stimulating environment for platelet aggregation which may trigger smooth muscle cell proliferation. Larger post interventional lumen size may allow more tissue mass (intimal hyperplasia) to grow during the healing process prior to reaching a hemodynamically significant stenosis. If tissue growth is self-limiting, this may result in only a partial stenosis rather than a clinically significant stenosis. It has been shown that some restenosis is due to elastic recoil rather than smooth muscle cell proliferation [4]. Tissue removal with atherectomy should reduce or prevent elastic recoil and thus may reduce restenosis. All this is speculation, and it is obvious that this needs to be confirmed with prospective clinical studies to evaluate whether atherectomy and angioplasty have different restenosis rates.

Currently, two devices have been used clinically: these are the directional coronary atherectomy (DCA) catheter (Fig. 1) and the transluminal extraction catheter (TEC) (Fig. 2). Although both devices were designed to remove obstructive tissue from lesions, their mechanisms of action are different. The DCA catheter is a side cutter enclosed in a housing, and excision of atheroma

P.W. Serruys, B.H. Strauss and S.B. King III (eds), Restenosis after Intervention with New Mechanical Devices, 237–240.
© 1992 *Kluwer Academic Publishers. Printed in the Netherlands.*

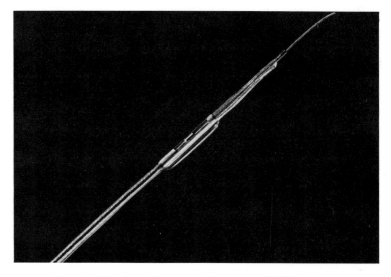

Figure 1. Directional Coronary Atherectomy (DCA) catheter.

is performed directionally by aiming the window of the housing toward the diseased segment of the vessel wall. In contrast, the TEC is an exposed front cutter and excises tissue in a concentric manner as the catheter is advanced. Although both devices have the same goal of tissue removal, the evaluation of the efficacy and safety must be evaluated separately because of their different cutting and tissue collection mechanisms.

Studies designed to compare restenosis rates between PTCA and new devices provide the opportunity to evaluate other procedure-related factors. These are: (1) acute outcome; (2) additional risk to the patient; (3) complexity of the procedure; (4) complexity of post procedure patient management, and; (5) cost. The procedure is not applicable for clinical use if the acute outcome is suboptimal regardless of the effectiveness for restenosis. In the multicenter trial for both DCA and TEC it has been shown that these procedures were safe and effective for the treatment of obstructive lesions despite inclusion of some high-risk lesions [5–7]. Compared to other new procedures, atherectomy may require more operator skill because of the relative complexity of the procedure. It may seem obvious but it should be emphasized that it is very important for the operator to clearly understand the concept and technique of atherectomy, as well as be trained appropriately before performing atherectomy to have a high success rate and low complication rate. Through this careful training process, the multicenter experience has shown that atherectomy can be safely performed by a new operator.

One of the advantages of atherectomy is that it does not require any special patient care prior to or following the procedure. The patient is usually treated similarly to PTCA patients. Prolonged heparinization and long-term anticoagulation are not required, and the patient can be discharged the

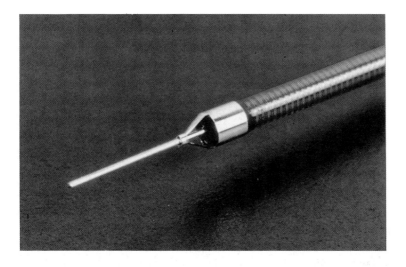

Figure 2. Transluminal Extraction Catheter (TEC).

following day in most cases. The other potential advantage of atherectomy is that it does not increase the cost significantly for the procedure and hospital stay. While the catheter is more expensive than the PTCA balloon, it does not require any other expensive equipment. In addition, the cost for the hospitalization is similar to PTCA because it does not require a prolonged hospitalization.

Information regarding restenosis is discussed in detail in the following chapters for DCA and TEC separately. There is no conclusive evidence at the present time that the post atherectomy restenosis rate is significantly different from PTCA [7, 8]. The overall restenosis rate documented by angiography was similar to PTCA; however, it is premature to conclude that the restenosis rate is the same as PTCA. The patient populations differ significantly from the general PTCA population since many of the patients are specifically referred for atherectomy because of recurrent restenosis following PTCA or high-risk lesions with complex angiographic appearance such as extreme eccentricity, ulceration or ostial lesions. Furthermore, the atherectomy procedure and equipment have continued to evolve and the current data are based on the early stage of the atherectomy experience. Atherectomy experts are currently divided as to whether aggressive therapy to try to achieve a larger post procedure lumen size or less aggressive therapy to avoid deep cuts should be utilized to provide the best chance of minimizing restenosis. Therefore, further analysis will be required to determine the "optimal atherectomy technique." One of the encouraging results following DCA is that restenosis seems to be low for large vessels, particularly those treated with a 7 French device, with a good post-DCA lesion diameter.

Since restenosis can occur following atherectomy, it is important to compare the restenosis rate to PTCA in a prospective randomized study. A multicenter trial (CAVEAT: Coronary Angioplasty Versus Excisional Atherectomy Trial; principal investigator Eric Topol, M.D.) has been organized and will start in the summer of 1991. The primary end-point of this study is to compare the incidence of angiographically documented restenosis between DCA and PTCA. Although the "best" technique for performing DCA remains controversial, the basic catheter design has evolved to a level of stability that should permit a useful comparison between an established and a new evolving technology. This study is likely to answer some of the questions regarding restenosis and could provide a model for comparison of many future technologies.

References

1. Simpson, J B (1988) Future interventional techniques. In: Califf R M, Mark D B, Wagner G S (eds) *Acute Coronary Care on the Thrombolytic Era.* Year Book Medical Publishers, Chicago, 392–404
2. Simpson J B, Selmon M R, Robertson G C, Cipriano P R, Hayden W G, Johnson D E, Fogarty T J (1988) Transluminal atherectomy for occlusive peripheral vascular disease. *Am J Cardio* 61:96G-101G
3. Johnson D E, Braden L, Simpson J B (1990) Mechanism of directed transluminal atherectomy. *Am J Cardio* 65:389–91
4. Waller B F, Pinkerton C A, Orr C M, Slack J D, VanTassel J W, Peters T (1991) Morphological observations late (> 30 days) after clinically successful coronary balloon angioplasty. *Circulation* 83(suppl I):I-28–I-41
5. U. S. Directional Coronary Atherectomy Investigator Group. Directional coronary atherectomy: multicenter experience (abstract). *Circulation* 82 (supp III)III-71
6. Hinohara T, Rowe M H, Robertson G C, Selmon M R, Braden L, Leggett J H, Vetter J W, Simpson J B (1991) Effect of lesion characteristics on outcome of directional coronary atherectomy. *JACC* Vol. 17, No. 5, April 1991:1112–20
7. Sketch M H, O'Neill W W, Tcheng J E, Walker C, Galichia J P, Sawchak S, Cress S, Phillips H R, Stack R S (1990) Early and late outcome following coronary transluminal extraction-endarterectomy: a multicenter experience. *Circulation* (supp III) Vol. 82, No. 4, October 1990
8. U. S. Directional Atherectomy Investigator Group. Restenosis following directional coronary atherectomy in a multicenter experience (abstract). *Circulation* 82 (supp III)III:679

11. Restenosis: Directional Coronary Atherectomy

TOMOAKI HINOHARA, JOHN B. SIMPSON, GREGORY C.
ROBERTSON and MATTHEW R. SELMON

Introduction

The concept of atherectomy was developed by J. B. Simpson to overcome
some of the limitations of PTCA with the hypothesis that removal of tissue
from an obstructed vessel would create a smooth and wide lumen [1, 2]. A
smooth, wide lumen without dissection may prevent acute occlusion or reduce thrombus formation, thus improving the acute outcome. Improved flow
pattern may prevent platelet aggregation or thrombus formation which are
potential triggers for smooth muscle cell proliferation. Furthermore, a wide
lumen following intervention may allow some intimal hyperplastic tissue to
grow during the healing process without creating a hemodynamically significant stenosis. There is, therefore, the potential that atherectomy may reduce
restenosis.

The directional coronary atherectomy (DCA) catheter was developed to
remove tissue from a lesion safely and effectively. Since the initial DCA
attempt in 1986, the catheter has been improved significantly through many
generations and the current device was approved by the Food and Drug
Administration (FDA) in September 1990. Through the multicenter investigation in the United States, the acute safety and efficacy of DCA have
been established [3, 4]. In addition, some information has become available
regarding restenosis through the investigation.

Multicenter experience in the United States demonstrates an overall restenosis rate of 40% for native arteries and 50% for saphenous vein grafts
[5]. The restenosis rate for primary stenoses in native coronary arteries was
26% with a trend for a lower restenosis rate in discrete lesions [6]. Although
these data include a moderate number of lesions, conclusions should not be
prematurely drawn based on these data if the restenosis rate differs from
that with PTCA. This was an observational study and was not intended to
be compared to PTCA. Patient populations may significantly differ from the
"general PTCA population" since the cases were often referred to investigators because of recurrent restenosis or "high-risk lesion." In addition,

P.W. Serruys, B.H. Strauss and S.B. King III (eds), Restenosis after Intervention with New Mechanical
Devices, 241–257.
© 1992 *Kluwer Academic Publishers. Printed in the Netherlands*

Table 1. Lesion characteristics and DCA outcome.

	No. of Lesions	DCA Success	DCA & PTCA Success	Major Complication
Simple Lesion	105	97%	97%	0%
Complex Lesion	342	87%	93%	3.8%
Eccentric	188	87%	93%	3.2%
Lesion >10 mm	97	88%	92%	6.3%
Calcification	70	70%	87%	5.7%
Abnormal contour	54	93%	94%	5.6%
Angulation	55	86%	91%	3.6%

DCA & PTCA Success: Combined success rate for DCA success and PTCA success for failed DCA attempts.

Table modified from "Effect of Lesion Characteristics on Outcome of Directional Coronary Atherectomy." Hinohara, T et al [7].

DCA evolved during this investigational period both in terms of equipment and method of procedure. Modification of the procedure and adjustment in case selection may change the restenosis rate further.

Acute Outcome and Indications

Before any procedure can be used to reduce restenosis, acute safety and efficacy with a new procedure needs to be established. New procedures are not clinically applicable unless their acute outcomes are adequate regardless of the effect on restenosis. In the multicenter investigation in the United States (June 1988 to September 1990) appproximately 2,000 cases of DCA were performed. This experience, as well as the Sequoia Hospital experience, demonstrated that atherectomy removed tissue from obstructed vessels and the acute outcome was satisfactory. The success rate was high despite inclusion of high-risk lesions. The success rate for 447 lesions treated at Sequoia Hospital was 90% (97% for simple lesions and 87% for complex lesions) [7]. Significant complications were infrequent and very similar to PTCA. Three percent of patients required emergency bypass surgery for either occlusive complication at the atherectomy site, guide dissection, nose cone injury at the distal vessel, or perforation. The risk of perforation, initially a major concern prior to the investigation, was observed infrequently, 0.8% (3 out of 447 lesions). Although acute tamponade may occur with a vessel perforation, this serious complication was very infrequent and only observed in 1 case out of approximately 2,000 cases in the multicenter investigation.

As demonstrated in Table 1, the outcome of DCA was good even among those relatively "high-risk lesions" except for lesions with calcification. The directional nature of this procedure helps treat extremely eccentric lesions or lesions with abnormal contour. In addition, removal of tissue with a low dissection rate may help treat left anterior descending artery ostial lesions.

Not only is DCA able to treat these lesions successfully, but the post-DCA angiographic appearance is usually superior to that with PTCA. Retrospective comparison of angiograms following DCA and PTCA revealed that DCA created a larger lumen without significant dissection. The incidence of dissection or flap was less frequent (DCA 11%, PTCA 37%) and quantitatively measured post procedure stenosis was significantly less (DCA 13%, PTCA 31%) when the lesion was treated with DCA [8].

Limitations of DCA should be recognized. The atherectomy procedure requires new skills and even those having extensive experience with PTCA need to go through the learning process. The guiding catheter is larger than the PTCA guiding catheter – 11 French for the left coronary artery and 9.5 French for the right coronary artery – and the handling of these guiding catheters needs to be extremely gentle to avoid guide-induced dissections, which were mostly observed in the right coronary artery. The profile and stiffness of the device prevent use of this procedure in tortuous or small vessels. In addition, the procedure is very limited in calcified lesions or lesions in a calcified vessel.

Case selection for DCA is summarized in Table 2. Currently, atherectomy is indicated for a lesion with vessel size greater than 2.5 mm in a non-tortuous vessel. Atherectomy can be performed in the left main, left anterior descending artery, right coronary artery, saphenous vein graft, and the circumflex artery if the origin of its takeoff is not steep from the left main. It seems to be particularly useful for the treatment of "bulky lesions" in relatively large vessels.

The removal of tissue rather than simple dilatation may help to treat these lesions with an excellent angiographic outcome without dissection. In addition to concentric and discrete "ideal PTCA lesions," DCA is extremely effective for eccentric lesions including extreme eccentricity, lesions with abnormal contour, lengthy lesions, or ostial lesions, particularly in the left anterior descending artery. In addition, DCA has been shown to be useful in selective cases for the treatment of lesions which were not effectively dilated by PTCA [9]. Calcified lesions or lesions in a diffusely calcified vessel or a diffusely diseased vessel are not ideal candidates since either the catheter will not reach or cross the lesion, or the cutter cannot cut the calcified lesion. Lesions with a spiral dissection should not be approached with DCA since there is the potential risk of perforation.

Restenosis Following DCA – Sequoia Experience

To document the incidence of restenosis following successful DCA, it is part of our protocol at Sequoia Hospital that the patient undergo repeat angiographic evaluation at approximately six months regardless of symptoms. If the patient becomes symptomatic, the patient will undergo angiography

Table 2. Case selection for DCA.

Vessel size:	>2.5 mm
Type:	primary lesion, restenosed lesion

Accessibility:
  Location of vessel
    – LM
    – LAD – ostial – proximal – mid
    – RCA – ostial – proximal – mid – distal
    – CX – ostial – proximal – mid – shallow takeoff
    – SVG – ostial – proximal – mid – distal anastomosis
    – Large branch (diagonal, marginal)

  Tortuosity: none or mild.
  Calcification of vessel: none or mild.
  Diffusely diseased: none.
  Peripheral vascular disease: none.

Lesion characteristics favorable for DCA:
  Eccentricity: eccentric, concentric
  Contour: normal, dissection, ulceration, flap
  Ostial involvement: non-aorta ostial (LAD, CX, branches)
                      aorta ostial (LM, RCA, SVG)
  Lesion length: discrete or tubular

Lesion characteristics unfavorable for DCA:
  Calcification: moderate, heavy
  Angulation: >45 degrees
  Lesion length: lengthy (>20 mm)
  Dissection: extensive or spiral
  Degenerative SVG

CX:	Circumflex artery
LAD:	Left anterior descending artery
LM:	Left main artery
RCA:	Right coronary artery
SVG:	Saphenous vein graft.

earlier. The definition of restenosis used in this chapter was greater than 50% stenosis at the DCA segment. This definition is used since many of the restenosis studies for the PTCA experience use this definition, and a stenosis greater than 50% is usually considered to be "clinically significant."

A. *Incidence of Restenosis*

The following results are based on angiographic evaluation of 282 lesions (angiographic compliance rate of 82%). The overall restenosis rate for the native artery was 37% (n = 225), and 63% (n = 57) (p < 0.001) for saphenous vein grafts. These data suggest that the native artery and saphenous vein graft were two different clinical groups and need to be evaluated separately. The reason for the high restenosis rate in the saphenous vein graft is not certain, although a similar tendency was observed for PTCA. The overall restenosis rate may not reflect the general population because of the referral pattern which contained more restenosed lesions (52% of cases were re-stenosed lesions). The restenosis rate for primary lesions in the native coronary artery was 31% (n = 90) whereas the restenosis rate for restenosed lesions in the native coronary artery was 41%: 28% (n = 46) for one previous PTCA, 49% (n = 55) for two previous PTCAs and 44% (n = 34) for three or more previous PTCAs. These data suggest that lesions with multiple previous PTCAs tend to have a higher restenosis rate. This is most likely due to selection of a patient who had a tendency to have recurrent restenosis, whatever the underlying mechanism was.

One of the strongest associations with recurrent restenosis in those lesions with previous PTCA was the number of days following previous PTCA (interval between PTCA and DCA). The shorter the duration following PTCA to DCA, the higher the recurrent restenosis following DCA: restenosis rate was 56% for intervals less than 120 days and 21% for intervals greater than 120 days (p < 0.001). Thus, restenosis following DCA remains a significant problem among those who had either multiple recurrent restenoses or patients who have lesions which tend to restenose quickly following intervention.

A similar effect of previous PTCA on recurrent restenosis following DCA was also observed among lesions in the saphenous vein graft. The restenosis rate in primary lesions in the saphenous vein graft was 54% (n = 28) and for restenosed lesions was 72% (n = 29).

The timing of restenosis following DCA seems similar to that of PTCA. Many restenoses (41%) occurred within four months following DCA and the majority (92%) were observed within eight months following DCA. A few cases had restenosis after eight months; however, these were in relatively asymptomatic patients and they had routine angiogram as part of the protocol. Although the timing of the restenosis pattern seems to be similar to that of PTCA, longer term follow-up is necessary to exclude late restenosis. Since lumen size following successful DCA is generally large with minimal residual stenosis, the restenosis process may be slower compared with PTCA. It may simply take more time to fill out the larger space with cell proliferation.

Restenosis following DCA can be treated with repeat DCA. Similar to re-do PTCA, re-do DCA is usually highly successful without significant complications. The success rate of those lesions which were previously treated by DCA was 98%. Although recurrent restenosis following repeat DCA may continue to be a significant problem, our current approach for restenosis following DCA is to repeat DCA and to perform a more aggressive atherectomy, attempting to retrieve a larger amount of tissue than the first time using either higher balloon inflation pressure or a larger device, if appropriate.

Table 3. Factors associated with restenosis following DCA.

CLINICAL FACTORS
Hypertension
Class IV angina
Age >65

ANGIOGRAPHIC FACTORS
Lengthy lesion (>10 mm)
Vessel size <3 mm

PROCEDURAL FACTORS
Use of smaller device (6 Fr)
Post-DCA diameter <3 mm

B. *Factors Associated With Restenosis*

The factors which may affect the incidence of restenosis are summarized in Table 3. Among the clinical factors, a history of Class IV angina and hypertension were associated with a high incidence of restenosis. The restenosis rate for patients with Class IV angina was 48%, while that for patients with Class I-III angina was 32%. The restenosis rate for patients with hypertension was 48%, and for patients without a history of hypertension was 29%.

Among pre-DCA angiographic appearances, a higher restenosis rate was associated with lengthy lesions and smaller vessels (vessel size <3 mm). The restenosis rate was 57% for lesion length >10 mm and 29% for lesion length <10 mm. This tendency was particularly more significant for restenosis lesions: restenosis rate was 64% for lesion length >10 mm and 32% for lesion length <10 mm. The restenosis rate was 44% for vessel size <3 mm and 29% for vessel size >3 mm.

Among procedural factors, use of small device (6 French rather than 7 French) and small post-DCA diameter was associated with high incidence of restenosis. The restenosis rate was 49% for the 6 French device and 27% for the 7 French device. The restenosis rate was 41% for post-DCA diameter <3 mm and 28% for a post-DCA diameter of >3 mm. Some data have suggested that overtreatment, either retrieval of media or angiographically overstretched appearance, may actually increase the incidence of restenosis. The restenosis rate was significantly higher for those with media retrieval among restenosis lesions; however, the restenosis rate was similar among primary lesions regardless of media retrieval [12]. The angiographic overstretched appearance (less than 10% residual stenosis) tended to have a higher restenosis rate (34% with no overdilatation versus 48% with overdilatation), although the difference was not statistically significant.

Although the overall restenosis rates may be similar to those with PTCA, certain subgroups treated by atherectomy were promising for reduction of restenosis. Restenosis seemed to be lower in larger vessels, with a good post-

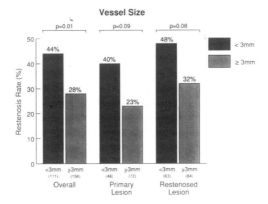

Figure 1. Vessel size and restenosis rate. Reference vessel size was quantitatively measured and divided into smaller vessel (<3 mm) and larger vessel (>3 mm).

DCA result using a large device. The restenosis rate for overall as well as for primary lesions and restenosis lesions in native coronary arteries is summarized in Figs 1, 2 and 3. Restenosis rates in primary lesion are encouraging; 23% for vessel size ≥3 mm, 16% for post DCA diameter ≥3 mm and 17% for lesion treated by French device.

C. Restenosis and Analysis of Excised Tissue

One of the unique features of DCA is that it excises tissue intact from obstructive lesions and the tissue can be analyzed. We routinely performed hematoxylin-eosin stain, trichrome stain and van Gieson's stain. In addition,

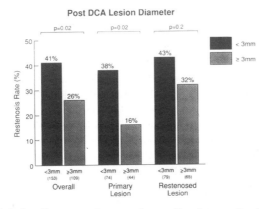

Figure 2. Post DCA lesion diameter and restenosis rate. Post intervention lesion diameter was quantitatively measured and divided into smaller post DCA diameter (<3 mm) or larger post DCA diameter (>3 mm).

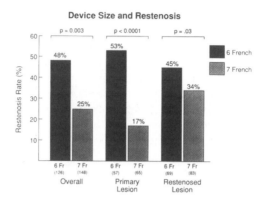

Figure 3. Maximum size of device used and restenosis rate.

some of the investigators have performed special antibody staining to identify the cells or matrix and also in situ hybridization to evaluate the concentration of the receptors [10]. Analysis of the excised tissue will be helpful in understanding the pathophysiology of atherosclerosis and restenosis. In addition, subsequent restenosis following DCA may be predicted based on the type of histology of the excised tissue examined.

The histology of the excised tissue has a significant variation from patient to patient and lesion to lesion [11, 12]. Although most of the primary lesions showed more classical atherosclerosis (fibrous plaque, cholesterol clefts, calcification, organized thrombus, foam cells), cellularity in fibrous plaque may differ significantly from one patient to another. In fact, some of the lesions were very similar to restenosis lesions with significant intimal hyperplasia rather than typical atheroma. Intimal hyperplasia without atherosclerosis was observed in 6% of the primary lesions [11]. Our preliminary experience suggests that lesions with high cellularity also act more like restenosis lesions: the restenosis rate following DCA was higher for fibrous plaque with high cellularity than plaque with typical old atheroma (Figs 4, 5) [13].

Histology from restenosis lesions revealed some important observations as to the cause of restenosis. As shown in most of the animal studies or limited autopsy analysis in humans, significant smooth muscle cell proliferation was observed in the majority of lesions. The cellularity, however, varied from extreme to minimal. In addition, in the same lesion the cellularity seemed to be significantly different from one location of the lesion to another. Also, some of the patients who had multiple atherectomy procedures revealed that the cellularity may significantly change during the process of multiple atherectomies (Fig. 6). The higher cellularity lesion may represent a more proliferative environment than those lesions with scanty cellularity. As observed in primary lesions, the restenosis rate following DCA is higher for those with higher cellularity compared to those with mild-to-moderate cellularity.

The preliminary results also suggest that some of the restenosis after PTCA may occur as a result of elastic recoil, as previously speculated [12, 14]. Although the incidence is relatively infrequent, a small number of lesions had only atherosclerosis without significant intimal hyperplasia, suggesting that these lesions represent elastic recoil as the main reason for restenosis. Pure elastic recoil is an example of one extreme and it can be speculated that restenosis occurs from a combination of elastic recoil and intimal hyperplasia on many occasions.

Our preliminary histological analysis demonstrated the potential importance of tissue analysis to expand our knowledge of atherosclerosis and intimal hyperplasia. Although technically demanding, some investigators were successful in performing in situ hybridization using a PDGF or FGF probe [10]. Further information may become available in the near future. In addition, some investigators have been successful in culturing smooth muscle cells from excised tissue from coronary or peripheral lesions. Dartsch, PC et al. successfully cultured cells from both a primary lesion and a restenosis lesion, and the cells were identified as smooth muscle cells based on cell characterization [15]. The cells' growth rate was faster in the restenosis lesion than the primary lesion. The cell growth rate was significantly stimulated when PDGF was added to the culture media for the restenosis lesion but not for the primary lesion. In contrast, when culture media from a restenosis lesion was added to the culture media of a primary lesion, cell growth of the primary lesion was significantly stimulated, suggesting that there are some growth factors other than PDGF which were secreted by the smooth muscle cell from the cultured restenosis cells.

Lessons from Our Experience

It was clear through our preliminary experience that DCA does not eliminate restenosis. Although DCA may effectively reduce restenosis in selected subgroups of patients such as those with lesions in large vessels, lesions treated with a 7 French device or a wide post-DCA luminal diameter, this procedure still faces the problem of restenosis, particularly in saphenous vein grafts or restenosed lesions previously treated with multiple PTCAs. Although restenosis is observed following DCA, it is premature to conclude that the restenosis rate following DCA does not differ from PTCA based on the current data. Many factors such as patient or lesion characteristics may alter the incidence of restenosis. In our experience many of the lesions were treated with multiple previous PTCAs and patients were referred for DCA because of a malignant form of restenosis. In addition, many primary lesions are also referred for DCA because of their being high-risk lesions rather than simple lesions. Furthermore, many of the procedure's features also have continued to evolve and the current data include the early stage of the

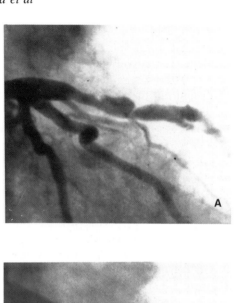

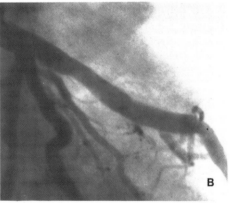

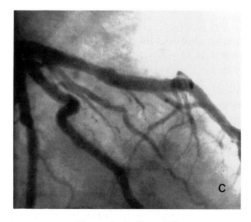

Figure 4. A, B and C.

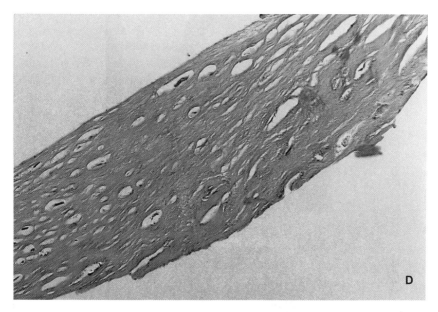

Figure 4. DCA of primary lesions in left anterior descending artery. A. Pre DCA angiogram. B. Post DCA angiogram. C. 6-month follow-up angiogram. There was no evidence of restenosis. D. Histology of excised tissue (trichrome stain). Typical atherosclerotic plaque with acellular fibrous plaque.

atherectomy experience rather than the current method of DCA using the most up-to-date device.

One of the most encouraging results is that the restenosis rate seemed to be lower in large vessels, particularly if treated with a large device (7 French) with a large post-DCA diameter. Although no information is available for the restenosis rate of PTCA on these large vessels, a restenosis rate of approximately 20% for primary lesions for native arteries following DCA in this particular subgroup may be lower than with PTCA. These preliminary results support the "large lumen concept." This concept is based on the hypothesis that the vessel wall following an intervention will undergo intimal hyperplasia as a healing process regardless of the type of intervention; however, this process will cease spontaneously following a certain number of cell cycles in many cases. By creating large lumen size with intervention, there is more space available for the tissue to grow; thus, tissue growth causes only partial obstruction without clinically significant restenosis. If only a small lumen size is achieved with an intervention, such as is often observed with PTCA, only a small amount of tissue growth will cause significant restenosis. It is interesting to observe a similar effect of vessel size on restenosis following the stent placement. It has been reported that post lumen diameter and vessel size are important predictors of restenosis following stent placement. Although many lesions in relatively small vessels in a mid or distal location can be effectively and safely treated with DCA, the current

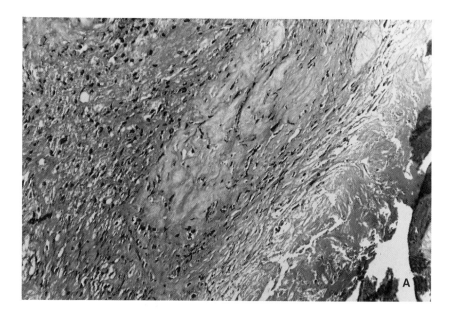

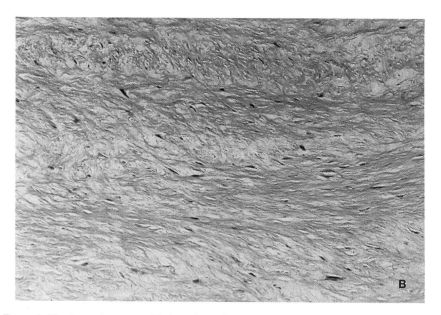

Figure 6. Histology of restenosed lesion of a saphenous vein graft. A. Excised tissue from the lesion of saphenous vein graft. This lesion was treated with PTCA 3 times prior to DCA. Restenosis occurred at 6 weeks following each intervention. Histology from 1st DCA showed organized thrombus and intimal hyperplasia with marked cellularity. B. Histology from 4th DCA for recurrent multiple restenosis. Following 3rd DCA this patient was placed on methotrexate; however, restenosis occurred 6 weeks later. Histology revealed fibrous plaque with minimal cellularity without typical intimal hyperplasia.

sary to maximize the atherectomy effect and minimize deep cuts which cause exposure of the media or adventitia. Although further study is necessary to evaluate the use of the imaging device to guide the atherectomy procedure, there is significant potential for the use of the device to improve the atherectomy procedure for better acute outcome as well as long-term outcome.

There are some advantages in performing DCA compared to some of the other new interventional technologies for primary intervention to potentially reduce restenosis. The atherectomy procedure is slightly more expensive than the PTCA procedure because of the cost of the catheter; however, it does not require extensive equipment to perform the procedure. In addition, the atherectomy patient can be handled almost the same as the PTCA patient. Prolonged hospitalization or anticoagulation following the procedure is not required and thus the patient does not require an extended hospital stay. Most of the patients following successful DCA can be discharged 24 hours following the procedure. Therefore, it does not add any risk of complication from anticoagulation and the cost of hospitalization is similar to PTCA. There are, however, some limitations of the atherectomy procedure which need to be recognized. Although the atherectomy procedure is somewhat similar to the PTCA procedure, DCA is more complex, and therefore some learning process is involved. The operator needs to be familiar with the device and guiding catheter manipulation to avoid potential complications, in addition to appropriate case selection. Compared to the other new technologies such as the stent, laser or rotablator, atherectomy seems to be the most complicated procedure from a technical point of view.

Current Method of DCA Procedure

We at Sequoia Hospital currently try to perform a more effective atherectomy with less Dotter or balloon dilatation effect. We usually select the appropriate sized device based on vessel size and currently we use a 7 French device if the vessel size is at least 3 mm or larger. If the vessel is less than 3 mm we often start with a 6 French device. Following placement of the device, we initially use minimal balloon inflation pressure (5–15 psi) to minimize balloon dilatation effect and to avoid deep cuts. Following the initial series of cuts (6–8 cuts) we evaluate the lesion with angiography. If there remains a greater than 20 or 30% stenosis, further atherectomy will be performed with higher balloon inflation pressure (20–30 psi) or use of a larger device if appropriate for the vessel size. We aim for no or minimal residual stenosis determined angiographically. We avoid overtreatment (overdilatation) of the lesion since overdilatation is often associated with media excision which may potentially increase the risk of restenosis in addition to the risk of perforation. We feel that it is important not to leave any residual stenosis; however, we also avoid overtreating the segment.

Future Prospects

Further investigation will help identify the procedure or lesion risk factors for restenosis following DCA. Although the current experience demonstrated a favorable outcome with a relatively low restenosis rate in large vessels, further analysis will help identify good candidates for DCA when this procedure is used for primary intervention for the reduction of restenosis. In addition, the "ideal DCA procedure" is not established at the present time, and should be established in the future based on our current technique. Devices for Vascular Intervention, Inc., the manufacturer of the coronary AtheroCath, is also currently working to improve some of the features of the atherectomy device. This includes a new nose cone with a lower profile using thinner balloon material, although the housing compartment is the same size as in the current device. This new design may prevent some of the nose cone-induced trauma and improve the crossing profile of the device. This improved version of the current device may help prevent some of the device-induced vessel damage or Dotter effect which may cause some of the restenosis.

Although the procedure and device have continued to evolve, we feel that the procedure is in a relatively steady phase. A randomized trial comparing DCA and PTCA (CAVEAT trial: Coronary of Angioplasty Versus Excisional Atherectomy Trial) has been organized. This is a multicenter trial involving both U.S. and European centers organized by Eric Topol, M.D. This study is designed to compare DCA and PTCA in a randomized fashion, with the primary end-point of the study being restenosis documented by six-month angiography. This trial will include approximately 1,000 randomized patients. With this study, many questions will be answered regarding restenosis as well as some of the acute outcome. Over the next few years the role of DCA as a primary intervention for both improvement of acute outcome and reduction of restenosis will become more clear through various studies.

References

1. Simpson J B (1988) Future interventional techniques. In: Califf R M, Mark D B, Wagner G S (eds) *Acute Coronary Care on the Thrombolytic Era.* Year Book Medical Publishers, Chicago, 392–404
2. Simpson J B, Selmon M R, Robertson G C, Cipriano P R, Hayden W G, Johnson D E, Fogarty T J (1988) Transluminal atherectomy for occlusive peripheral vascular disease. *Am J Cardio* 61:96G–101G
3. U. S. Directional Coronary Atherectomy Investigator Group (1990) Directional coronary atherectomy: multicenter experience. (abstract) *Circulation* 82:III–71
4. U. S. Directional Coronary Atherectomy Investigator Group (1990) Complications of directional coronary atherectomy in a multicenter experience. (abstract) *Circulation* 82:III–311
5. U. S. Directional Coronary Atherectomy Investigator Group (1990) Restenosis following

directional coronary atherectomy in a multicenter experience. (abstract) *Circulation* 82:III–679

6. Simpson J B, Baim D S, Hinohara T, Cowley M J, Smucker M L, Williams D O and the U. S. Directional Coronary Investigator Group (1991) Restenosis of de novo lesions in native coronary arteries following directional coronary atherectomy: multicenter experience. *J Am Coll Cardiol* 17:346A

7. Hinohara T, Rowe M H, Robertson G C, Selmon M R, Braden L, Leggett J H, Vetter J W, Simpson J B (1991) Effect of lesion characteristics on outcome of directional coronary atherectomy. *J Am Coll Cardiol* 17:1112–20

8. Rowe M H, Hinohara T, White N W, Robertson G C, Selmon M R, Simpson J B (1990) Comparison of dissection rates and angiographic results following directional coronary atherectomy and coronary angioplasty. *Am J Cardiol* 67:49–53

9. Whitlow P L, Robertson G C, Rowe M H, Douglas J S, Cowley M J, Kereiakes D J, Smucker M L, Hartzler G O, Hinohara T (1990) Directional coronary atherectomy for failed percutaneous transluminal coronary angioplasty. (abstract) *Circulation* 82:III–1

10. Leclerc G, Weir L, Simons M, Safian R, Kearney M, Baim D, Isner, J (1991) In Situ hybridization of human atherosclerotic material from coronary arteries and saphenous vein graft biopsied with an atherectomy catheter. *J Am Coll Cardiol* 17:73A

11. Johnson D E, Hinohara T, Simpson J B (1990) Pathology of coronary atherectomy. *J Am Coll Cardiol* 15:196A

12. Johnson D E, Hinohara T, Selmon M R, Braden L J, Simpson J B (1990) Primary peripheral arterial stenoses and restenoses excised by transluminal atherectomy: a histopathologic study. *J Am Coll Cardiol* 15:419–425

13. Johnson D, Hinohara T, Selmon M, Robertson G, Braden L, Simpson J (1991) Histologic predictors of restenosis after directed coronary atherectomy. *J Am Coll Cardiol* 17:53A

14. Waller B F, Pinkerton C A, Orr C M, Slack J D, VanTassel J W, Peters T (1991) Morphological observations late (>30 days) after clinically successful coronary balloon angioplasty. *Circulation* 83(supplI)I–28–I–41

15. Dartsch P C, Voisard R, Bauriedel G, Hofling B, Betz E (1990) Growth characteristics and cytoskeletal organization of cultured smooth muscle cells from human primary stenosing and restenosing lesions. *Arteriosclerosis* 10:62–75

12. Transluminal Extraction Endarterectomy

ROGER S. GAMMON, MICHAEL H. SKETCH JR. and
RICHARD S. STACK

Introduction

Coronary balloon angioplasty has been established as an effective means of
treating coronary artery disease in selected patients. The procedure continues
to grow in popularity, with more than 300,000 procedures performed each
year [1]. However, despite more than 10 years experience and major technical
improvements, the success of the procedure continues to be limited by two
major problems. First, balloon expansion within an atherosclerotic artery
often results in intimal dissection and this, with attendant vasospasm and
thrombus formation, results in acute thrombosis in 3–5% of cases [2–5].
Second, despite alterations in angioplasty technique and multiple trials with
systemic adjunctive drug therapy, restenosis rates remain unchanged at 30–
43% [6–13]. These limitations of PTCA have prompted development of
many new devices for coronary intervention [14].
  Our understanding of the mechanism of balloon angioplasty and the resulting complications continues to evolve. Original reports by Dotter and Judkins
[15], and subsequently Gruentzig [16], attributed improvement in luminal
diameter to compression and redistribution of plaque. However, the major
component of human coronary plaque is dense fibrocollagenous tissue with
varying amounts of calcific deposits, and deformation of this tissue with
balloon inflation would be unlikely. Subsequent studies from cadaver specimens [17, 18] and human coronaries examined after successful angioplasty
[19–22] revealed plaque fracture as a more important mechanism of improving luminal cross-sectional area. Stretching of plaque-free arterial segments, particularly with eccentric lesions, also contributes to a larger lumen
[23–27].
  Restenosis following angioplasty represents an overzealous reparative response to the injury created by balloon inflation [28–30]. Distinct from
primary atherosclerosis, the lesion of restenosis is typically a fibrocellular
intimal proliferation composed of smooth muscle cells which have migrated
from the media and changed to a synthetic phenotype [14, 31–36]. Increased

*P.W. Serruys, B.H. Strauss and S.B. King III (eds), Restenosis after Intervention with New Mechanical
Devices, 259–272.*
© 1992 *Kluwer Academic Publishers. Printed in the Netherlands.*

extracellular matrix composed of proteoglycans is also seen [37]. Restitution of vascular tone, or elastic recoil, after overstretching during balloon dilatation may also contribute to restenosis [14, 38–42]. The stretch injury itself may be a stimulus to the smooth muscle cell proliferation seen following angioplasty [43–45].

Atherectomy

The concept of transluminal atherectomy was introduced by John Simpson in an effort to overcome some of the limitations of PTCA [46, 47]. It was reasoned that by avoiding the excessive vessel distention required to effect plaque fracture, intimal dissections and acute occlusion might be reduced, and the stimulus for smooth muscle cell proliferation would be lessened [43–45]. By actually excising the plaque a greater vessel lumen and more favorable rheologic environment would be created. Postangioplasty residual stenosis is a strong determinant of restenosis. Numerous studies have found lower restenosis rates when residual stenosis was reduced [48–52]. Similarly, the rate of restenosis is inversely correlated with the improvement in luminal area during the intervention [49, 53, 54].

The Transluminal Extraction-endarterectomy Catheter

The transluminal extraction-endarterectomy catheter (TECTM) is an atherectomy device invented by Interventional Technologies, Inc. (San Diego, California) and developed at Duke University Medical Center. The device is a percutaneously introduced flexible torque tube designed to both excise and extract atherosclerotic plaque (Fig. 1). Plaque is excised by two stainless steel blades at the conical head of the catheter which rotate at 750 rpm

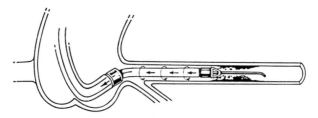

Figure 1. Diagrammatic illustration of the transluminal extraction-endarterectomy catheter excising atherosclerotic plaque as it tracks over a steerable 0.014–inch guidewire. (From Stack RS, et al (1988) Interventional cardiac catheterization at Duke University Medical Center. Am J Cardiol 62:3F–24F, with permission).

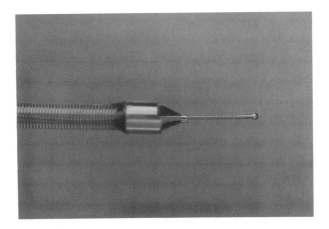

Figure 2. Close-up view of the distal end of the torque tube showing the cutter head with two
stainless steel blades, tracking over a 0.014–inch guidewire.

(Fig. 2). The excised fragments are extracted through the central lumen by
continuous vacuum suction. The proximal end of the TEC is connected to a
catheter drive unit. This unit houses the motor and trigger with a site for
attachment of a remote battery power source and a glass reservoir for retrieval of excised debris (Fig. 3). The trigger simultaneously activates the cutting
blade rotation and the vacuum system. A lever on top of the catheter drive
unit controls both the antegrade and retrograde excursion of the cutter over
a 0.014–inch guidewire.

Initial testing of safety and efficacy of the device was performed in human

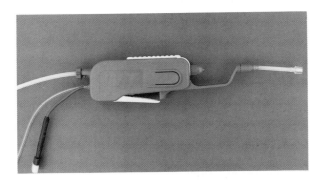

Figure 3. The TEC drive unit which houses the motor and trigger with sites for attachment of
a remote battery power source and vacuum bottle for retrieval of excised material.

cadaveric arterial segments and in vivo in canine arteries [55–57]. These studies demonstrated that the TEC could be easily maneuvered percutaneously in canine peripheral and coronary arteries. Histologic examination following operation of the TEC in normal arteries revealed focal intimal disruption with occasional excision limited to 25 percent of the medial thickness. The TEC was found to successfully remove atherosclerotic plaque from human cadaveric arterial specimens. The depth of the excision was typically limited to the media, although occasional disruption of the external elastic lamina was seen. No angiographic or histologic evidence of intimal dissection or vessel perforation were seen. These studies led to approval for clinical investigation of this device in human peripheral arteries.

The first peripheral TEC procedure was performed at Duke University Medical Center in 1987. Early experience with the TEC in peripheral arteries demonstrated a high success rate (94%) without perforation or distal embolization [58]. This study demonstrated a lesion restenosis rate of 20% and a patient restenosis rate of 32%. In 1989 this device was approved by the FDA for market release in the United States for treatment of obstructive disease in peripheral vessels.

In July 1988, clinical investigation of the TEC in coronary arteries was begun at Duke University Medical Center. After the initial 50 clinical cases at Duke, 18 additional investigational sites in the United States participated in the FDA multicenter investigation. To date, over 900 TEC procedures have been performed in the United States.

Case Selection Criteria

Initial selection criteria included patients meeting standard clinical criteria for angioplasty revascularization with proximal, discrete, concentric lesions in nontortuous vessels. With improvements in technology and growing operator experience, the selection criteria were expanded to include more diffuse and complex lesions often unfavorable for PTCA, including ostial lesions and vein graft lesions with thrombus present. Current exclusion criteria include: 1) bleeding diathesis including thrombolytic drug therapy; 2) severe peripheral vascular disease; 3) tortuous anatomy proximal to the target lesion; 4) major side branch (>2 mm) involvement at the target lesion; 5) heavily calcified lesion; 6) severe eccentricity or angulation of the target lesion; 7) coronary ectasia; or 8) aspirin allergy. As with other wire-based systems, total occlusions that cannot be crossed with the guidewire are not amenable to TEC atherectomy.

Several investigators have reported a favorable outcome with the use of the TEC in the presence of thrombus [59, 60]. The device also appears effective in treating ostial lesions. With continued operator experience and further catheter refinements, the indications for TEC atherectomy should expand.

TEC Procedure

All patients are pretreated with 325 mg of aspirin, 75 mg of dipyridamole, and a calcium channel blocker. The procedure is performed via a percutaneous transfemoral technique similar to PTCA. A #10.5 French arterial sheath is placed to allow insertion of a #10 French guide catheter. After insertion of the sheath, 10,000 units of heparin are administered; additional boluses are given hourly as needed to maintain an activated clotting time greater than 300 seconds.

The guide catheter is advanced to the ascending aorta over a 0.063–inch guide wire to prevent trauma to the vessel wall. The guide catheter is positioned in the coronary orifice and a 0.014–inch guidewire is advanced through the catheter, across the stenosis, and into the distal portion of the vessel as far as possible. The torque tube cutter is then advanced over this wire to the origin of the lesion and connected proximally to the catheter drive unit. Intracoronary nitroglycerin (0.1–0.3 mg) is administered prior to activation of the cutter to prevent coronary spasm.

Five cutter sizes are currently available: #5.5 French (1.8 mm), #6 French (2.0 mm), #6.5 French (2.2 mm), #7 French (2.3 mm), and #7.5 French (2.5 mm). Cutter size selection is based on the severity of stenosis and the adjacent normal vessel diameter. In severe stenoses, a smaller cutter is used initially, with progression to larger cutters as necessary to achieve maximal resection of the lesion. An average of three passes across the lesion are made with each cutter. A lactated Ringer's solution is infused through the guide catheter during periods of cutter activation to enhance return of excised debris. If significant residual stenosis (>25% luminal narrowing) remains after TEC, adjunctive PTCA is performed to optimize the angiographic appearance. This is frequently necessary in large coronary arteries and saphenous vein grafts, where the maximal cutter size available (2.5 mm) may not be able to remove all residual stenosis.

Following the procedure, heparin is discontinued (unless there is angiographic evidence of dissection or thrombus) and the arterial sheath is removed as soon as possible. The patient is discharged on 325 mg of aspirin daily with arrangements for clinical and 6–month angiographic follow-up.

TEC Results

With the initial 50 clinical cases at Duke University Medical Center as a foundation, the Duke Multicenter Coronary TEC Registry was initiated. In addition to Duke, this registry includes: William Beaumont Hospital in Royal Oak, Michigan (William W. O'Neill, M.D.); Wichita Institute for Clinical Research in Wichita, Kansas (Joseph P. Galichia, M.D.); Samuel Merritt Hospital in Oakland, California (Robert C. Feldman, M.D.); and Cardiovascular Institute of the South in Houma, Louisiana (Craig M. Walker, M.D.).

In a preliminary series from this registry, coronary extraction-endarterectomy with the TEC was performed on 223 lesions in 201 patients [61]. The TEC was used exclusively in 76 (34%) lesions and in conjunction with balloon angioplasty in 147 (66%). Lesion distribution included: protected left main (8), left anterior descending (53), circumflex (23), right coronary (55), and saphenous vein grafts (84). The primary success rate (<50% residual diameter stenosis by digital analysis) was 94% (130/139) in native coronary and 98% (82/84) in vein graft lesions.

Procedural complications in this initial series included: major dissection (3), coronary thrombosis (1), and perforation (4). Emergency coronary bypass surgery was required in seven (4%) patients. One patient suffered a Q-wave myocardial infarction. There were no procedural deaths. Distal embolization was not seen in any patient following use of the TEC alone.

Restenosis Following TEC Atherectomy

To date, six-month angiographic follow-up (with digital analysis) is available on 95 of 102 (93%) of eligible patients [61]. Restenosis has been defined as >50% luminal diameter narrowing at the site of previous treatment as measured by quantitative digital analysis. Forty-two out of 95 patients have angiographic restenosis, yielding a restenosis rate of 44%. These results are similar to the patient restenosis rate of 43% recently reported in 2,191 consecutive patients undergoing PTCA at Duke University Medical Center during a similar time period with 84% catheterization follow-up [13].

TEC Atherectomy in Saphenous Vein Grafts

The preliminary results of a study examining the safety and efficacy of the TEC in the management of patients with saphenous vein graft stenosis were presented at the 40th Annual Scientific Session of the American College of Cardiology in March 1991 [61]. In this study the TEC was used on 125 vein graft lesions in 98 patients. The mean vein graft age was 8.8 years with range of 1 to 18 years. Thirty percent of the lesions had been considered unsuitable for PTCA due to diffuse disease or intraluminal thrombus. The procedural success rate (<50% residual stenosis) was 96% (120/125). There was no evidence of distal embolization with myocardial infarction.

Discussion

A large number of new interventional devices have been introduced in an effort to reduce the complications of balloon angioplasty. The transluminal extraction-endarterectomy catheter is still in the early phases of evaluation.

Less than three years have passed since the first TEC procedure was performed in a human coronary artery. The initial experience with the TEC device demonstrated its ability to excise and extract atheromatous plaque percutaneously from a wide variety of sites in native vessels and vein grafts without distal embolization. The device continues to evolve, and this, combined with increased operator experience, has led to success and complication rates comparable to PTCA.

Despite theoretical reasons why atherectomy might decrease restenosis, preliminary results indicate restenosis rates following TEC atherectomy are similar to PTCA. Presently available cutter sizes necessitate use of adjunctive PTCA in two-thirds of lesions to attain desired results. This complicates the comparison of restenosis after TEC vs. PTCA. Other atherectomy devices currently under clinical investigation thus far have not shown a significant reduction in restenosis rates [62–66].

Balloon angioplasty of diffusely diseased saphenous vein grafts is associated with frequent complications, including distal embolization and myocardial infarction [67, 68]. The TEC catheter, by applying constant vacuum evacuation of excised debris, may obviate this problem. While 30% of bypass graft lesions in the initial TEC series were considered unsuitable for PTCA due to diffuse disease or intraluminal thrombus, the primary success rate was high (96%) without evidence of distal embolization or infarction. An example of TEC use in a totally occluded vein graft is shown in Fig. 4.

During TEC operation, the catheter traverses the lesion for approximately 15 seconds with each pass. This results in minimal disruption of coronary blood flow and can be shown to induce less ischemia than standard angioplasty. In the future, this feature may prove beneficial in the management of patients with multivessel disease or severe left ventricular dysfunction who do not tolerate prolonged balloon inflation.

Comparison with Other Atherectomy Devices

Two other atherectomy devices have undergone or are currently undergoing clinical investigation in coronary artery disease. The AtherocathTM (Devices for Vascular Intervention, Inc., Redwood City California) was developed by John Simpson and consists of a cylindrical unit housing a rotational cutter over a guide wire, with a small support balloon attached to the housing unit [69]. Preliminary results with this device in proximal large native coronaries are promising [70]. However, design characteristics of this device may prohibit its use in tortuous or small vessels. The Rotablator™ (Heart Technology, Inc., Bellevue, WA) consists of an oblong metal burr which rotates at approximately 180,000 rpm over a central guide wire [71]. The distal half of the burr has fine diamond abrasive particles to emulsify plaque rather than extracting it. This system is flexible and may have special utility in the treatment of distal lesions in tortuous vessels.

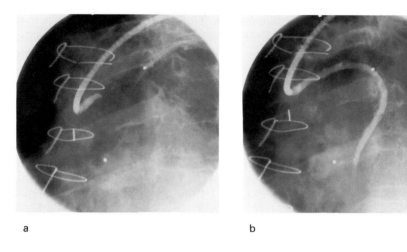

a   b

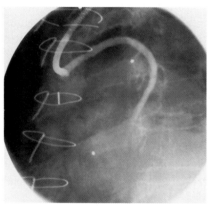

Figure 4. A: Total occlusion of a saphenous vein graft to the left anterior descending artery. A guidewire is present across the lesion. B: Result after treatment with the TEC alone. C: Final result after both the TEC and adjunctive balloon angioplasty.

c

In comparison with these devices, a unique feature of the TEC is its ability to continuously remove excised material, thereby reducing the risk of distal embolization. Since the head of the TEC cuts as it advances, it can successfully cross tight lesions despite a higher profile than balloon catheters.

The exact indications for each atherectomy device can only be determined through further use of these devices and from comparative clinical trials. Each device may play a complementary role in different types of lesions, in various locations in coronary arteries and bypass grafts.

Combining the TEC With Other Technology

Increasingly sophisticated new interventional devices may permit the combination of different technologies and enhance our ability to effectively and permanently treat atherosclerotic lesions. New imaging technologies, such as intravascular ultrasound and angioscopy, allow more accurate assessment of plaque burden and composition, and detect intraluminal thrombus and dissection [72, 73]. Intravascular ultrasound has lead to insights about the mechanism of atherectomy [74, 75] and can be used to assess the result and guide decisions regarding the need for further cuts [73, 75, 76].

Despite all the new technologies available for treating coronary artery disease, to date no device has significantly reduced restenosis. In addition, systemic adjuvant drug therapy has not been effective in controlling restenosis [77–88]. Despite success in animal models of restenosis, comparable dosing in humans would often lead to systemic toxicity. A much more efficient means of treatment would be through local drug therapy. Endovascular stents could perform as a vehicle for local drug delivery. Ideally, the stent would be placed at the site of coronary intervention and release a therapeutic agent to limit the healing process, then be absorbed by the vessel wall [56]. Bioabsorbable polymers can be fashioned into stents with excellent mechanical performance [89], and implantation of these devices into canine arteries has been successful [90]. Local drug therapy is most likely to be effective after plaque burden has been decreased. The combination of atherectomy for lesion "debridement", followed by local drug therapy, could potentially reduce restenosis.

Analysis of excised atherectomy specimens is rapidly expanding our understanding of the restenosis process [91]. Cell cultures of the excised material allow insight into the numerous mitogenic substances that may fuel the restenosis process [92–94]. A clearer understanding of the role of these substances could allow manipulation of this milieu through genetic manipulation of vascular cells at the site of intervention [95]. In vivo gene transfer has been shown to be possible [96, 97], and recently interventional techniques have been used to accomplish gene transfer in canine coronary arteries in vivo [98].

Future Developments

Evolution of the TEC design over the past several years has resulted in improved device performance. However, the major limitation of the current design is a maximum cutter size of #7.5 French (2.5 mm), often necessitating adjunctive balloon angioplasty to obtain optimal angiographic appearance in large vessels. To overcome this limitation, both an expandable cutter and eccentric cutter are being developed. In addition, alterations in cutter angle and cutter sharpness are being examined, as well as a bidirectional cutter, which could provide a more favorable rheologic environment with better laminar flow.

After completion of the developmental phases of the TEC, further studies will be necessary to evaluate the efficacy of this device for both acute and long-term outcome. Randomized trials comparing the TEC to PTCA, other new devices, and coronary artery bypass grafting, will be necessary to define the specific role of this device in myocardial revascularization.

References

1. Califf R M, Fortin D F, Frid D J, et al (1991) Restenosis after coronary angioplasty: An overview. *J Am Coll Cardiol* 17:2B–13B
2. Cowley M J, Dorros G, Kelsey S, Van Roden K, Detre K M (1984) Acute coronary events associated with percutaneous transluminal coronary angioplasty. *Am J Cardiol* 53:12C–16C
3. Bredlau C E, Roubin G S, Leimgruber P P, et al (1985) In-hospital morbidity and mortality in patients undergoing elective coronary angioplasty. *Circulation* 72:1044–1052
4. Detre K, Holubkov R, Kelsey S, et al (1988) Percutaneous transluminal coronary angioplasty in 1985–86 and 1977–81. *N Engl J Med* 318:265–270
5. Simpefendorfer C, Belardi J, Bellamy G, et al (1987) Frequency, management and follow-up of patients with acute coronary occlusion after percutaneous transluminal angioplasty. *Am J Cardiol* 59:267–269
6. McBride W, Lange R A, Hillis D L (1988) Restenosis after successful coronary angioplasty: pathology and prevention. *N Engl J Med* 318:1734–1737
7. Ernest S M, Feltz T A, Bal E T, et al (1987) Long term angiographic follow up, cardiac events and survival in patients undergoing percutaneous transluminal coronary angioplasty. *Br Heart J* 57:220–225
8. Roubin G S, King S B, Douglas J S Jr (1987) Restenosis after percutaneous transluminal coronary angioplasty: The Emory University Hospital experience. *Am J Cardiol* 60:39B–44B
9. Holmes D R Jr., Vliestra R E, Smith H C, et al (1984) Restenosis after percutaneous transluminal coronary angioplasty (PTCA): A report from the PTCA registry of the National Heart, Lung, and Blood Institute. *Am J Cardiol* 53:77C–81C
10. Pepine C J, Hirshfeld J W, MacDonald R G, et al (1990) A controlled trial of corticosteroids to prevent restenosis after coronary angioplasty. *Circulation* 81:1753–1761
11. Blackshear J L, O'Callaghan W G, Califf R M (1987) Medical approaches to prevention of restenosis after coronary angioplasty. *J Am Coll Cardiol* 9:834–848
12. Nobuyoshi M, Kimura T, Nosaka H, et al (1988) Restenosis after successful percutaneous transluminal coronary angioplasty: serial angiographic follow-up of 299 patients. *J Am Coll Cardiol* 12:616–623
13. Tcheng J E, Fortin D F, Frid D J, et al (1990) Conditional probabilites of restenosis following coronary angioplasty. *Circulation* 82:III-1
14. Waller B F (1989) "Crackers, breakers, stretchers, drillers, scrapers, shavers, burners, welders, and melters" – the future treatment of atherosclerotic coronary artery disease? A clinical-morphologic assessment. *J Am Coll Cardiol* 13:969–987
15. Dotter C T, Judkins M P (1964) Transluminal treatment of atherosclerotic obstructions: Description of new technique and a preliminary report of its application. *Circulation* 30:654–670
16. Gruentzig A R (1978) Transluminal dilatation of coronary artery stenosis. *Lancet* 1:263–266
17. Baughman K L, Pasternak R C, Fallon J T, Block P C (1981) Transluminal coronary angioplasty of postmortem human hearts. *Am J Cardiol* 48:1044–1047
18. Castaneda-Zuniga W R, Formarek A, Todavarthy M, Edwards J E (1980) The mechanism of balloon angioplasty. *Radiology* 135:565–569
19. Block P C, Myler R K, Stertzer S, Fallon J T (1981) Morphology after transluminal angioplasty in human beings. *N Engl J Med* 305:382–385

20. Mizuno K, Jurita A, Imazeki N (1984) Pathologic findings after percutaneous transluminal coronary angioplasty. *Br Heart J* 52:588–590
21. Soward A L, Essed C E, Serruys P W (1985) Coronary arterial findings after accidental death immediately after successful percutaneous transluminal coronary angioplasty. *Am J Cardiol* 56:794–795
22. Waller B F (1987) Pathology of transluminal balloon angioplasty used in the treatment of coronary heart disease. *Human Pathol* 18:476–484
23. Saner H E, Gobel F l, Salomonowitz E, Erlien D A, Edwards J E (1985) The disease-free wall in coronary atherosclerosis: its relation to degree of obstruction. *J Am Coll Cardiol* 6:1096–1099
24. Waller B F (1985) Coronary luminal shape and the arc of disease-free wall: morphologic observations and clinical relevance. *J Am Coll Cardiol* 6:1100–1101
25. Waller B F (1989) The eccentric coronary atherosclerotic plaque: morphologic observations and clinical relevance. *Clin Cardiol* 12:14–20
26. Sanborn T A, Faxon D P, Haudenschild C G, Gottsman S B, Ryan T J (1983) The mechanism of transluminal angioplasty: evidence for aneurysm formation in experimental atherosclerosis. *Circulation* 68:1136–1140
27. Faxon D P, Weber V J, Haudenschild C, et al (1982) Acute effects of transluminal angioplasty in three experimental models of atherosclerosis. *Arteriosclerosis* 2:125–133
28. Ip J H, Fuster V, Badimon L, et al (1990) Syndromes of accelerated atherosclerosis: role of vascular injury and smooth muscle cell proliferation. *J Am Coll Cardiol* 15:1667–1687
29. Hollman J (1991) What does pathology teach us about recurrent stenosis after coronary angioplasty? *J Am Coll Cardiol* 17:440–441
30. Forrester J S, Fishbein M, Helfant R, Fagin J (1991) A paradigm for restenosis based on cell biology: clues for the development of new preventive therapies. *J Am Coll Cardiol* 17:758–769
31. Liu M W, Roubin G S, King S B III (1989) Restenois after coronary angioplasty. Potential biologic determinants and role of intimal hyperplasia. *Circulation* 79:1374–1387
32. Essed C D, Brand M V D, Becker A E (1983) Transluminal coronary angioplasty and early restenosis. *Br Heart J* 49:393–396
33. Austin G E, Norman N B, Hollman J, Tabei S, Phillips D F (1985) Intimal proliferation of smooth muscle cells as an explanation for recurrent coronary stenosis after percutaneous transluminal angioplasty. *J Am Coll Cardiol* 6:369–375
34. Garratt K M, Edwards W D, Kaufmann U P, Vlietstra R E, Holmes D R Jr. (1991) Differential histopathology of primary atheroscletotic and restenotic lesions in coronary arteries and saphenous vein bypass grafts: analysis of tissue obtained from 73 patients by directional atherectomy. *J Am Coll Cardiol* 17:442–448
35. Clowes A W, Reidy M A, Clowes M M (1983) Mechanisms of stenosis after arterial injury. *Lab Invest* 49:208–215
36. Manderson J A, Mosse P R, Safatrom J A, Young S B, Campbell G R (1989) Balloon catheter injury to rabbit carotid artery. I. Changes in smooth muscle phenotype. *Arteriosclerosis* 9:289–298
37. Nobuyoshi M, Kimura T, Ohishi H, et al (1991) Restenosis after percutaneous transluminal coronary angioplasty: pathologic observations in 20 patients. *J Am Coll Cardiol* 17:433–439
38. Fischell T A, Derby G, Tse T M, Stadius M L (1988) Coronary artery vasoconstriction routinely occurs after percutaneous transluminal coronary angioplasty. A quantitative arteriographic analysis. *Circulation* 78:1323–1334
39. Rensing B J, Hermans W R, Beatt K J, et al (1990) Quantitative angiographic assessment of elastic recoil after percutaneous transluminal coronary angioplasty. *Am J Cardiol* 66:1039–1044
40. Rensing B J, Hermans W R, Strauss B H, Serruys P W (1991) Regional differences in elastic recoil after percutaneous transluminal coronary angioplasty: a quantitative angiographic study. *J Am Coll Cardiol* 17:34B–38B

41. Lehmann K G, Feuer J M, Kumamoto K S, Le H M (1990) Elastic recoil following coronary angioplasty: magnitude and contributory factors. *Circulation* 82:III–313
42. Waller B F, Pinkerton C A, Orr C M, Slack J D, VanTassel J W (1990) Two distinct types of restenosis lesions after coronary balloon angioplasty: intimal proliferation and therosclerotic plaques only. An analysis of 20 necropsy patients. *Circulation* 82:III–314
43. Leung D Y, Glagov S, Mathews M B (1976) Cyclic stretching stimulates synthesis of matrix components by arterial smooth muscle cells in vitro. *Science* 191:475–477
44. Clowes A W, Clowes M M, Fingerle J, Reidy M A (1989) Kinetics of cellular proliferation after arterial injury. V. Role of acute distension in the induction of smooth muscle cell proliferation. *Lab Invest* 60:360–364
45. Webster M W, Chesebro J H, Heras M, et al (1990) Effect of balloon inflation on smooth muscle cell proliferation in the porcine carotid artery. *J Am Coll Cardiol* 15:165A
46. Simpson J B (1988) Future interventional techniques. In: Califf RM (ed) *Acute Coronary Care in the Thrombolytic Era.* Year Book Medical Publishers, Chicago, 392–404
47. Simpson J B, Robertson G C, Selmon M R (1988) Percutaneous coronary atherectomy. *J Am Coll Cardiol* 11:110A
48. Lambert M, Bonan R, Cote G, et al (1988) Multiple coronary angioplasty: a model to discriminate systemic and procedural factors related to restenosis. *J Am Coll Cardiol* 12:310–314
49. Guiteras V P, Bourassa M G, David P R, et al (1987) Restenosis after successful percutaneous transluminal coronary angioplasty: the Montreal Heart Institute experience. *Am J Cardiol* 60:50B–55B
50. Mata L A, Bosch X, David P R, et al (1985) Clinical and angiographic assessment 6 months after double vessel percutaneous coronary angioplasty. *J Am Coll Cardiol* 6:1239–1244
51. Rapold H J, David P R, Guiteras V P, et al (1987) Restenosis and its determinants in first and repeat coronary angioplasty. *Eur Heart J* 8:575–586
52. Ellis S G, Roubin G S, King S B III, Douglas J S Jr, Cox W R (1989) Importance of stenosis morphology in the estimation of restenosis risk after elective percutaneous transluminal coronary angioplasty. *Am J Cardiol* 63:30–34
53. Levine S, Ewels C J, Rosing D R, Kent K M (1985) Coronary angioplasty: clinical and angiographic follow-up. *Am J Cardiol* 55:673–676
54. DiSciascio G, Cowley M J, Vetrovec G W (1986) Angiographic patterns of restenosis after angioplasty of multiple coronary arteries. *Am J Cardiol* 58:922–925
55. Perez J A, Hinohara T, Quigley P J, et al (1988) In-vitro and in-vivo experimental results using new wire-guided concentric atherectomy device. *J Am Coll Cardiol* 11:109A
56. Stack R S, Califf R M, Phillips H R, et al (1988) Advances in cardiovascular technologies: Interventional cardiac catheterization at Duke University Medical Center. *Am J Cardiol* 62:1F–44F
57. Sketch M H Jr, Phillips H R, Lee M, Stack R S (1991) Coronary transluminal extraction-endarterectomy. *J Inv Cardiol* 3:23–28
58. Sketch M H Jr, Newman G E, McCann L, et al (1989) Transluminal extraction-endarterectomy in peripheral vascular disease: late clinical and angiographic follow-up. *Circulation* 80:II–305
59. Rosenblum J, Pensabene J F, Kramer B (1991) The TEC divice: distal atherectomy and removal of an intracoronary thombus. *J Inv Cardiol* 3:41–43
60. O'Neill W W, Meany T B, Kramer B, et al (1991) The role of atherectomy in the management of saphenous vein graft disease. *J Am Coll Cardiol* 17:384A
61. Sketch M H Jr, O'Neill W W, Galichia J P, et al (1991) The Duke Multicenter Coronary Transluminal Extraction-Endarterectomy Registry: acute and chronic results. *J Am Coll Cardiol* 17:31A
62. Rogers P J, Garratt K N, Kaufmann U P, et al (1990) Restenosis after atherectomy versus PTCA: initial experience. *J Am Coll Cardiol* 15:196A

63. Holmes D R, Garratt K N, Bell M R (1990) Follow-up events after directional coronary atherectomy. *Circulation* 82:III–493

64. Robertson G C, Selmon M R, Hinohara T, et al (1990) The effect of lesion length on outcome of directional coronary atherectomy. *Circulation* 82:III–623

65. U.S. Directional Coronary Atherectomy Investigator Group (1990) Restenosis following directional coronary atherectomy in a multicenter experience. *Circulation* 82:III–679

66. Buchbinder M, Warth D, O'Neill, et al (1991) Multi-center registry of percutaneous coronary rotational ablation using the rotablator. *J Am Coll Cardiol* 17:31A

67. Saber R S, Edwards W D, Holmes D R Jr, Vlietstra R E, Reeder G S (1988) Balloon angioplasty of aortocoronary saphenous vein bypass grafts: a histopathologic study of six grafts from five patients, with emphasis on restenosis and embolic complications. *J Am Coll Cardiol* 12:1501–1509

68. Margolis J R, Mogensen L, Mehta S, Chen C Y, Krauthamer D (1991) Diffuse embolization following percutaneous transluminal coronary angioplasty of occluded vein grafts: the blush phenomenon. *Clin Cardiol* 14:489–493

69. Simpson J B, Selmon M R, Robertson G B, et al (1988) Transluminal atherectomy for occlusive peripheral vascular disease. *Am J Cardiol* 61:96G–101G

70. Simpson J B, Rowe M H, Selmon M R, et al (1990) Restenosis following atherectomy in de novo lesions of native coronary arteries. *Circulation* 82:III–313

71. Hansen D D, Auth D C, Hall M, Ritchie J L (1988) Rotational endarterectomy in normal canine coronary arteries: preliminary report. *J Am Coll Cardiol* 11:1073–1077

72. White N W, Webb J G, Rowe M H, et al (1989) Atherectomy guidance using intravascular ultrasound: quantitation of plaque burden. *Circulation* 80:II–374

73. Yock P G, Fitzgerald P J, Linker D T, Angelsen B A J (1991) Intravascular ultrasound guidance for catheter-based coronary interventions. *J Am Coll Cardiol* 17:39B–45B

74. Smucker M L, Howard P F, Scherb D E, Kil D, Saranat W S (1991) Is intracoronary ultrasound a valid means to assess the mechanism of atherectomy? *J Am Coll Cardiol* 17:126A

75. Keren G, Pichard A D, Satler L F, et al (1991) Intravascular ultrasound of saphenous vein grafts after PTCA and investigational angioplasty procedures. *J Am Coll Cardiol* 17:126A

76. Keren G, Pichard A D, Satler L F, et al (1991) Intravascular ultrasound of coronary atherectomy. *J Am Coll Cardiol* 17:157A

77. Thornton M A, Gruentzig A R, Hollman J, et al (1984) Coumadin and aspirin in prevention of recurrence after transluminal coronary angioplasty: a randomized study. *Circulation* 69:721–727

78. White C W, Knudson M, Schmidt D, et al (1987) Ticlopidine Study Group: neither ticlopidine nor aspirin-dipyridamole prevents restenosis post PTCA: results from a randomized placebo-controlled multicenter trial. *Circulation* 76:IV–213

79. Mufson L, Black A, Roubin G, et al (1988) A randomized trial of aspirin in PTCA: effect of high vs. low dose aspirin on major complications and restenosis. *J Am Coll Cardiol* 11:236A

80. Schanzenbacher P, Grimmer M, Maiasch B, Kochsiek K (1988) Effect of high dose and low dose aspirin on restenosis after primary successful angioplasty. *Circulation* 78:II–99

81. Slack O D, Van Tassel J, Orr C M, et al (1987) Can fish oil supplement minimize restenosis after percutaneous transluminal coronary angioplasty? *J Am Coll Cardiol* 9:64A

82. Grigg L E, Kay T W, Valentine P A, et al (1989) Determinants of restenosis and lack of effect of dietary supplementation with eicosapentaenoic acid on the incidence of coronary artery restenosis after angioplasty. *J Am Coll Cardiol* 13:665–672

83. Reis G S, Sipperly M E, Boucher T M, et al (1988) Results of a randomized double-blind placebo-controlled trial of fish oil for prevention of restenosis after PTCA. *Circulation* 78:II–291

84. Corcos T, David P R, Val P G, et al (1985) Failure of diltiazem to prevent restenosis after percutaneous transluminal coronary angioplasty. *Am Heart J* 109:926–931
85. Whitworth H B, Roubin G S, Hollman J, et al (1986) Effect of nifedipine on recurrent stenosis after percutaneous transluminal coronary angioplasty. *J Am Coll Cardiol* 8:1271–1276
86. Klein W, Eber B, Fluch N, Dusleag J (1989) Ketanserin prevents acute occlusion but not restenosis after PTCA. *J Am Coll Cardiol* 13:44A
87. Ellis S G, Roubin G S, Wilentz J, et al (1989) Effect of 18– to 24–hour heparin administration for prevention of restenosis after uncomplicated coronary angioplasty. *Am Heart J* 117:777–782
88. O'Keefe J H, McCallister B D, Bateman T M, et al (1991) Colchicine for the prevention of restenosis after coronary angioplasty. *J Am Coll Cardiol* 17:181A
89. Gammon R S, Chapman G D, Agrawal G M, et al (1991) Mechanical features of the Duke biodegradable stent. *J Am Coll Cardiol* 17:235A
90. Chapman G D, Gammon R S, Bauman R P, et al (1990) A bioabsorbable stent: initial experimental results. *Circulation* 82:III–72
91. Johnson D E, Hinohara T, Selmon M R, Braden L J, Simpson J B (1990) Primary peripheral arterial stenoses and restenoses by transluminal atherectomy: a histopathologic study. *J Am Coll Cardiol* 15:419–425
92. Windstetter U, Bauriedel G, Uberfuhr P, et al (1991) Cell culture of human coronary plaques obtained by percutaneous and intraoperative atherectomy. *J Am Coll Cardiol* 17:194A
93. Leclerc G, Weir L, Simons M, et al (1991) In situ hybridization of human atherosclerotic material from coronary arteries and saphenous vein graft biopsied with an atherectomy catheter. *J Am Coll Cardiol* 17:73A
94. Flugelman M Y, Correa R, Zu-Xi Y, et al (1991) Fibroblast growth factors are expressed in coronary lesions of patients with unstable angina pectoris and those who have post angioplasty restenosis. *J Am Coll Cardiol* 17:73A
95. Swain J L (1989) Gene therapy. A new approach to the treatment of cardiovascular disease. *Circulation* 80:1495–1496
96. Nabel E G, Plautz G, Nabel G J (1990) Site-specific gene expression in vivo by direct gene transfer into the arterial wall. *Science* 249:1285–1288
97. Lim C S, Chapman G D, Gammon R S, et al (1991) Direct in vivo gene transfer into the coronary and peripheral vasculature of the intact dog. *Circulation* 83:2007–2011
98. Chapman G D, Lim C S, Swain J L, Gammon R S, Bauman R P, Stack R S (1991) In vivo cardiovascular gene transfer via interventional technique: Initial experimental results. *J Am Coll Cardiol* 17:25A

PART FIVE

Rotational Ablation

Introduction: Angioplasty with High Speed Rotary Ablation

DAVID C. AUTH

Scientific Rationale

Barotrauma and Debulking: *Two Methods of Increasing Luminal Diameter*

There are two commonly accepted methods of increasing the luminal dia-meter of a vessel using percutaneous techniques. The first method is baro-trauma. Barotrauma is a term used to describe either dottering (with a fixed diameter, wedge shaped instrument) or angioplasty using a balloon catheter. Barotrauma results in the circumferential enlargement of the vessel to facili-tate increased blood flow through the occluded arterial segment.

Barotrauma increases the luminal space within a vessel by expanding the diameter of an artery. In the early days of angioplasty it was believed that plaque could be physically compressed against the artery wall. It was later realized that this assumption was erroneous because atheromatous plaque is generally incompressible. Thus, in order to provide more luminal space for blood to flow through the stenotic segment, dottering and balloon angioplasty must either open up fissures and cracks in the plaque or stretch the wall to expand the residual opening of the stenosis. These methods of increasing luminal diameter create a permanent distortion of the architecture of the artery. Such permanent restructuring of the arterial wall is accomplished by rupturing the muscular structure within the wall and by creating voids in the plaque itself. This also causes physical displacement of the plaque relative to the underlying medial substrate which results in dissection between the plaque and the artery (Fig. 1). Such physical displacement of the plaque relative to the medial underpinnings creates flaps which can lead to abrupt closure of the artery if the flap falls across the lumen. Deep rupture of the media must occur for a permanent stretch distortion of the artery. Such deep medial injury is thought to promote intimal hyperplasia.

Another problem associated with barotrauma is elastic recoil. This occurs when the arterial segment has not been enlarged sufficiently to cause perma-nent muscular distention. Over time, the artery will attempt to regain its

P.W. Serruys, B.H. Strauss and S.B. King III (eds), Restenosis after Intervention with New Mechanical Devices, 275–288.
© 1992 *Kluwer Academic Publishers. Printed in the Netherlands.*

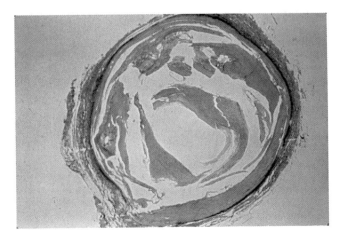

Figure 1. Photomicrograph of the cross-section of an artery treated with balloon angioplasty showing multiple flaps and dissections.

normal muscular tone. As this occurs, the artery "recoils" to its original size and shape, once again reducing blood flow.

The second method of increasing the luminal diameter and the flow rate of blood through a stenosed arterial segment is to debulk or remove the plaque. Debulking has a number of intuitive advantages over dottering and balloon angioplasty. The arterial injury resulting from stretching and baro-trauma is reduced or eliminated. In addition, the offending material is re-moved along with a theoretically reduced propensity for abrupt closure caused by flaps and dissections suddenly occluding blood flow.

In order to avoid the arterial trauma necessarily associated with permanent stretching and distortion of the artery, several approaches have been pro-posed and evaluated during the past decade to physically remove plaque from within an artery. Lasers and various mechanical atherectomy devices have been suggested and in many cases clinically tested. Many laser catheters achieve improvement of the lumen angiographically by a combination of dottering and debulking. The way that lasers accomplish debulking is by using light energy to break up plaque into particles which are subsequently washed away in the blood. Unfortunately, the particles that are produced with laser energy can be quite large, in some cases larger than 50 microns. Contrary to common beliefs, lasers do not have the energy available at the catheter tip to "vaporize" plaque. Instead, they rely on rapidly boiling pockets of water based materials which in turn cause small micro explosions. These micro explosions disrupt and break off particles of plaque. Excimer lasers produce particles in the range of 20 microns in diameter. Various mechanical atherectomy devices have been employed which use sharp cutting blades of steel to slice away plaque and either store the plaque fragments in a chamber which is subsequently emptied outside of the body or attempt to

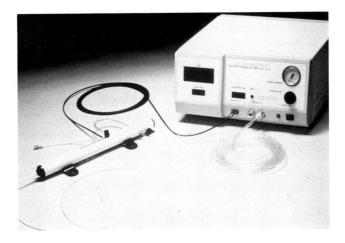

Figure 2. Rotablator® advancer and console.

evacuate the plaque through a luminal conduit to which a vacuum is applied. Lesion composition, shape, and size can have an effect on the effectiveness of these methods.

One "atherectomy" device, the Rotablator, is predicated on the concept that fragments of plaque can be disposed of by the body's own disposal mechanism provided the fragments are predictably small enough to pass through the capillary network and be ingested by phagocytes.

Rotablator System

The Rotablator is a gas powered mechanical angioplasty system. The system is comprised of the Rotablator advancer/catheter, the guide wire, the console and a source of air or nitrogen to power the device (Fig. 2).

The Rotablator advancer/catheter contains a small turbine. When the device is activated with a foot pedal, the flexible drive shaft rotates the catheter tip at a speed of 150,000–190,000 rpm. The drive shaft spins within a 4FR Teflon® sheath. This sheath protects the arterial tissue from potential injury caused by the spinning shaft and also acts as a conduit for a flush of saline. The low pressure flush flows at approximately 10 cc/min. The catheter tip is precisely advanced across the lesion using the small knob on the top of the advancer.

The catheter tip is coated with hundreds of tiny diamond crystals (Fig. 3). With each revolution the diamond crystals remove tiny scoops of plaque from the artery. The particles removed are smaller than a red blood cell and so pass from the body via the reticuloendothelial system. The removal of these tiny particles, at high speed produces an extremely smooth, polished

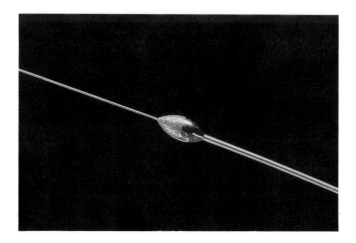

Figure 3. Rotablator catheter, burr tip and drive shaft.

surface. In addition because the cutting surfaces are made of diamonds, they can remove even the hardest calcified plaque.

The Rotablator catheter tracks over a steerable 0.009 inch diameter guide wire with a 0.017 inch atraumatic spring tip (Fig. 4).

The console is used to monitor and control the speed of rotation of the drive shaft and catheter tip. Fiber optic cables from the advancer/catheter connect to the console to measure and display the speed of rotation of the burr. The speed of the advancer turbine is controlled by the pressure and volume of gas passing from the console to the advancer.

Physical Principles and Design Characteristics

The Rotablator is based on several basic principles of physics. These principles combined with specific design features have produced an effective clinical device.

Differential Cutting

Of all of the features of the Rotablator, none is more important than differential cutting. Figure 5 illustrates this concept. When a sharp knife or cutting surface is passed over an elastic material at an oblique angle it deforms the material without cutting it. By contrast when the same knife is passed over inelastic material it cuts the surface. The elastic tissue is able to move away from the knife while the inelastic material can not. This inelastic material is cut but the elastic material is spared. This is commonly demonstrated in the act of shaving wherein the elastic skin and tissue of the face escapes injury

Figure 4. Rotablator .009 inch (.017 inch tip) guide wires.

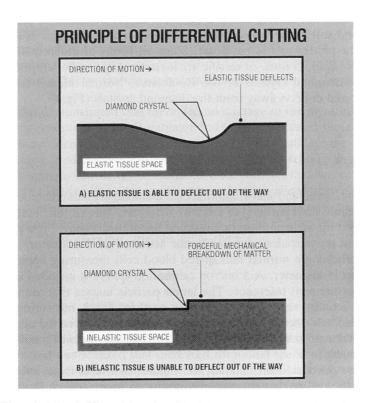

Figure 5. The principle of differential cutting: Elastic material moves away from the cutting surfaces. Inelastic material can not move away and is therefore cut.

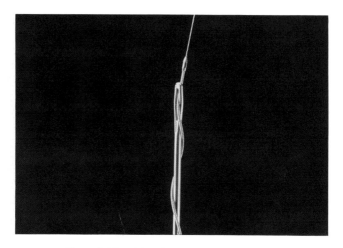

Figure 8. The drive shaft is small and flexible.

negotiate severely tortuous arterial segments. Figure 8 is a photograph of a Rotablator drive shaft wound around and through a needle. The Rotablator can negotiate curves with a radius of curvature less than 5 mm.

Orthogonal Displacement of Friction

Orthogonal displacement of friction is a principle of physics referring to the change in the effective friction in one direction between two adjacent sliding surfaces that results from relative motion between the two surfaces in a plane perpendicular to that direction. Friction normally occurs between sliding surfaces in contact and opposes the relative motion between them. However, when the available friction is used up by a large sliding motion in one direction, then little friction is available at 90° (i.e., perpendicular or ortho-gonal) to the sliding motion direction.

This principle is easily demonstrated by pulling a cork out of a bottle. If the cork is twisted as it is pulled, the frictional force is reduced and the cork comes out much easier. The faster the cork is turned, the more easily the cork is withdrawn. This phenomenon is also experienced when lateral resistance to sliding is lost in an automobile as excessive forward spinning of tires is produced. Common examples include "fishtailing" of a car spinning its wheels in the snow, or a dragster fishtailing as it leaves the starting gate. This physical principle is useful in the exchange over the guide wire of one size Rotablator for another because it grossly reduces the longitudinal friction whenever the system is operating in excess of a few thousand RPM. When the Rotablator spins at 60,000 RPM and above, the longitudinal friction vector is virtually eliminated. When the Rotablator is spinning, the reduction of the longitudinal friction vector provides for extremely low drag of the

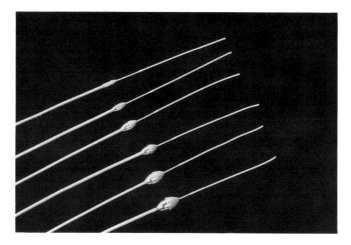

Figure 9. The Rotablator is available in a range of catheter tip sizes.

drive shaft over the guide wire. This facilitates smooth exchange over a guide wire even when tortuosity would normally impair trackability.

This characteristic provided by the principle of the orthogonal displacement of friction is a great convenience to the physician when treating distal and hard to reach atheromatous lesions.

Arterial Sizing

Matching the correct catheter tip diameter for the arterial diameter is crucial to the success of the procedure. A catheter tip that is too small results in an inadequate luminal diameter. A tip that is too large can cause damage to the arterial wall. Arterial injury occurs when the tip stretches the artery past its elastic limit. When the artery is no longer elastic, the diamond crystals will tend to ablate it. This is analogous to exerting too much pressure with a razor against the skin while shaving. If the elastic potential of the skin is exceeded by the razor, the blade will nick the skin. Similar to balloon angioplasty, sizing the catheter is an important aspect of the procedure. With sizes ranging from 1.25 mm to 2.5 mm in small increments for coronary devices (and up to 4.5 mm for peripheral devices) it is possible to select an appropriately sized burr for each artery and lesion of interest (Fig. 9). Because of the exchangeable guide wire, it is possible to produce a small initial channel through a very tight occlusion and change to a larger catheter tip while leaving the guide wire in place for safety and convenience. The wide range of burr sizes and the ready exchangeability enable the Rotablator to effectively treat lesions in very narrow vessels as well as large coronary arteries.

The features of diamond cutting surfaces, differential cutting, excellent

References

1. Zacca N M, Raizner A E, Noon G P, Short III D H, Weilbaecher D G, Gotto Jr, A M, Roberts R (1988). Short term follow up of patients treated with a recently developed rotational atherectomy device and in vivo assessment of the particles generated. *JACC* II:2, 109A

2. Fourrier J L, Stankowiak C, LaBlanche J M, Prat A, Brunetaud J M, Bertrand M E (1988). Histopathology after rotational angioplasty of peripheral arteries in human beings. *JACC* II:2,IO9A

3. Fourrier J L, Auth D, LaBlanche J M, Brunetaud J, Gommeaux A, Bertrand M E (1988) Human percutaneous coronary rotational atherectomy: preliminary results. *Circulation,* Supplement II, 78:4, II–82

4. Ginsburg R, Jenkins N, Wright A, Wexler L, McCowan L, Mehighan J (1988) Transluminal peripheral vessel angioplasty: clinical experience with new therapeutic devices. *Circulation,* Supplement II, 78:4, II–270

5. Thorpe, P E, Ginsburg R, Wright A M, Kusnick C A, Baxter R, Wittich G R, Jenkins N, Wexler L (1988) Evolution of lower extremity angioplasty: Stanford experience comparing the use of Laser, Kensey Catheter, Rotablator^{TM}, and Atherectomy Catheter as adjuncts to balloon angioplasty for vascular occlusions. *Radioloy*, Volume 169P, Supplement 306

6. Kusnick C A, Wright A M, Ginsburg R, Thorpe P E, Jenkins N, Wexler L (1988) High speed rotary atherectomy in the lower extremities: early results with the Rotablator^{TM}. *Radiology*, Volume 169P, Supplement 306

7. Hatfield S, (1989) Research reporting preliminary success with Rotablator^{TM}. *Advance*, Volume 2, No 1, 1

8. Zacca N M, Raizner A E, Noon G P , Short III, D, Weilbaecher D, Gotto Jr. A, Roberts R (1989) Treatment of symptomatic peripheral atherosclerotic disease with a rotational atherectomy device. *AJC* 63, 77–80

9. O'Neill W W, Bates R E, Kirsh M, Bassett J, Sakwa M, Elliott M, Doppke D (1989) Mechanical transluminal coronary endarterectomy: initial clinical experience with the Auth mechanical rotary catheter. *JACC* 13:2, 227A

10. Fourrier J L, Auth D, Lablanche J M, Brunetaud J M, Gommeaux A, Bertrand M E (1989) Human percutaneous coronary rotational atherectomy: results and short follow up. *JACC* 13:2, 228A

11. Erbel R, Dietz U, Auth D, Haude M, Nixdorf U, Meyer III J (1989) Percutaneous transluminal coronary rotablation during heart catheterization. *JACC* 13:2, 228A

12. Erbel R, O'Neill W, Auth D, Haude M, Nixdorf U, Dietz U, Rupprecht H J, Tschollar W, Meyer J (1989) Hochfrequenz-Rotationsatherektomie bei koronarer Herzkrankheit (High frequency rotational atherectomy in coronary heart disease). *Deutsche Medizinische Wochenschrift* 114:13, 487–495

13. Erbel R, O'Neill W, Auth D, Haude N, Nixdorf U, Rupprecht H J, Dietz U, Meyer J (1989) High-frequency rotablation of occluded coronary artery during heart catheterization. *Cathet Cardiovasc Diagn* 17:56–58

14. Fourrier J L (1989) Atherectomie Coronaire Par "Rotablator. *Ann. Cariol. Angeiol.* 38:505–508

15. Fourrier, J L, Bertrand M E, Auth D C, LaBlanche J M, Gommeaux A, Brunetaud J M, Percutaneous coronary rotational angioplasty in humans: preliminary report. *ACC* 11–89, (in press)

16. Ginsburg R, Teirstein P S, Warth D C, Haq N, Jenkins N S, McCowan L C (1989) Percutaneous transluminal coronary rotational atheroblation: clinical experience in 40 patients. *Circulation*, Supplement II, 80:4

17. O'Neill W W, Friedman H Z , Cragg D, Strzelecki M R, Gangadharan V, Levine A B, Ramos R G (1989) Initial clinical experience and early follow-up of patients undergoing mechanical rotary endarterectomy. *Circulation*, Supplement II, 80:4

18. Fourrier J L, Auth D, Lablanche J M, Brunetaud J M, Gommeaux A, Bertrand M E First percutaneous coronary rotational atherectomies in man. *European Heart Journal*, Vol 9,

19. Pannen B, Dietz U, Erbel R, Iversen S, Nixdorf U, Meyer J, Auth D (1989) Ultrastructural changes in coronary arteries after rotational angioplasty: possible relevance of dotter effects. *European Heart Journal*, Vol 10

20. Erbel R, Dietz U, Auth D, Oner E, Haude M, Nixdorf U, Meyer J (1989) Percutaneous transluminal coronary rotablation: efficacy and safety analysis. *European Heart Journal*, Vol 10

21. Rupprecht H J, Erbel R, Brennecke R, Stadtfeld M, Meyer J (1989) Measurement of coronary flow reserve using a Doppler catheter after rotational coronary angioplasty. *European Heart Journal*, Vol 10

22. Niazi K, Brodsky M, Friedman H, Gangadharan, V, Choksi N, O'Neill W (1990) Restenosis after successful mechanical rotary atherectomy with the Auth Rotablator. *JACC*, Vol 15, No 2, 57A

23. Tierstein P S, Ginsburg P, Warth D, Hoq N, Jenkins N, McCowan L (1990) Complications of human coronary rotablation. *JACC*, Vol 15, No. 2: 57A

24. Zacca N, Heibig J, Harris S, Kleiman N, Staudacher R, Smith S, Khalil J A, Roberts R (1990) Percutaneous coronary high speed rotational atherectomy. *JACC*, Vol 15 No. 2, 58A

25. Buchbinder M, O'Neill W, Warth D, Zacca N, Dietz U, Bertrand M E, Fourrier J L, Leon M B (1990) Percutaneous coronary rotational ablation using the Rotablator: results of a multicenter study. *Circulation*, Supplement III, Vol 82, Number 4, III–309

26. Bertrand M E, Fourrier J L, Dietz U, DeJaegere P (1990) European experience with percutaneous transluminal coronary rotational ablation. Immediate results. *Circulation*, Supplement III, Vol 82, Number 4, III–310

27. Rodriguez A R, Zacca N, Heibig J, Warth D, Harris S, Staudacher R, Smith G S, Minor S T, Abukhalil J M, Raizner A E, Kleiman N S (1990) Coronary rotary ablation using a single large burr and without balloon assistance. *Circulation*, Supplement III, Vol 82, Number 4, III–310

28. Schieman G, McDaniel M, Fenner J, Mehl J K, Rivera I, Podolin R A, Peterson K L, Buchbinder M (1990) Quantitative angiographic assessment of percutaneous transluminal coronary rotational ablation. *Circulation*, Supplement III, Vol 82 Number 4, III–493

29. Cheirif J B, Heibig J, Harris S, Staudacher R, Brown D, Quinones M A, Zacca N (1990) Rotational ablation is associated with less myocardial ischemia than PTCA. *Circulation*, Supplement III, Vol 82, Number 4, III–493

30. Fourrier J L, Lefebvre J M, Henry M, Dorros G, Ginsburg R, Zacca N M, Walker C M (1990) Rotational atherectomy in complex and long peripheral lesions – multicentric study. *International Course on Peripheral Vascular Intervention*

31. Dorros G (1990) Percutaneous rotational atherectomy (Rotablator) in peripheral lesions. *International Course on Peripheral Vascular Intervention*

32. Zaitoun R, Dorros G, Iyer S S, Lewin R F (1990) Percutaneous high speed rotational atherectomy (Rotablator) of a restenosed ostial renal artery: A case report. *Cathet Cardiovasc Diagn* 20:254–256

33. Bertrand M E, Lablanche J M, Fourrier J L, Bauters C, Leroy F (1990) Percutaneous coronary rotary ablation, abstract from article in *Herz* 15(5):285–91

34. Zotz R, Stahr P, Erbel R, Auth D, Meyer J (1991) Analysis of high-speed frequency rotational angioplasty-induced echo contrast. *Cathet Cardiovasc Diagn* 22:137–144

35. Bertrand M, Fourrier J, Buchbinder M, Warth D, O'Neill Wm, Zacca N, Erbel R, Leon M (1991) Abrupt closure following rotational ablation with the rotablator – short term clinical follow-up. *JACC*, Vol. 17, No. 2, 22A

36. Buchbinder M, Warth D, O'Neill Wm, Zacca N, Ginsburg R, Bertrand M, Erbel R, Fourrier J, Leon M (1990) Multi-center registry of percutaneous coronary rotational ablation using the rotablator. *JACC*, Vol 17, No. 2, 31A

37. Harris S L, Staudacher R A, Heibig J P, Minor S T, Abukhalil J M, Kleiman N S, Raizner A E, Zacca N M (1991) Rotational coronary ablation achieves lumen size comparable to balloon angioplasty without stretching the arterial wall. *JACC*, Vol. 17, No. 2, 124A

38. Warth D, Buchbinder M, O'Neill Wm, Zacca N, Bertrand M, Fourrier J, Erbel R (1990)

Rotational ablation using the rotablator for angiographically unfavorable lesions. *JACC*, Vol. 17, No. 2, 125A

39. Pavlides G S, Hauser A M, Dudlets P I, O'Neill Wm (1991) The value of transesophageal echocardiographic imaging during high-risk coronary intervention. *JACC*, Vol.17, No. 2, 127A

40. Keren G, Pichard A D, Satler L F, Hansch E C, Oblon C, Leon M B, Kent K K (1991) Intravascular ultrasound of coronary atherectomy. *JACC*, Vol. 17, No. 2, 157A

41. Niazi K, Cragg D R, Strzelecki M, Friedman H A, Gangadharan V, O'Neill Wm (1991) Angiographic risk factors for coronary restenosis following mechanical rotational atherectomy. *JACC*, Vol 17, No. 2, 218A

42. Erbel R, Stahr P, Dietz U, Zotz R, Brennecke R, Meyer J (1991) High frequency rotational angioplasty induced echocardiographic contrast. *JACC*, Vol. 17, No. 2, 259A

13. Percutaneous Transluminal Coronary Rotary Ablation with Rotablator: European Experience

MICHEL E. BERTRAND, JEAN M. LABLANCHE, FABRICE
LEROY, CHRISTOPHE BAUTERS, PETER DE JAEGERE,
PATRICK W. SERRUYS, JURGEN MEYER, ULRICH DIETZ
and RAIMUND ERBEL

Introduction

Over the past decade, it has been recognized that percutaneous transluminal coronary angioplasty [1] is a very effective method of myocardial revascularization. Nevertheless, in spite of real advances in technique and equipment, there are still several limitations: These include the treatment of ostial lesions, diffuse disease and complex lesions with surface irregularity or marked eccentricity etc. Lastly, restenosis of the dilated segment can occur in 30 to 35% [2] particularly when multiangioplasties are performed [3]. These problems have driven engineers and interventional cardiologists to develop and to explore new methods of recanalization including laser angioplasty, implantation of endovascular prostheses and atherectomy. This term, now applied to any catheter-based mechanical device removing atherosclerotic material from the vessel wall in situ, includes directional or excisional atherectomy (J. Simpson), transluminal extraction atherectomy (R.Stack)[4] and rotary ablation (RA) with the Rotablator (D. Auth)[7–17].

In this chapter, we present the results obtained in three European centers with high speed rotary ablation.

Material and Methods

Description of the Rotary Ablation Device

The Rotablator^{TM} (Heart Technology,Inc.,Bellevue, Washington, USA) consists of an abrasive tip welded to a long flexible drive shaft tracking along a central flexible guide wire (Fig. 1). The ablation tip is an elliptically shaped burr of various sizes (1.0, 1.25, 1.50, 1.75, 2.00, 2.15, 2.25 and 2.5 mm in diameter). The distal portion of the burr is coated with diamond chips of 30–50 microns. Rotational energy is transmitted by a disposable compressed air-motor driving the flexible helical shaft at very high speed up to 190,000

P.W. Serruys, B.H. Strauss and S.B. King III (eds), Restenosis after Intervention with New Mechanical Devices, 289–296.
© 1992 *Kluwer Academic Publishers. Printed in the Netherlands.*

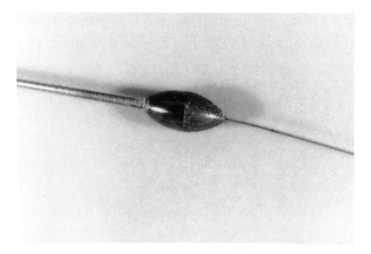

Figure 1. Distal aspect of the Rotablator™ and the burr.

rpm. The number of revolutions per minute is measured by a fiberoptic light probe and displayed on a control panel. The speed of rotation is controlled by the air pressure, which itself is controlled by a pedal. During rotation a small volume of sterile saline solution irrigates the catheter sheath to lubricate and cool the rotating system. The burr and the drive shaft track along a central coaxial guide wire (0.009″) with a flexible radioopaque platinum distal part (20 mm). The central guide wire can be controlled and moved with a pin vise. The wire and abrasive tip can be advanced independently; thus, the wire could be placed in the selected artery,thereby directing the burr safely into the diseased artery. The steerable guide wire does not rotate with the burr during abrasion.

Protocol

The patients receive Nifedipine (60 mg) and Aspirin (500 mg) the day before the procedure. Sedation is obtained with an IV injection of 50 mg of Chlorodiazepate. After local anesthesia, a sheath is inserted into the femoral artery. A guiding catheter is placed into the ostium of the coronary artery to perform an initial angiogram made in 3 different projections after IC injection of 2 mg of isosorbide dinitrate. Then, ten thousand units of Heparin are intravenously injected. Rotary ablation begins with the placement of the small guide wire across the lesion to a safe distal vessel location, sometimes guided by a 3F infusion catheter which was positioned first. Then, the burr and the drive shaft are manually advanced over the guide wire to the lesion site. The motor is activated and rotation starts. When the adequate speed of rotation is reached (175,000 rpm) the abrasive tip is advanced gently over the guidewire.

If a resistance is encountered, the tip is successively pulled back and advanced to maintain a high speed rotation. Several slow passes are required to achieve the maximal plaque removal.

This protocol was approved by the individual local Ethical Committees. All the patients gave their written informed consent. The angiographic results of Lille and Rotterdam were assessed with automatic computerized quantitative coronary angiography. Primary success of rotary ablation was defined as a significant reduction ($>20\%$) of stenosis without complications. When the residual stenosis after rotational atherectomy remained significant ($>50\%$), a percutaneous transluminal balloon angioplasty completed the procedure.

Within the in-hospital period, several electrocardiograms and repeat creatine kinase measurements were performed during the first 48 hours. The patients were discharged with a regimen of Aspirin (100 or 500 mg) and Nifedipine (60 mg). and underwent coronary angiography 3 to 6 months after the procedure.

Study Population

One hundred and twenty-nine patients (107 males, 22 females), mean age: 57 yrs (range 33 to 68), underwent rotary ablation (RA). Sixty five patients were treated in Lille (France), fifty four in Mainz (Germany) and ten in Rotterdam (The Netherlands). Thirty-six patients had a history of prior myocardial infarction. Six patients had prior PTCA and underwent RA for restenosis.

All patients, except twelve, complained of chest pain. Sixty eight patients had severe angina on effort (Canadian Heart Class III or IV). Thirteen patients had mixed angina and fifteen patients had unstable angina. Fifteen patients had some episodes of angina pectoris at rest,and six had atypical chest pain. Coronary angiography showed single vessel disease in 87 patients. Thirty-three patients had two-vessel disease and 9 had triple-vessel disease. The treated vessel was the right coronary artery in 47 patients, the left anterior descending artery(LAD) in 63 cases and, in 19 patients, the circumflex branch.

Statistical Analysis

All the data are presented as mean ± standard deviation. Comparisons between vessel diameters and percentage of reduction of luminal diameters were analyzed with paired t test. A difference of $p < 0.05$ was considered as statistically significant.

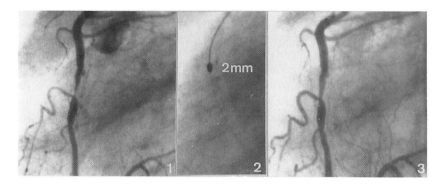

Figure 2. Rotary ablation as a stand alone procedure for treatment of a lesion of the right coronary artery.

Results

Rotary ablation was performed in 128 patients since the guide wire was unable to pass across a very tight and tortuous narrowing in one case. Eighty-eight patients were treated with rotary ablation alone (Stand alone procedure).In 40 patients rotary ablation was completed by adjunctive balloon angioplasty. This was due to abrupt closure post RA in 10 patients and insufficient results (residual stenosis >50%) in 30 patients. Primary success (gain of at least 20% with residual stenosis <50% and without complications) was achieved by rotary ablation as a stand alone procedure in 73 patients (57%). This relatively small proportion of primary success was mainly the result of the small size of the channel created by rotary ablation, the limited size of the burrs and guiding catheters at the beginning. In the group of patients treated by RA followed by conventional angioplasty primary success was achieved in 38 patients. Thus, at the end of the procedure, for the whole group, the primary success was 86% (111 of 129 patients). Figures 2 and 3 show typical result after rotary ablation. Minor complications were observed within the procedure: A transient (few seconds) reversible bradycardia was

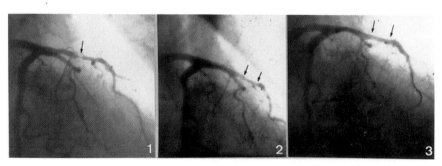

Figure 3. Lesion of the mid portion of the left anterior descending coronary artery treated by Rotablator[TM].

Table 1. Quantitative coronary analysis after rotary ablation.

		Before RA	After RA	After RA + Ballon
RA	mm	0,72 ± 0,30	1,46 ± 0,43*	–
Stand alone procedure	%	73 ± 12	42 ± 13*	–
RA + PTCA	mm	0,49 ± 0,37	1,14 ± 0,36*	2,2 ± 0,46*
	%	80 ± 12	61 ± 13*	31 ± 9*

RA: Rotary ablation
PTCA: Percutaneous transluminal coronary angioplasty
*: $p < 0.01$.

recorded in 6 cases: Rotary ablation was applied to the right coronary artery in three of them and one can suspect possible microembolization in the A-V node artery; Thus, in the following RCA cases a pacing catheter was inserted into the right ventricle. After the procedure, we oberved in 8 cases a long diffuse coronary spasm which was easily relieved by intracoronary injection of isosorbide dinitrate.

Transient abrupt closure was observed during the procedure in 10 cases: Seven were easily recrossed with a balloon and successfully dilated, and two cases required emergency by-pass surgery; in one case recanalization of the abrupt closure was not attempted and there was no complication nor enzyme rise (CPK max: 96 units). No perforations were observed: Three patients developed late occlusion (6, 24 hours and 6 days after the procedure). Finally, major complications were represented by three Q-wave myocardial infarction and 7 non Q wave MI. There were no deaths related to the procedure.

Quantitative coronary angiography was performed in 69 cases. Table 1 shows the results of rotary ablation as a stand-alone procedure:In absolute values the minimal luminal diameter increased from 0.72 ± 0.30 mm to 1.46 ± 0.43 mm (p < 0.0001). The degree of percentage stenosis decreased from 73 ± 12% to 42 ± 13%. If rotary ablation was completed by adjunctive PTCA the residual stenosis was 31 ± 9% and the residual luminal diameter was measured at 2.2 ± 0.46 mm.

Follow-up

Seventy four patients were restudied with coronary angiography, 3 to 6 months after the procedure.

Restenosis was defined as the recurrence of a significant narrowing (reduction of luminal diameter >50%).The angiographic results at follow up were analyzed in two groups of patients: Group A (n = 37) where rotary ablation was performed as a stand-alone procedure and Group B (n = 37) including rotary ablation with adjunctive PTCA.

Seventeen patients (46%) of group A had typical restenosis.In group B restenosis was observed in 29.7% of cases. For the whole group, the restenosis rate was 37.8%.

Discussion

The main mechanism of action of Rotablator is the abrasion of occlusive material allowing restoration of lumen patency. The diamond chips of the burr remove material in millions of tiny particles. Previous experimental studies, and observations made on iliac segments treated by rotary ablation showed that the resulting arterial lumen was smooth and polished. Nevertheless, endothelium and different portions of the atherosclerotic tissue were missing. In most cases the media was not damaged (Dietz).

Several problems related to this technique are of concern. It is well known that most of the atherosclerotic plaques are eccentric. Therefore, abrasion could cause severe injury of the normal part of the wall. Moreover, when the spinning burr is moving inside the vessel, some damages could occur in the adjacent part of the narrowing.

However, it has been shown that rotary micropulverization selectively removes firmer non compliant material while the normal elastic tissue, deflecting beneath the knife, is only displaced. The differential removal, limited to diseased surfaces, with particular affinity for harder materials including calcium is obviously of interest.

It is indubitable that the endothelium of segments next to stenosis, is removed. This could explain vasospasm seen after rotational abrasion. However, in our experience, spasm can be observed 2 to 3 cm beyond the treated segment and could be related to some vibrations transmitted to the guide wire during the rotation. A similar type of spasm has been reported by Hansen [5] in rabbit atherosclerotic arteries treated by rotational atherectomy.

No-flow phenomenon, transient bradycardia and A-V blocks may be related to microcavitation production. As a result of high velocity, at the burr surface, cavitations are produced according to the Bernouilli phenomenon and were documented in experimental studies [18].

The second concern is related to the size of the particles created by rotary abrasion. Hansen et al [5] collected the perfusate of segments of aorta treated by rotary ablation. The particles were sized and counted with a FACS analyzer (Becton Dickinson) while standard sized beads were analyzed for comparison. Large macroscopically visible debris were not seen and only 1.5 to 2% of particles generated by the device were >10 microns: On average, the particles size was <5 microns. Similar observations were made by Ahn et al [6]. Furthermore injection of technetium 99 m labeled particles into the femoral artery in dogs revealed that vey few were lodged in the lower extremity and most of them were found in spleen, liver etc.

Finally, scanning electronic microscopy of human iliac arteries treated by

Rotablator, showed than 75% of the particles on the surface were less than 10 to 15 microns. Thus, in most cases, the debris are most often too small to clog capillaries.

The size of the burr is a limitation of the Rotablator™: the abrasive tips are manufactured in various sizes up to 4.5 mm. To insert the device in coronary artery, we must use large guiding catheters. But, even with the largest lumen guiding catheter, the inside luminal diameter is only 2.2 or 2.5 mm. so that in the coronary arteries the size of the burr cannot exceed 2 to 2.5 mm. Therefore, for a coronary vessel of 3 to 3.5 mm, a significant residual stenosis is frequently observed after treatment.

Moreover, when one compares with quantitative coronary angiography, the size of the burr and the diameter of the channel resulting of coronary ablation, a Dottering effect is in part responsible of the results.

From these observations two types of strategy could be developed: The first consists to start with a small, intentionally undersized burr, with stepwise increments in abrasive tip sizes until the optimal result can be obtained. The second strategy involves the use of a small burr (1.75 to 2 mm) to "debulk" the vessel with a smooth residual surface and to systematically complete the procedure with a balloon inflated at a very low pressure. The lower rate of restenosis observed in our small series of patients supports the latter strategy. Nevertheless, these problems require further investigation and longer periods of follow-up.

Currently, the high-speed rotary ablation appears to be most useful for 1) small vessels (2 to 2.5 mm in diameter); 2) distal locations of the lesions 3) calcified or non distensible lesions; 4) eccentric lesions.

Diffuse disease, large coronary vessels (>3.7 mm), intracoronary thrombus, degenerated saphenous vein grafts with friable atherosclerotic materials should be avoided.

Acknowledgement

We are grateful to Catherine Feucherolles for expert secretarial assistance.

References

1. Gruentzig A R, Senning A, Siegenthaler W E (1979) Non operative dilatation of coronary artery stenosis. Percutaneous transluminal coronary angioplasty. *N Engl J Med* 301: 61–3
2. Kent K M, Bentivoghio L G, Block PC et al (1984) Long term efficacy of percutaneous transluminal coronary angioplasty (PTCA): report from the NHLBI-PTCA registry. *Am J Cardiol* 27 c–31 c
3. Simpson J B, Robertson G C, Selmon M R (1988) Percutaneous coronary atherectomy. *J Am Coll Card* (abst) 11:110A
4. Stack R S, Quigley P J, Sketch M H (1989) Treatment of coronary artery disease with the

transluminal extraction-endarterectomy catheter: initial results of a multicenter study (abst). *Circulation* 80(suppl II):II–852

5. Hansen D D, Auth D C, Vrocko R, Ritchie J L (1988) Rotational atherectomy in atherosclerotic rabbit iliac arteries. *Am Heart J* 115:160–165

6. Ahn S S, Auth D C, Marcus D R, Moore W S (1988) Removal of focal atheromatous lesions by angioscopically guided high speed rotary atherectomy. *J Vasc Surg* 7:292–9

7. Fourrier J L, Stankowiak C, Lablanche J M, Prat A, Brunetaud J M, Bertrand M E (1988) Histopathology after rotational angioplasty of peripheral arteries in human beings. *J Am Coll Card* (abst) 11:109A

8. Zacca N M, Raizner A E, Noon G P,Short H D, Weilbaecher D G, Gotto A M, Roberts R (1988) Short term follow up of patients treated with a recently developed rotational atherectomy device and in vivo assessment of the particules generated. *J Am Coll Card* (abst) 11:109A

9. Hansen D D, Auth D C, Hall M, Ritchie J L (1988) Rotational endarterectomy in normal canine coronary arteries. Preliminary report. *J Am Coll Card* 11:1073–7

10. Fourrier J L, Auth D C, Lablanche J M, Brunetaud J M, Gommeaux A, Bertrand M E (1988) Human percutaneous coronary rotational atherectomy: preliminary results. (abstract) *Circulation* 78:II–82

11. Fourrier J L, Bertrand M E, Auth D C, Lablanche J M, Gommeaux A, Brunetaud J M (1989) Percutaneous coronary rotational angioplasty in humans: Preliminary report. *J Am Coll Cardiol* 14:1278–82

12. Ginsburg R, Teirstein P S, Warth D C, Hocq N, Jenkins N S, McCowan L C (1989) Percutaneous transluminal coronary rotational atheroablation: clinical experience in 40 patients. (abst) *Circulation* 80 (suppl II):II–584

13. Teirstein P S, Ginsburg R, Warth D C, Hoq N, Jenkins N S, McCowan L C (1990) Complications of human coronary rotablation (abst). *J Am Coll Cardiol* 15:57a

14. Bertrand M E, Lablanche J M, Fourrier J L, Bauters C, Leroy F (1990) Percutaneous rotary ablation. *Herz* 15:285–7

15. Buchbinder M, O'Neill W, Warth D, Zacca N, Dietz U, Bertrand M E, Fourrier J L, Leon M (1990) Percutaneous coronary rotational ablation using the Rotablator: Results of a multicenter study (abst). *Circulation* 82:III–309

16. Bertrand M E, Jean L. Fourrier, David Auth, Jean M. Lablanche, Antoine Gommeaux (1990) Percutaneous coronary rotational angioplasty. In: Eric J. Topol (ed) *Textbook of Interventional Cardiology*, Philadelphia: W. B Sauders, 580–589

17. Bertrand M E, Fourrier J L, Dietz U, De Jaegere (1990) European experience with percutaneous transluminal coronary rotational ablation (abst). *Circulation* 82, III–310

18. Zotz R, Stahr P, Erbel R, Auth D, Meyer J (1991) Analysis of high-frequency rotational angioplasty-induced echo contrast. *Cath Cardiovasc Diagn* 22:137

14. Percutaneous Coronary Rotational Atherectomy: The William Beaumont Hospital Experience

MARK S. FREED, KHUSROW NIAZI and
WILLIAM W. O'NEILL

Introduction

Percutaneous transluminal coronary angioplasty (PTCA) is an effective and important alternative to continued medical treatment or coronary artery bypass grafting in the management of patients with obstructive coronary artery disease. Symptom relief, increased exercise capacity, reduced antianginal requirements and a shortened hospitalization for unstable angina are benefits attributable to PTCA.

However, the overall effectiveness of balloon angioplasty has been limited by the later development of restenosis. Occurring in 35–40% of over 200,000 individuals requiring PTCA annually, restenosis results in re-exposure to the risks associated with subsequent revascularization procedures and in additional health care expenditures of up to 500 million.

Various strategies have been implemented in the hope of reducing the incidence of restenosis. Yet, despite advances in the design of PTCA hardware, optimization of procedural variables and use of adjunctive pharmacotherapy, restenosis rates remain unacceptably high. Indeed, improved PTCA materials now allow operators to successfully cross and dilate increasingly complex lesions with higher intrinsic restenosis rates, magnifying the importance of this problem.

The proliferation of non-balloon devices provides yet another strategy aimed at reducing the incidence of restenosis. It is hoped that by minimizing or modifying the mechanical injury signals responsible for intimal thickening and incomplete dilatation, restenosis will be effectively reduced. We now report our experience with one such device, the Auth Rotablator™ (manufactured by Heart Technology, Bellevue, Washington) a high-speed rotational atherectomy catheter which preferentially ablades atheromatous wall segments. A description of the device, proposed mechanisms by which use of the Rotablator may limit restenosis, case illustrations, overall restenosis rate and risk factors for restenosis in 100 patients having percutaneous coron-

P.W. Serruys, B.H. Strauss and S.B. King III (eds), Restenosis after Intervention with New Mechanical Devices, 297–311.
© 1992 *Kluwer Academic Publishers. Printed in the Netherlands.*

ary rotational atherectomy at William Beaumont Hospital will now be described.

Description of the Device

The Rotablator (Fig. 1) consists of a brass burr coated with 40 μ diamond chips and welded to a flexible drive shaft. Housed in a Teflon sheath, the drive shaft is connected to a compressed air-powered turbine. Activated and controlled by a foot pedal, the drive shaft and burr rotate at 150–200,000 rpm (fiberoptic light probe records rotational speed) as they are advanced over a guidewire. The 0.009 inch stainless steel guidewire has a flexible 0.017 inch spring tip at its terminal portion to prevent distal embolization of the burr should tip fracture occur.

A saline flush solution is injected into the plastic sheath around the drive shaft to minimize frictional heat during use. After the guidewire is steered into proper position as with balloon angioplasty, the atherectomy burr is advanced to the lesion and the turbine is activated. A control knob on the top of the plastic casing allows the operator to slowly advance the burr over the guidewire and through the lesion, resulting in harmless micropulverization of the obstructing atheroma. Technical details concerning use of the Rotablator have been previously described.[1]

Potential Advantages to Rotational Atherectomy in Limiting Restenosis

As with other non-balloon percutaneous revascularization devices, the Rotablator has been designed to modify and minimize injury to both atheromatous and contralateral plaque-free wall segments. The proposed mechanisms by which balloon angioplasty leads to restenosis and the steps in which these injury signals may be attenuated by use of the Rotablator are seen in Fig. 2.

Balloon angioplasty-induced transmural stretch results in radial coronary artery expansion which injures both atheromatous and contralateral plaque-free wall segments[2]. Plaque fracture, circumferential splitting of the tunica intima and deep fracture of the tunica media create new channels for coronary blood flow. However, in the process, several potent activators of the coagulation cascade and platelets are released or exposed including tissue factor [3] (a lipoprotein concentrated around cholesterol crystals in the plaque core which initiates the extrinsic pathway of the clotting system) and subendothelial collagen (a potent platelet aggregator and the main constituent of the extracellular matrix of the plaque).

Consequently, thrombus formation, coronary artery spasm (mediated by thromboxane and serotonin secretion) and growth factor release occur (e.g. platelet, macrophage and fibroblast-derived growth factors). These biological

ROTABLATOR

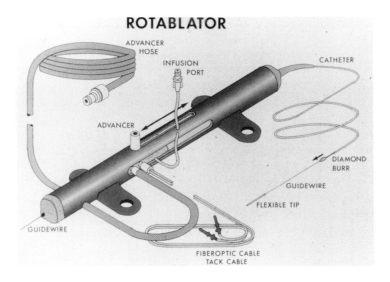

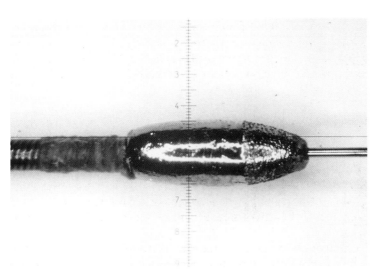

Figure 1. The Rotablator™ device and a close-up of a 2.0 mm diamond-coated atherectomy burr.

pathways result in restenosis through incomplete dilatation and neointimal hyperplasia.

In addition to creating new channels for coronary flow, balloon angioplasty improves luminal diameter by transmural stretching and radial expansion of both atheromatous and contralateral plaque-free wall segments. However,

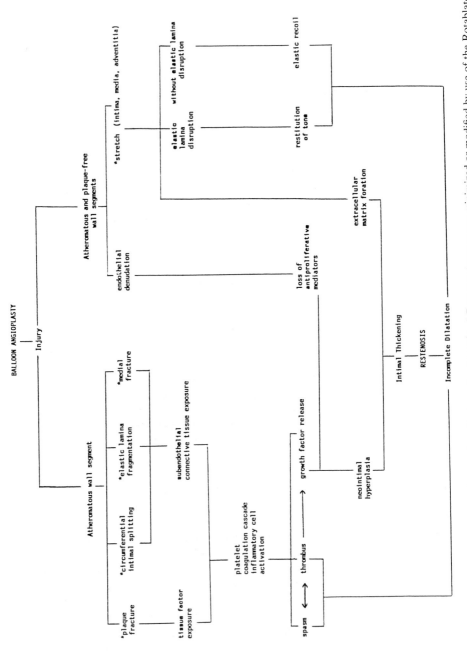

Figure 2. Proposed pathophysiologic mechanisms and medicators of restenosis.   * Represents processes minimized or modified by use of the Rotablator.

balloon-induced coronary artery expansion has been directly implicated in incomplete dilatation and the subsequent development of intimal thickening. In vitro studies indicate that transmural stretch can potentiate the migratory and proliferative capacity of smooth muscle cells and stimulate the synthesis of extracellular matrix components found in restenosis lesions[4, 5]. In addition to these effects on intimal thickening, transmural stretch may initiate vessel responses which result in incomplete dilatation and limit the gain achieved in luminal expansion during balloon angioplasty. In this regard, when stretching is accompanied by elastic lamina disruption as occurs in atheromatous wall segments, restitution of tone in the media and adventitia result in early loss of luminal diameter. Likewise, when stretching occurs without significant elastic lamina fragmentation, as may be seen in plaque-free wall segments and ostial stenoses, elastic recoil limits the effectiveness of balloon dilatation. Restitution of tone, elastic recoil, thrombus formation and spasm result in incomplete dilatation and may be responsible for very early restenosis following balloon angioplasty[6, 7].

The Rotablator, which ablates tissue to generate an expanded arterial lumen, theoretically attenuates many of the mechanical injury mechanisms implicated in restenosis (Fig. 2). Experimental studies using the Rotablator have confirmed that injury to both atheromatous and contralateral plaque-free wall segments is modified and minimized. In cadaver arteries with atheromatous lesions involving the superficial femoral, popliteal and tibial arteries, use of the Rotablator routinely led to widely patent, smooth, polished surfaces. Unlike balloon angioplasty, angioscopic and histologic evaluation of treated specimens demonstrated removal of obstructing atheroma and diseased intima in the absence of significant intimal flaps or medial fracture[8]. Early experimental studies using the Rotablator in 11 normal canine coronary arteries resulted in a reliable loss and fragmentation of the internal elastic membrane, theoretically limiting the potential for elastic recoil. Importantly, unlike balloon angioplasty in which radial coronary artery expansion results in circumferential splitting of the intima and medial dissections, no intimal cracks or medial fractures were seen[9]. These histologic findings were again observed following rotational atherectomy of atherosclerotic rabbit iliac arteries. The new lumen was found to be smooth walled; atheroma, diseased intima and internal elastic membrane were largely removed. Intimal splits and medial dissections again were not seen[10].

Percutaneous revascularization using this high-speed rotational atherectomy device pulverizes obstructing atheroma into microparticles, which pass harmlessly into the capillary circulation. Compared to conventional balloon angioplasty, the Rotablator preferentially ablades inelastic atheromatous tissue, minimizing trauma to plaque-free wall segments which retain their visco-elastic properties and are deflected around the diamond-coated rotary burr. The result is an expanded, circular arterial lumen with a smooth, polished, less thrombogenic surface (Figs 3 and 4). This final result is frequently obtained without significant residual atheroma, internal elastic lamina, in-a   b

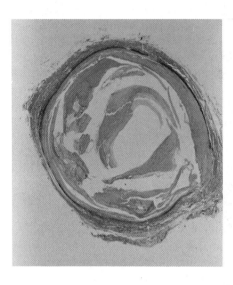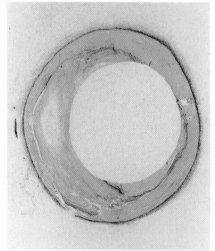

Figure 3. a. Cross-sectional photomicrograph following successful balloon angioplasty demonstrating plaque fracture and circumferential splitting of the intima. b. Successfully atherectomized artery demonstrating a smooth circular expanded lumina devoid of significant residual atheroma or diseased intima. Reprinted with permission from Samual Ahn, M.D.

timal splitting or medial dissection (Figs 5 and 6). These selective effects attenuate the mechanical injury signals which activate the cellular mechanisms responsible for restenosis.

Methodology

Patient Population and Procedure. The study group consisted of patients who underwent percutaneous coronary rotational atherectomy in the William Beaumont Hospital cardiac catheterization laboratory from September 1988 to July 1990. Briefly, the inclusion criteria for patients were age over 18 years, exertional angina or objective of ischemia, a target lesion of at least 70 percent of the luminal diameter and patients who were otherwise good candidates for coronary bypass surgery if required. Patients were excluded if they were unable to give informed consent, were evolving an acute myocardial infarction or had angiographic evidence of either thrombus, unprotected left main coronary artery disease, lesions greater than 25 mm in length or occlusions through which a guidewire would not pass.

All patients received aspirin, nitrates and calcium channel blockers prior to their procedure. Upon obtaining arterial and venous access, heparin

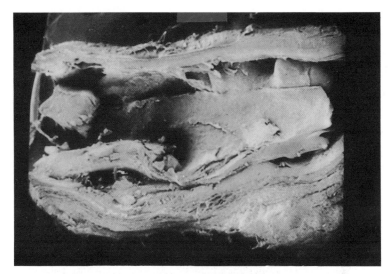

a

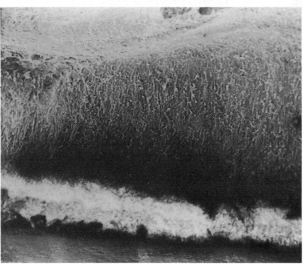

b

Figure 4. a. Scanning electron micrograph following balloon angioplasty demonstrating marked disruption of underlying vessel architecture. b. Following rotational atherectomy, a smooth, polished, less thrombogenic surface is seen. Reprinted with permission from Samual Ahn, M.D.

(10,000 units IV) was administered and continued for 24 hours. Additional adjunctive therapy included verapamil (5 mg IV bolus), low-molecular weight dextran and nitroglycerin (continuous 24 hour IV infusion followed by oral therapy).

Orthogonal views of the culprit lesion were obtained pre- and post-procedure. Adjunctive balloon angioplasty was performed if the post-Rotablator

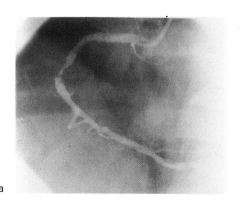
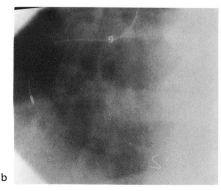

a   b

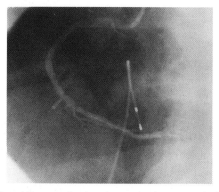

c

Figure 5. a. Left anterior oblique projection demonstrating an: a. Isolated mid-right coronary artery stenosis. b. Rotablator burr seen crossing the lesion. c. Final result demonstrating a widely patent vessel without residual stenosis or dissection.

angiographic result was felt to be suboptimal. Following the procedure, patients were monitored for 24–48 hours and then followed clinically at 1,3 and 6 months. All patients were scheduled to have repeat catheterization at 6 months or earlier if clinically necessary. Quantitative arteriography was performed on all patients utilizing the Artrek method.[11]

Definitions

Procedural success was defined as a final residual stenosis less than 50% of the luminal diameter and lack of major complications (need for emergency bypass surgery, coronary perforation, myocardial infarction and death).

The definition of restenosis remains a subject of considerable controversy. Depending on which definition is used, restenosis rates will vary. We have elected to express our data using both mechanistic (Thoraxcenter II; loss of absolute gain in luminal diameter of 0.72 mm) and functional definitions (Thoraxcenter I: >50% stenosis at the site of previous intervention). These

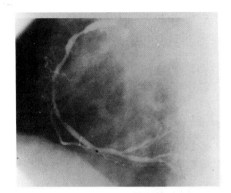
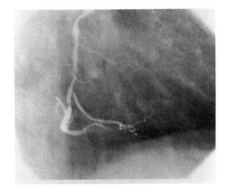

a

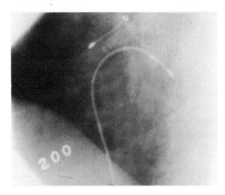

b

Figure 6. A and B.

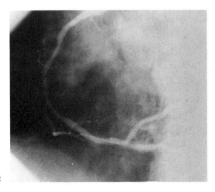
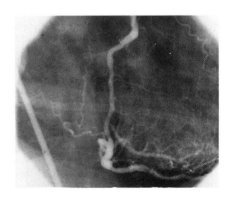

c

Figure 6. a. Left anterior oblique (LAO) and right anterior oblique (RAO) projections of a right coronary artery demonstrating multiple stenoses. b. Rotablator burr and drive shaft shown tracking over guidewire. c. LAO and RAO projections demonstrating an excellent final result with small dissection seen following adjunctive balloon angioplasty.

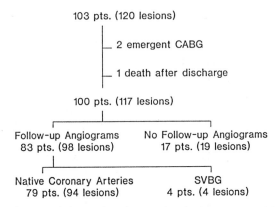

Figure 7. Total patient population undergoing rotational atherectomy and follow-up angiography at William Beaumont Hospital.

definitions reflect the actual amount of intimal thickening which occurs and the likelihood of developing a clinically important stenosis following rotational atherectomy, respectively.

Each definition, however, has its limitations; in large caliber vessels, loss of 0.72 mm in luminal diameter, although a significant proliferative response, may represent only 20–30% stenoses at follow-up and therefore be clinically unimportant. Likewise, a post-procedural residual stenosis of 40% which at re-cath is 55% may qualify as restenosis yet actually represent trivial intimal thickening. We believe that using both mechanistic and functional definitions are complementary and assist us in understanding the fate of coronary stenoses following rotational atherectomy.

Results

As previously reported[12] and seen in Fig. 7, there were 103 patients (120 lesions) who underwent rotational atherectomy. Two patients required emergency coronary artery bypass surgery for abrupt vessel closure, one directly related to the Rotablator and the other related to balloon angioplasty. One of these patients died 2 weeks following bypass surgery. In the follow-up period, 1 patient died of unknown cause. Of the remaining 100 patients (117 lesions), there were 17 patients (19 lesions) who refused follow-up angiograms because they were asymptomatic. Overall, 83 patients (98 lesions) had follow-up angiograms (83% angiographic follow-up) at a mean time of 5.3 months (range 0.8– 9.6 months). Saphenous vein bypass graft rotational atherectomy was performed on 4 patients (4 lesions). Acute closure occurred in 3 patients, two of whom required emergency bypass surgery (one death, one myocardial infarction) and the third case resulting in a myocardial infarction. Overall periprocedural event rate (Q-wave MI, death, emergency bypass surgery) was 2.9%.

Procedural success was achieved in 93% of lesions attempted. In the small number of SVBG lesions attempted, restenosis occurred in 75% (3/4). The following data presentation reflects our experience using the Rotablator in native coronary arteries. Overall minimal luminal diameters (mean ± standard deviation) pre- and post-Rotablator and at follow-up were 1.05 ± 6.1 mm, 1.95 ± 0.66 mm, 1.51 ± 0.76 mm respectively. Of 98 lesions successfully treated (less than 50% residual stenosis) and available for follow-up angiography, 25% had a coronary stenosis more than 50% (functional restenosis definition) whereas 29% had an absolute loss of 0.72 mm in luminal diameter (mechanistic restenosis definition). The impact of several clinical, angiographic and procedural variables on restenosis rates were considered, including gender, tobacco use, diabetes, hypertension, history of a previous MI, unstable angina at presentation, angina at re-cath, lesion location, involved vessel (LAD vs non-LAD), de novo versus restenosis lesions, residual stenosis more than 30% and use of adjunctive balloon angioplasty (Table 1). Considering the recurrence of a more than 50% stenosis at follow-up, the presence of angina at the time of re-cath, ostial/proximal lesions and stenosis in the LAD proved to be a significant risk factors (Fig. 8). Considering the absolute loss of 0.72 mm at follow-up, both the presence of angina at re-cath and diabetes mellitus were significant risk factors with a tendency toward restenosis following rotational atherectomy of the LAD coronary artery.

Finally, and quite interestingly, the overall recurrent restenosis rate (restenosis rate following rotational atherectomy of lesions which had previously developed restenosis following balloon angioplasty) was strikingly low, both by functional (5/31: 17%) and mechanistic definitions (7/31: 22%).

Conclusions

Conventional balloon angioplasty is an effective and important therapy in the management of patients with obstructive coronary artery disease. However, primary procedural success rates remain problematic especially for certain anatomic substrates (e.g. chronic total occlusions, intracoronary thrombus, ostial stenoses, degenerated saphenous vein grafts, diffuse disease). Additionally, the later development of restenosis has limited the long-term benefit of balloon angioplasty. Indeed, advances in the design of PTCA hardware allow increasingly complex lesions to be successfully dilated, perhaps accounting for what appears to be an overall trend toward higher restenosis rates in recent balloon angioplasty series.

Rotational atherectomy, as with other nonballoon percutaneous coronary revascularization devices, must ultimately be evaluated in terms of its primary procedural success and restenosis rates before defining its value in the treatment of obstructive coronary artery disease. Preliminary results obtained

opment of restenosis. Neither gender, tobacco use, hypertension, history of a previous MI, unstable angina at presentation or use of adjunctive balloon angioplasty were risk factors for restenosis, although small numbers of treated patients preclude definitive conclusions.

An interesting outcome from our data was the strikingly low recurrent restenosis rate. Treating lesions which have already restenosed with subsequent balloon dilatations have yielded disappointing results, with re-restenosis rates up 40–50%. In our small series, only 5 of 31 restenotic lesions treated with the Rotablator developed a subsequent restenosis for an overall recurrent restenosis rate of only 17%. The mechanism responsible for this result may relate to the minimal disruption of underlying vessel architecture likely to occur with passage of the high-speed diamond-coated rotary burr through the soft fibrocellular lesion typical of restenosis. Despite this intriguing observation and promising initial results, the ultimate role of the Rotablator in the therapeutic armamentarium available to the interventional cardiologist will depend on the results of prospective randomized trials comparing this and other devices to balloon angioplasty in both de novo and restenotic coronary artery lesions.

References

1. Meany T B, Friedman H Z, O'Neill W W (1991) Coronary rotational atherectomy: clinical applications. *J Invasive Cardiol* 3:19–24
2. Waller B F (1989) Crackers, breakers, stretchers, drillers, scrapers, shavers, burners, welders and melters. The future treatment of atherosclerotic coronary artery disease. A clinical assessment. *JACC* 13,5:969–987
3. Wilcox J N, Smith K M, Schwartz S M, Gordon D (1989) Localization of tissue factor in the normal vessel wall and in the atherosclerotic plaque. *Proc Natl Acad Sci USA* 86:2839–2843
4. Grünwald J, Haudenschild C C (1984) Intimal injury in vivo activates vascular smooth muscle cell migration and explant outgrowth in vitro. *Arteriosclerosis* 4:183–188
5. Leung D, Glagov S, Mathews M (1976) Cyclic stretching stimulates synthesis of matrix components by arterial smooth muscle cells in vitro. *Science* 6:475–477
6. El-Tamim H, Davies G J, Hackett D, Fragasso G, Crea F, Maseri A (1990) Very early production of restenosis after successful coronary angioplasty: anatomical and functional assessment. *J Am Coll Cardiol* 15:259–264
7. Nobuyosh M, Kimura T, Nosaka H et al (1988) Restenosis after successful PTCA: serial angiographic follow-up of 299 patients. *J Am Coll Cardiol* 12:616–623
8. Ahn S, Auth D C, Marcus D, Moore W (1988) Removal of focal atheromatous lesions by angioscopically guided high-speed rotary atherectomy. *J Vasc Surg* 7:292–300
9. Hansen D D, Auth D C, Hall M, Ritchie J L (1988) Rotational endarterectomy in normal canine coronary arteries: preliminary report. *J Am Coll Cardiol* 11:1073–1077
10. Hansen D D, Auth D C, Vracko R, Ritchie J L (1988) Rotational atherectomy in atherosclerotic rabbit iliac arteries. *Am Heart J* 115;1:160–165
11. LeFree M T, Simon S B, Lewis R J, Bates E R, Vogel R A (1987) Digital radiographic coronary artery quantitation. In: proceeding of the IEEE Computer Society. Computers in Cardiology. IEEE Computer Society, Long Branch, CA 99–102

12. Niazi K, Freed M S, O'Neill W W (1991) Angiographic risk factors for restenosis following mechanical rotational atherectomy. (submitted)
13. Tcheng J E, Frid D J, Fortin D F, Nelson C L, Stack R K, Peter R H, Stack R S, Califf R M (1991) Anatomic propensity for restenosis following coronary angioplasty. *J Am Coll Cardiol* 17:2:345A
14. Hinoharra T, Selmon M R, Robertson G C et al (1991) Angiographic predictions of restenosis following directional coronary atherectomy. *JACC* 17:2,385A
15. Sketch M H, O'Neill W W, Galichia J P et al (1991) The Duke Multicenter coronary transluminal extraction-endarterectomy catheter: acute and chronic results. *JACC* 17:2,31A
16. Rothbaum D, Linnemeier T, Landin R et al (1991) Excimer laser coronary angioplasty restenosis rate at six-month follow-up. *JACC* 17:2,205A

15. Percutaneous Transluminal Coronary Rotational Ablation: Serial Follow-up by Quantitative Angiography

KIRK L. PETERSON, ISABEL RIVERA, MARTIN MCDANIEL, JOHN LONG, ALLAN BOND, MIKKI BHARGAVA and the Clinical Investigators* of the Multicenter Trial of the Rotablator™

Introduction

Fourteen years after its first use in man [1], percutaneous transluminal coronary angioplasty by balloon dilation has now been widely accepted as a useful and alternative form of therapy for the symptomatic patient with coronary heart disease [2]. Nevertheless, the technique's value in improving luminal patency is dependent upon the characteristics of the lesion dilated and the reparative response to the traumatic injury created by the balloon [3]. Moreover, balloon dilation does not lead to direct ablation of tissue responsible for coronary artery obstruction and has now been documented to have restenosis rates as high as 50 percent [4–7].

These limitations have inspired the design and development of new catheter procedures, e.g., excimer laser angioplasty [8], laser balloon angioplasty [9], and directional coronary atherectomy [10], all aimed at coronary plaque ablation. For this same purpose, a high-speed rotational catheter (Rotablator), manufactured by Heart Technology, Inc. of Seattle, Washington, is undergoing clinical investigation [11]; the Rotablator has been found safe and effective in animal models of coronary and peripheral vascular atherosclerotic disease [12, 13]; moreover, it has now been applied to well over seven hundred patients with coronary heart disease in cardiovascular centers of both North America and Western Europe.

One year after the initiation of these clinical trials, a core laboratory image processing laboratory was retained to assess quantitatively the effect of coronary rotational ablation on coronary vasomotion, lesion geometry, and immediate and long-term vessel patency. Reported herein are the initial results from the first fifty-two patients where quantitative measurements

*Maurice Buchbinder, San Diego, Calif.; Gerald Dorros, Milwaukee, Wisconsin; Richard Podolin, San Diego, Calif.; Todd Sherman, Los Angeles, Calif.; Simon Stertzer, San Francisco, Calif.; David Warth, Seattle, Washington; Nadim Zacca, Houston, Texas; USA.

P.W. Serruys, B.H. Strauss and S.B. King III (eds), Restenosis after Intervention with New Mechanical Devices, 313–328.

were performed on serial coronary cineangiograms recorded before and over twenty-four hours to six months after rotational ablation.

Device Description

The Rotablator is a rotating catheter with a nickel burr tip which has 15–25 micron diamond microchips studded over its distal one-half, creating an abrasive surface. The burr is energized by a helical drive shaft capable of rotating up to a speed of 200,000 revolutions per minute. The drive shaft itself is housed in a 4-French teflon catheter through which saline is infused to cool and lubricate the system. Rotablator burrs for coronary ablation range from 1.25 to 2.25 mm. in diameter; any burr less than 2.15 mm in diameter can be introduced via a 9F guiding catheter. The catheter is delivered to the site of the lesion over a 0.009 inch stainless steel, steerable guidewire with a 2 cm radio-opaque platinum spring tip.

Patient and Cinefilm Selection

Once the Rotablator quantitative analysis program was established, all investigators were encouraged to contribute patient information along with cinefilms to a registry. An investigator worksheet was devised which enabled the angiographer or his assistant to record carefully the geometric position of the radiographic imaging chain as well as the catheters for each contrast injection. All angiographers were urged to choose projections which imaged optimally the treated lesion for purposes of edge recognition and quantitation, avoiding overlap of adjacent arteries and vessel foreshortening. Views utilized for diagnostic evaluation were repeated 1) immediately after the burr ablation, 2) immediately after any adjunctive use of balloon dilation, 3) 24 hours later before the vascular sheaths were removed, and 4) at six-month's post-ablation unless recurrence or signs of myocardial ischemia mandated an earlier angiographic restudy.

Despite these efforts, not all cinefilms submitted for quantitation were suitable for analysis. Rejection of films occurred for the following reasons: 1) catheter positioning or imaging was not satisfactory for calibration of the coronary artery lesion (e.g., injection catheter poorly centered or over the spine; visualization of only the tapered portion of the injection catheter; injection catheter opacified through the full cine-run), 2) cinefilm quality was insufficient (e,g, oversaturation or "blooming", excessive panning) for edge detection either by an automatic edge detection algorithm or with operator override, 3) problems with cine acquisitions including varying magnification or lesion projection at different times of filming (e.g., "diagnostic" versus "24 hours" versus "6-months"), obscurity of lesion by diaphragm or other vessels, inadequate opacification of vessel, or choice of only one view for quantitation. As of May 1, 1991, 173 lesions at the diagnostic study, 155 lesions post-burr ablation, 84 lesions post-burr and balloon adjunct therapy, 142 lesions at 24 hour follow-up study, and 52 lesions at 3–6 months post-ablation had been found suitable for quantitative analysis. It is the latter groups of lesions, i.e., those filmed serially at the time of diagnostic angiography, and at 24 hours, and, finally, at 3–6 months which form the basis for this report. Of these 52 lesions, 30 were treated by rotational ablation alone (Group A), and 22 were treated by rotational ablation followed by adjunctive balloon dilation (Group B).

Hardware, Procedures and Methods for Cinefilm Quantitation

All films are mounted on a CAP-35 (General Electric) cinefilm projector and optically magnified up to four times by an interposed optical lens. With this system, the iris, zoom, and mirrors are all remotely controlled and used to optimize the size of any given coronary artery segment. The video camera can be rotated so as to align the lesion at any angle desired with respect to the raster lines of a television image. The magnified images are recorded by a mounted, switchable videocamera (Cohu), digitized as an interlaced television image (512×512 pixels, 8 bits and 256 shades of gray) and stored in a Gould-DeAnza IP-8500 image processor interfaced to a Digital Equipment Corportion VAX 11/780 computer. The operator chooses the proximal and distal ends of the segment of vessel to be analyzed, allowing for a significant length of reference vessel in order to compute percentage diameter and area stenosis (vide infra).

The coronary artery quantification software provides the following general features: a) automatic edge detection with manual override, b) correction for pincushion distortion based on radial symmetric transformation and bilinear approximation to determine non-distorted from distorted intensity values, c) three alternative methods for estimation of lesion cross-section area including i) a geometric method based upon either single or biplane orthogonal views of the lesion, ii) a videodensitometric method based upon background subtracted, log-transformed videointensities, and iii) a combined geometric-video-densitometric method. For the analysis of patients undergoing rotational ablation with the Rotablator, we have chosen to utilize the geometric approach because it could be applied to the largest proportion of patient films submitted to the Core Laboratory; moreover, it was most suitable for images archived on cinefilm.

The automatic edge detection routine involves a two-dimensional search where an edge likelihood matrix is created based upon two-dimensional gradients from Sobel operators. Local edge correction is then accomplished from derivative thresholds (first and second derivatives) and image weighted by the Laplacian; the image is then inverted so that small values are likely edge points. Finally, each edge is obtained as the least cost path through the modified gradient image with the starting and ending points provided by the operator. This heuristic argument assumes that the slope of the edge will not change drastically at any edge point, i.e., that successor points on the edge make an angle of no more than 90 degress with the last path segment.

Once edges have been established, a centerline is calculated based upon the shortest distance between successive points on either edge as the computer interrogates down the path of the coronary artery segment chosen. Once the centerline is established, the algorithm then recalculates perpendicular chords based upon intersections with the inner and outer edges of the arterial segment. These perpendicular chords are then plotted as successive diameters along the centerline; in addition, ten diameters from the proximal reference segment and ten diameters from the distal reference segment are averaged, and a linear fit of these two average values over the length of the coronary artery lesion serves to establish theoretical normal diameters within an area of plaque. Division of the average of a minimum of three successive diameters by their corresponding theoretical (interpolated) normal diameters serves to provide a measure of the percent diameter and percent area obstruction of the atherosclerotic plaque. The area subtended by the edge of the lumen and the theoretical normal edge (calculated from the linear fit of the proximal and distal segments) can also provide an estimate of plaque area.

If only one view is available, minimal luminal cross-sectional area is derived from minimal luminal diameter by assuming a circular model. If two views are available, the final vessel cross-section is calculated from the average of the two views. Of the 52 lesions evaluated serially after coronary rotational ablation, 22 were satisfactorily visualized in two relatively orthogonal projections at the time of all three angiograms, i.e., diagnostic, 24-hour, and 3–6 months. When one view only was utilized, it was accepted for quantitation of lesion severity when it met the following criteria: a) near perpendicularity to the direction of imaging, b) no significant overlap of adjacent vessels, c) no evidence of foreshortening of part of the vessel due to significant tortuosity, d) ready use of automatic edge detection without operator override.

In order to assess the accuracy of one view only for assessment of lesion severity, we compared by linear regression the single view minimal diameter (SV-MLD) versus the average of two views (AV-MLD) in the 66 instances where both methods of measuring lesion severity were available (Fig. 1).

The correlation coefficient (R) of this relation was 0.964 (Standard Error of Estimate = 0.143) and with

$$SV\text{-}MLD = 1.028 \ (AV\text{-}MLD) - 0.056.$$

Quantitative Results

For the 52 patients where quantitative coronary angiography was accomplished upon diagnostic, 24-hour post-burr or burr/balloon, and 3–6

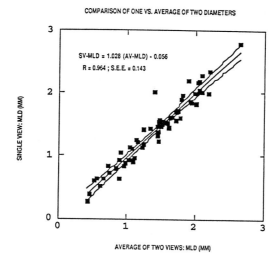

COMPARISON OF ONE VS. AVERAGE OF TWO DIAMETERS

Figure 1. Plot of minimal luminal diameter obtained from a single view (SV-MLD, vertical axis, in millimeters) as opposed to the average of two nearly orthogonal views (AV-MLD, horizontal axis, in millimeters). The least squares linear regression line, and associated 95% confidence intervals, are shown.

months follow-up cinefilms, the average serial measurements (and the associated standard deviations, maximum and minimum values) are displayed in Table 1. Measurements are given for a proximal reference segment, at the minimum diameter, and for a distal reference segment. Calculations are also given for the percentage diameter stenosis and percentage area stenosis. As shown in Fig. 2, the minimum diameter improved significantly between the diagnostic and 24-hour studies from 0.75 ± 0.27 mm to $1.70 \pm$ mm ($p < 0.001$, by ANOVA); by 3–6 months there was some loss of this improved patency to an average of 1.45 ± 0.48 mm ($p < 0.001$ vs both diagnostic and 24-hour determinations). Some of the improvement in patency between diagnostic and 24-hour studies is relief of vasoconstriction as evidenced by an improvement in the proximal and distal reference segments from 2.62 ± 0.59 to 2.71 ± 0.61 mm and 2.36 ± 0.54 to 2.53 ± 0.48 mm, respectively. However, most of the observed reduction in minimal luminal diameter between 24-hours and 3–6 months was undoubtedly the result of a restenotic process. In fact, at three-six months followup angiography, 1 of 52 lesions was calculated as greater than 70% stenotic, 8/52 greater than 60% stenotic, and 19/52 greater than 50% stenotic. A total of 10 of the 52 patients exhibited minimal luminal diameters of less than 1.0 mm. at the time of their late follow-up study.

The total group of 52 lesions were segregated into those where rotational ablation only (Group A, 30 lesions) was utilized and those where rotational ablation followed by adjunctive balloon dilation (Group B, 22 lesions) was used. Serial quantitative data for group A are shown in Table 2 and diagrammatically displayed in Figs 3 and 4. The minimum luminal diameter improved

Table 1. Group A and B – rotational ablation with or without adjunctive balloon angioplasty.

	Diagnostic					24-hr Follow-up					3–6 Month Follow-up				
	Mean	SD	Max	Min	N	Mean	SD	Max	Min	N	Mean	SD	Max	Min	N
PDia1	2.62	0.59	4.03	1.28	52	2.71	0.61	4.46	1.70	52	2.69	0.68	4.71	1.49	52
MDia1	0.75	0.27	1.43	0.24	52	1.70	0.32	2.53	1.07	52	1.45	0.48	2.78	0.24	52
DDia1	2.36	0.54	3.77	1.40	52	2.53	0.48	3.40	1.54	52	2.49	0.59	3.90	1.38	52
%Dia1	70.25	8.83	89.60	54.80	52	33.37	12.69	53.00	6.90	52	43.63	16.47	89.60	10.70	52
%Are1	89.71	6.25	98.90	61.90	52	54.28	17.43	77.90	13.50	52	65.75	18.49	98.90	20.30	52

PDia1 = Proximal Diameter, One View; MDia1 = Minimal Diameter, One View; DDia1 = Distal Diameter, One View; %Dia1 = percentage diameter stenosis; %Are1 = percentage area stenosis, One View; SD = Standard deviation; N = Number of lesions.

ROTATIONAL ABLATION MULTICENTER DATA: SERIAL ANGIOGRAPHIC
ANALYSIS UP TO SIX MONTHS

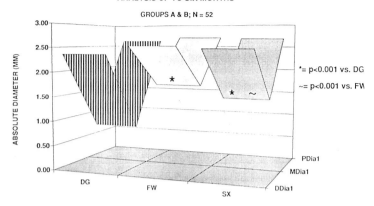

Figure 2. Three dimensional plot of the absolute diameter in mm (Y axis) at the proximal reference segment (PDial), at the minimum diameter (MDial), and the distal reference segment (DDial)(Z axis), taken from coronary arteriographic cinefilms recorded before rotational ablation (DG), at 24 hours after ablation (FW) and then again at 3–6 months later (SX) axis). Data is taken from patients undergoing both rotational ablation alone (Group A) and combined rotational ablation and balloon dilation (Group B).

significantly between the diagnostic and immediately post-burr state from 0.75 ± 0.31mm to 1.37 ± 0.24 mm ($p < 0.001$, by ANOVA); by 24 hours later, the minimum diameter had improved further to 1.57 ± 0.23 mm; however, by 3–6 months there was some loss of this improved patency to an average of 1.33 ± 0.45 mm ($p < 0.001$ vs both diagnostic and 24-hour determinations). The sizes of the proximal and distal reference diameters did not change significantly over this period. Understandably, the percentage diameter and area stenosis calculations revealed a measurable increase from 36 ± 13 to 45 ± 18 and 58 ± 17 to 67 ± 20, respectively, Fig. 4. Of the 30 patients in Group A, 22 exhibited a minimum luminal diameter of greater than 1 mm at their 3–6 month follow-up film.

The serial quantitative data for group B are shown in Table 3 and diagrammatically displayed in Figs 4 and 5. The minimum luminal diameter improved significantly between the diagnostic and immediately post-burr state from 0.78 ± 0.22mm to 1.16 ± 0.30 mm ($p < 0.01$ versus diagnostic, by ANOVA) and increased even further to 1.68 ± 0.34 mm post balloon adjunct dilation ($p < 0.01$ vs post-burr); by 24 hours later, the minimum diameter had improved further to 1.89 ± 0.32 mm($p < 0.001$ vs diagnostic); however, by 3–6 months there was some loss of this improved patency to an average of 1.63 ± 0.48 mm. ($p < 0.001$ vs both diagnostic and 24-hour determinations). The sizes of the proximal and distal reference diameters did not change significantly between the 24-hour and 3–6 month follow-up study. Therefore, the percentage diameter and area stenosis calculations revealed a measurable increase from 29 ± 12 to 42 ± 15 and 48 ± 22 to 64 ± 19, respectively, Fig. 4, bottom panel. Of the 22 patients in Group B, 20 exhibited a minimum luminal diameter of greater than 1 mm at their 3–6 month follow-up film.

Table 2. Group A – rotational ablation alone.

	Dg					Br					Fw					Sx				
	Mean	SD	Max	Min	N	Mean	SD	Max	Min	N	Mean	SD	Max	Min	N	Mean	SD	Max	Min	N
PDial	2.54	0.64	3.77	1.28	30	2.47	0.66	3.75	1.41	30	2.62	0.61	4.37	1.79	30	2.51	0.72	4.71	1.49	30
MDial	0.75	0.31	1.43	0.24	30	1.37	0.24	1.90	0.90	30	1.57	0.23	2.19	1.23	30	1.33	0.45	2.27	0.24	30
DDial	2.30	0.64	3.77	1.40	30	2.22	0.52	3.53	1.34	30	2.44	0.51	3.40	1.59	30	2.36	0.64	3.90	1.38	30
%Dial	69.46	9.26	89.60	54.80	30	39.40	12.61	59.90	13.30	30	35.52	12.59	53.00	13.90	30	44.16	17.60	89.60	10.70	30
%Are1	89.83	5.27	98.90	79.60	30	62.00	15.78	84.30	25.00	30	57.11	16.79	77.90	26.00	30	66.04	18.92	98.90	20.30	30

PDial = Proximal Diameter, One View; MDial = Minimal Diameter, One View; DDial = Distal Diameter, One View; %Dial = percentage diameter stenosis; %Are1 = percentage area stenosis, One View; N = Number lesions; Dg = Diagnostic; Br = post-burr; Bl = post burr and balloon; Fw = 24-hour follow-up; Sx = 3–6 month follow-up; SD = Standard deviation.

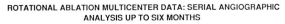

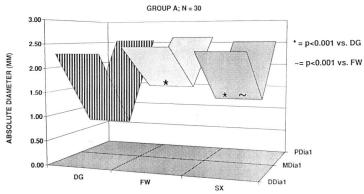

Figure 3. Three dimensional plot of the absolute diameter in mm (Y axis) at the proximal reference segment (PDial), at the minimum diameter (MDial), and the distal reference sement (DDial)(Z axis), taken from coronary arteriographic cinefilms recorded before rotational ablation (DG), at 24 hours after ablation (FW) and then again at 3–6 months later (SX)(X axis). Data is taken from patients undergoing rotational ablation alone (Group A).

Recently, we have been working on new approaches for graphic display of the differences in luminal patency brought about by rotational ablation. One approach is to simply show the relevant coronary artery segments in a side-by-side display after the edge recognition and plaque fill-in algorithms have been applied (Fig. 6, top panel). However, in some instances the anatomical changes are subtle and not so readily apparent to the eye. Thus, we are now beginning to plot histograms of the total population of diameters calculated perpendicular to the centerline, Fig. 6, bottom panel. When these histograms are either superimposed in different colors, or, alternatively, demonstrated on top of one another in black and white, the greater uniformity of luminal patency post-plaque ablation is more readily appreciated. The topographic location of the individual diameters is missing, however, in such a display. Two other examples of coronary artery diameter histograms (before, at 24 hours after, and at 6 months after rotational ablation) are shown in Fig. 7, left and right panels.

Conclusions

These early, serial quantitative angiographic observations suggest that rotational ablation is an effective mode of improving and sustaining luminal patency when used to ablate hemodynamically significant coronary artery stenoses. Although the patients reported herein were neither a randomly-assigned or consecutively-analyzed cohort (nigh impossible conditions to fulfill when using serial, quantitative coronary angiographic indices as endpoints), nevertheless the conclusion is strongly suggested that this new ap-

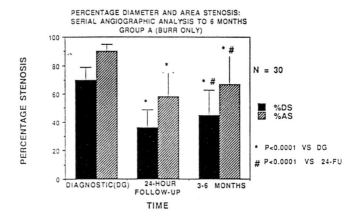

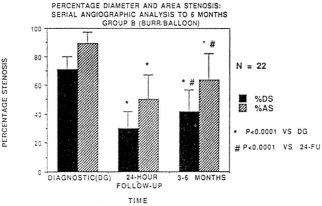

Figure 4. Plots of percentage diameter and area stenosis before, at 24 hours after, and at 3–6 months after rotational ablation. Group A (rotational ablation alone) is shown in the top panel; Group B (combined rotational ablation and balloon dilation) is shown in the bottom panel.

proach to coronary angioplasty is associated with an acceptably low restenosis rate and is not associated with significant induction of new atherosclerotic disease on either side of the treated lesion.

Any interventional technique for plaque ablation has the potential for inciting the complex mechanisms underlying restenosis. Since intimal abrasion in an experimental animal fed a high-cholesterol diet is known to produce atherosclerosis, there is obvious concern that the abrasive action of the diamond-studded Rotablator burr might induce disease, particularly in areas formerly free of significant luminal obstruction. However, thus far in our quantitative registry, we have not encountered patients where reference segments, i.e., areas of the coronary arterial tree on either side of an obstructive lesion, manifested significant diminution of luminal diameter on the six-month post-rotablation angiogram.

In this early comparison of patients treated with the rotablator alone

Table 3. Group B – rotational ablation followed by balloon angioplasty.

	Dg					Br					Bl					Fw					SX				
	Mean	SD	Max	Min	N	Mean	SD	Max	Min	N	Mean	SD	Max	Min	N	Mean	SD	Max	Min	N	Mean	SD	Max	Min	N
PDia1	2.70	0.49	4.03	1.72	22	2.60	0.59	3.87	1.62	22	2.75	0.57	4.15	1.76	22	2.77	0.50	3.95	1.70	22	2.93	0.54	4.00	1.91	22
MDia1	0.78	0.22	1.18	0.36	22	1.16	0.30	1.64	0.56	22	1.68	0.34	2.44	1.02	22	1.89	0.32	2.53	1.36	22	1.63	0.48	2.78	0.79	22
DDia1	2.46	0.40	3.06	1.78	22	2.28	0.54	3.16	1.48	22	2.39	0.52	3.80	1.57	22	2.65	0.41	3.38	1.54	22	2.65	0.46	3.49	1.77	22
%Dia1	70.56	8.52	85.50	58.80	22	51.48	13.85	72.10	22.20	22	32.14	13.64	61.90	1.00	22	28.84	11.68	46.20	6.90	22	41.74	15.36	68.40	13.60	22
%Are1	88.87	7.73	97.40	61.90	22	74.59	14.41	92.20	40.10	22	52.56	19.23	85.50	1.00	22	48.35	22.10	71.00	13.50	22	63.98	18.63	90.20	25.30	22

PDia1 = Proximal Diameter, One View; MDia1 = Minimai Diameter, One View; %Dia1 = Distal Diameter, One View; DDia1 = percentage diameter stenosis; %Are1 = percentage area stenosis, One View; N = Number of lesions; Dg = Diagnosic; Br = post-burr; Bl = post burr and balloon; Fw = 24-hour follow-up; Sx = 3–6 Month follow-up; SD = Standard deviation.

ROTATIONAL ABLATION MULTICENTER DATA: SERIAL ANGIOGRAPHIC
ANALYSIS UP TO SIX MONTHS

GROUP B; N= 22

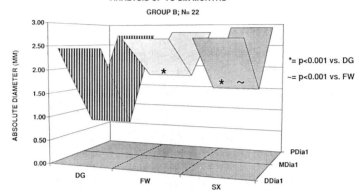

Figure 5. Three dimensional plot of the absolute diameter in mm (Y axis) at the proximal reference segment (PDial), at the minimum diameter (MDial), and the distal reference segment (DDial)(Z axis), taken from coronary arteriographic cinefilms recorded before rotational ablation (DG), at 24 hours after ablation (FW) and then again at 3–6 months later (SX)(X axis). Data is taken from patients undergoing combined rotational ablation and balloon dilation (Group B).

(Group A), as opposed to rotablator followed by adjunctive balloon dilation (Group B), it appears that the ultimate absolute minimal diameter, although not the percentage stenosis, is greater at 6 months follow-up in the latter group. Whether this difference represents a true superiority of the combined rotational ablation/balloon dilation approach, however, remains questionable. Since the size of the proximal reference segment in Group B (2.93 + 0.54 mm) appeared to be trending toward a larger size than in Group A (2.51 + 0.72 mm), the differences between the two groups may simply represent a difference in intrinsic vessel size. Alternatively, the operator may be influenced to use balloon adjunctive dilation by the appearance of the heated segment, as compared to the reference segment, following ablation with a burr which is relatively small compared to the nominal vessel size. It is too early in our analysis to know whether the final burr size used has a significant influence on the ultimate quantitative result at follow-up angiography. Our early analysis would suggest that when lesions are grouped into two categories, those where a burr size of less than 1.75 mm and those greater than 1.75 mm were utilized, there was no difference noted in the amount of plaque removed. In all cases the ratio of minimal luminal diameter to burr size increased significantly after ablation, and approximated unity (0.85 + 0.16) on the twenty-four hour follow-up film, indicating that the final patency achieved approached final burr size used during the procedure. The fact that this ratio is less than unity, however, indicates that there is some degree of "watermelon seed" slippage of the burr as it traverses through an area of narrowing.

Presently, we are interpreting these serial angiographic analyses with cau-

A.

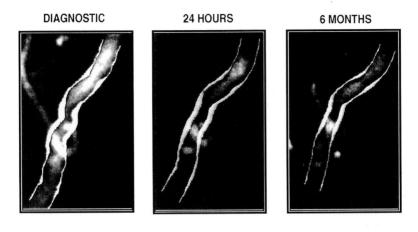

DIAGNOSTIC   **24 HOURS**   **6 MONTHS**

B.

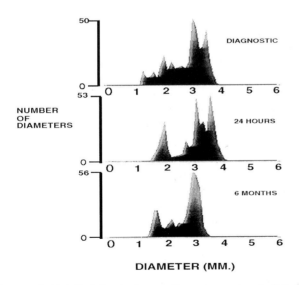

NUMBER
OF
DIAMETERS

DIAMETER (MM.)

Figure 6. Top panel: End-diastolic cineframes of coronary artery before (diagnostic), at 24 hours after, and at 6 months after rotational ablation. An edge recognition algorithm has been applied to the vessels, and the plaque area as been hypothetically determined based upon a linear decrement in size between the proximal and distal reference segments. Bottom panel: Histograms of the number of diameters against the absolute diameter in mm for each of the coronary artery segments shown in the top panel. Note the change in the profile of the diameters between diagnostic and 24 hours; also note the greater uniformity of diameter size post-rotational ablation. Full vasodilation was not accomplished at the time of the 6 month angiogram, believed to account for the absence of diameters in the 3.5 to 4.0 mm range.

A.

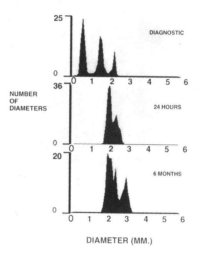

Figure 7A.

tious optimism. Only the accumulation of further experience will provide guidelines for technique, choice of burr size, and the ultimate wisdom of using balloon adjunctive dilation. Since a significant proportion of the lesions in this series were, in fact, eccentric, calcified, and relatively long, we see even greater reason to be enthused about the ultimate utility of this device for improving the clinical results of coronary angioplasty.

Acknowledgement

The authors gratefully acknowledge the expert help of Ian Gocka, M.S., in the statistical analysis of the data included in this report.

B.

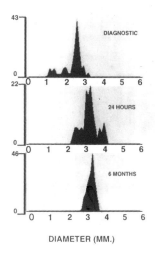

DIAMETER (MM.)

Figure 7. A: Histograms of the number of diameters against the absolute diameter in mm for the same coronary artery segment before, 24 hours after, and at 6 months after rotational ablation. Note the change in the profile of the diameters between diagnostic and 24 hours; also note the greater uniformity of diameter size post-rotational ablation. In this instance, full vasodilation was accomplished immediately before each coronary artery injection. Note the increase in diameters in the 2.75 to 3.0 mm range at 6 months, presumably related to vessel expansion in areas of atherosclerotic involvement. B: Histograms of a further patient, presented in the same format as the left panel. Note in this case that the profile of the diameters in the treated coronary segment have become quite uniform at the time of the 6 months follow-up study.

References

1. Gruentzig A R, Senning A, Sigenthaler W E (1979) Nonoperative dilaton of coronary artery stenosis – percutaneous transluminal coronary angioplasty. *N Engl J Med* 01:61–68
2. Detre K, Holubkov R, Kelsey S, Cowley M, Kent K, Williarns D, Myler R, Faxon D, Holmes D R Jr, Bourassa M, Block P, Gosselin A, Bentivoglio, Leatherman L, Dorros G, King S, Galichia J, Al-Bassam M, Leon M, Robertson T, Passamani E (1988) Percutaneous transluminal coronary angioplasty in 1985–1986 and 1977–1981. The National Heart, Lung, and Blood Institute Registry. *N Engl J Med* 318:265– 270
3. Ryan T J, et al (1988) Guidelines for percutaneous transluminal coronary angioplasty: A report of the American College of Cardiology/American Heart Association Task Force on assessment of diagnostic and therapeutic cardiovascular procedures (Subcommittee on percutaneous transluminal coronary angioplasty). *J Am Coll Cardiol* 12:529–545
4. Serruys P W, Luijten H E, Beatt K J, Geuskens R, De Feyter P J, Van Den Brand M, Reiber J H C, Ten Katen H J, vas Es G A, Hugenholtz P G (1988) Incidence of restenosis after successful coronary angioplasty: a time-related phenomenon: a quantitative angiographic study in 342 consecutive patients at 1, 2, 3 and 4 months. *Circulation* 77:361–371
5. Nobuyoshi M, Kimura T, Nosaka H, Mioka S, Ueno K, Yokoi H, Hamasaki N, Horiuchi H,

Ohishi H (1988) Restenosis after successful percutaneous transluminal coronary angioplasty: serial angiographic follow-up of 229 patients. *J Am Coll Cardiol* 12:616–523

6. Guiteras V P, Bourassa M G, David P R, Bonan R, Crepeau J, Dyrda I, Lesperance J (1987) Restenosis after successful percutaneous transluminal coronary angioplasty: the Montreal Heart Institute experience. *Am J Cardiol* 60:50B-55B

7. Holmes D R Jr, Vlietstra R E, Smith H C, Vetrovec G W, Kent K M, Cowley M J, Faxon D P, Gruentzig A R, Kelsey S F, Detre K M (1984) Restenosis after percutaneous transluminal coronary angioplasty (PTCA): a report from the PTCA registry of the National Heart, Lung, and Blood Institute. *Am J Cardiol* 53:77C-81C

8. Litvack F, Eigler N L, Margolis J R, Grundfest W S, Rothbaum D, Linnemeier T, Hestrin L B, Tsoi D, Cook S L, Krauthamer D, Goldenberg T, Laudenslager J R, Segalowitz J, Forrester J S (1990) Percutaneous excimer laser coronary angioplasty. *Am J Cardiol* 66:1027–1032

9. Spears J R, Reyes V P, Wynne J, Fromm B S, Sinofsky E L, Andrus S, Sinclair I N, Hopkins B E, Schwartz L, Aldridge H E, Plokker H W Thijs, Mast E G, Rickards A, Knudtson M L, Sigwart U, Dear W E, Ferguson J J, Angelini P, Leatherman L L, Safian R D, Jenkins R D, Douglas J S, King S B III (1990) Percutaneous coronary laser balloon angioplasty: initial results of a multicenter experience. *J Am Coll Cardiol* 16:293–303

10. Safian R D, Gelbfish J S, Erny R E, Schnitt S J, Schmidt D A, Baim D S (1990) Coronary atherectomy: clinical, angiographic, and histological findings and observations regarding potential mechanisms. *Circulation* 82:69–79

11. Fourrier J L, Bertrand M E, Auth D C, LaBlanche J M, Gommeaux A, Brunetaud J M (1989) Percutaneous coronary rotational angioplasty in humans: preliminary report. *J Am Coll Cardiol* 14:1278–1282

12. Hansen D D, Auth D C, Vrocko R, Ritchie J L (1988) Rotational atherectomy in atherosclerotic rabbit iliac arteries. *Am Heart J* 115:160–165

13. Hansen D D, Auth D C, Hall M, Ritchie J L (1988) Rotational endarterectomy in normal canine coronary arteries: preliminary report. *J Am Coll Cardiol* 11:1073–1077

PART SIX

Lasers

Introduction

WARREN S. GRUNDFEST, FRANK LITVACK,
JAMES MARGOLIS, JAMES LAUDENSLAGER and
TSVI GOLDENBERG

Excimer Laser Angioplasty: Initial Experience and Restenosis Rates

The goal of this section is to present a brief explanation of the biophysical considerations involved in applying the technology of excimer laser angioplasty. A brief discussion of laser physics, fiberoptics, catheter design, and guidance systems is included to assist the reader in understanding the physical and biological foundations for excimer laser angioplasty. This introduction will provide the reader the information necessary to comprehend the rationale for our investigation of this method of angioplasty. The following section will present our initial restenosis findings following excimer laser angioplasty. The technique of excimer laser angioplasty is still in its preliminary stages of investigation, and significant changes in lasers, delivery systems or ablation parameters may have a significant impact on the acute and long-term outcome of the procedure. The reader is urged to view this technology as an evolving adjunct to the treatment of coronary artery disease rather than the final solution to the problem of obstructed arteries.

Lasers generate intense light (monochromatic radiation) which can be delivered to defined tissue areas with great precision through fiber optics. The laser/tissue interaction is affected by seven major processes: absorption, reflection, scattering, transmission, defraction, refraction, and reemission as fluorescence. Once absorption has occurred the light energy may be converted to heat, may break chemical bonds, may form a plasma, or be reemitted as fluorescence. Each of these pathways results in a different biologic effect on the tissue. Thus, the choice of laser depends upon the desired application, the tissue encountered, and the biologic constraints placed on the laser delivery system.

Initial clinical application of lasers for angioplasty were based on primitive delivery systems and poorly understood laser/tissue interactions [1, 2]. The disappointing clinical results from these initial trials reflected both a lack of experience in system design and a primitive notion that laser energy could "burn out" the atheroma. Despite the experimental nature of these initial

P.W. Serruys, B.H. Strauss and S.B. King III (eds), Restenosis after Intervention with New Mechanical Devices, 331–345.
© 1992 Kluwer Academic Publishers. Printed in the Netherlands.

systems, they were touted as miracle cures and purchased to attract patients. The combination of poor system design, minimal understanding of the laser/ tissue interaction, and minimal training with poor patient selection led to a negative impression of laser technology for laser angioplasty [3–5]. Delivery of laser energy was accomplished through crude single fiber optic systems without the benefit of guidance mechanisms. The preliminary results of laser angioplasty reported in the literature [6–8] were often used to compare laser systems to other more mature technologies (balloon angioplasty).

The Interaction of Light with Matter

Our research has shown that for laser angioplasty there is an optimal set of energy delivery parameters to achieve a desired result. This result, a smoothly recanalized non-thrombogenic artery, can only be achieved if the process of ablation is understood for each given wavelength. Prior to application in patients, this set of energy delivery parameters must be clearly defined. These parameters include the energy delivered per unit time at the target, the area of the target irradiated, the time of irradiation, and, if a pulsed laser is used, the duration of the laser pulse and the number of pulses per second. When pulsed lasers are employed, knowledge of the pulse duration becomes critical to controlling the laser's biologic effects. These pulse durations can range from a few milliseconds to a few picoseconds (10^{-12} seconds).

Laser power can be described in terms of average power or peak power. The average power is the energy delivered per unit of time. For pulsed lasers the peak power is the energy of a single pulse divided by its pulse width. The pulse width of the laser is determined by the lasers' electronics and the laser medium and is measured using photodiodes and an oscilloscope. Two lasers operating at an average power of 5 Watts will have distinctly different effects on the tissue if one is operating in the continuous-wave mode and the other operates in a pulsed mode. Unfortunately, there is a lack of clarity in the literature when describing laser power parameters. Descriptions of average power without knowing the spot size or pulse characteristics of the laser are inadequate and insufficient for characterization of the biologic effects.

The following example is used to illustrate the difference between average power and peak power. If a pulsed laser emits light with an energy of 100 millijoules at 100 pulses per second with a pulse duration of 10 nanoseconds and this energy is delivered to a $1\,cm^2$ spot, the average power density is 100 millijoules $\times$ 100 pulses per second per cm^2 or 10 Watts per cm^2 in average power terms. However, the peak power is calculated as 100 millijoules divided by 10×10^{-9} seconds/cm^2 or 10 megawatts (MW) per cm^2. In this example the peak power is enormous while the average power is much lower. High peak powers in the megawatt range tend to produce nonlinear effects such as photochemical rearrangements, photoplasmas, and photoacoustic shock waves. The pulse duration becomes a critical factor in the process of selecting the optimal laser for laser angioplasty. If the pulse duration is too short, damage to fiberoptics and generation of shock waves may limit the effectiveness of a particular laser angioplasty system. If pulse durations are too long, heating of adjacent tissue and subsequent rupture of the arterial wall may occur.

For pulsed lasers the term "energy fluence" is used to describe the irradiance level of the tissue. Energy fluence is the energy per pulse divided by the area under irradiation and is expressed in joules/cm^2 or millijoules/mm^2. For a continuous-wave laser the energy fluence equals the laser output power in Watts $\times$ the exposure time in seconds divided by the irradiated area. Thus, tissue effects are related to the energy per unit area delivered to the tissue. These effects, including heating, vaporization, ablation (layer by layer removal of tissue), and fragmentation, are a function of the wavelength of light, the laser pulse duration, the energy density at which the light is delivered, and the properties of the tissue.

The combination of pulsed delivery and spatial confinement of energy (due to intense absorption and resultant minimal depth of penetration) provide a unique opportunity to produce precise controllable tissue ablation and is the basis for pulsed ultraviolet laser angioplasty. The short pulse duration limits the time available for heat transfer to occur during irradiation, and the spatial confinement produced by the use of ultraviolet light limits the area irradiated. Understanding this process requires a brief description of the mechanisms of laser action on tissue.

The Process of *Tissue Ablation* by Laser Light

The absorption of laser light by tissue may cause tissue destruction and removal through three basic pathways: Photothermal, Photochemical, and Photoacoustic ablation. These three processes are not necessarily exclusive, and may occur simultaneously. With each process, energy may leak into the surrounding tissue. This "leakage" results in damage to adjacent tissue in the form of thermal coagulation injury, mechanical membrane rupture from shock waves, and photochemical damage to proteins and other biologic molecules. Energy that is not absorbed can be scattered or transmitted through the tissue and produce effects remote from the site of energy application. The extent of scattering depends upon the organization structure and particulate size within a given tissue, the depth of penetration of a particular wavelength within the tissue, and the presence of molecules which weakly or strongly absorb the light (chromophores). Energy delivered in short, intense pulses can generate a photoplasma. Alternatively, rapid deposition of energy can lead to almost instantaneous conversion of solid or liquid to the gas phase. From either process explosive ejection of material occurs and is accompanied by acoustic transients or shock waves. These shock waves can disrupt the tissues [9, 10].

Thermal Processes

The first and most common mechanism, conversion of light to heat, results when continuous-wave or pulsed infrared lasers are used to irradiate tissue. The absorbed photons increase the rotational/vibrational levels of the molecules which increase molecular motion. As tissue temperature rises, water vaporizes and proteins denature. If water is the absorbing chromophore, the tissue undergoes rapid dehydration as the water is converted to steam. The resulting shock wave from the conversion of water to steam can be quite pronounced. As energy delivery continues, heat is conducted to the surrounding tissues. Direct conversion of light to heat may also occur as proteins, lipids, and other tissue chromophores absorb light. Coagulation can be prominent, particularly in the infrared wavelengths.

As the tissue is heated to 43–50°C, the collagen helices uncoil, resulting in reversible tissue denaturation. If the heating is not prolonged, cooling may occur and the coils may actually fuse together. This annealing process is the basis for laser welding and laser tissue fusion experiments. Efforts to control this process are complicated by the enormous number of variables involved. The clinical application of laser welding has been slow to evolve due to the inability to predict the outcome of the process. As temperature of the tissue increases beyond 60°C irreversible protein denaturation occurs. If exposure to this level of heat is short, the cells are injured; prolonged heating results in cell death. As temperatures exceed 80°C the underlying structural elements of the tissue, collagen, elastin and proteoglycans, begin to degrade. At 100°C water within the tissue boils leading to a potentially explosive release of steam. When temperatures exceed 150°C pyrolysis of the tissue is observed (Fig. 1). At temperatures above 200°C the tissue begins to carbonize. Only the carbon particles are left behind as the rest of the organic material is oxidized. With continuous-wave lasers, attempts to ablate calcified tissue can result in temperatures in excess of 500°C.

When laser energy is converted to heat in the tissues, thermal diffusion begins. Diffusion of heat through the tissue depends on the thermal properties of the irradiated material. The thermal diffusion constants which govern the conduction of heat through vascular tissue are in part a function of the composition of the vascular wall and its hydration state. Pulses longer than several microseconds will allow thermal energy to diffuse over 10–100 microns in a few milliseconds. Pulses in the millisecond range are sufficiently long to allow for heat generated to diffuse between 100 and 1000 microns away from the zone of irradiation. The thermal relaxation (cooling) phenomenon is influenced by 1) the thermal coefficient of the tissue, 2) the properties of the surrounding tissue or fluids, and 3) the temperature differential be-

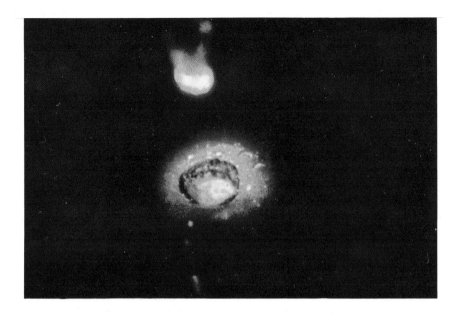

Figure 1. Aortic tissue ablation by Nd:YAG laser. This single image was obtained during high speed filming of an Nd:YAG laser beam ablating human atherosclerotic aortic tissue. The 600 micron fiberoptic delivery system delivered 38 Watts/mm^2 for a 2-second pulse. This frame obtained at 1.2 seconds shows a well defined crater with a carbonized rim. The crater diameter is 1.4 mm and the surrounding tissue is thermally altered. Note the boiling tissue components at the crater rim.

tween the irradiated and nonirradiated tissue [11–13]. The fundamental process, the conversion of light to heat, occurs during tissue ablation with all continuous-wave lasers and at pulse durations greater than 10 microseconds, regardless of the wavelength chosen and the energy delivery parameters. To minimize the lateral spread of energy it is necessary to select a pulsed laser with a pulse duration that is significantly shorter than the average thermal conduction time of the tissue.

Laser ablation produced by pulsed, mid-infrared lasers such as Holmium or Thulium YAG lasers, is a result of rapid thermal vaporization of water and subsequent mechanical processes. When energy is absorbed water is converted to steam, forming vapor bubbles. These vapor bubbles can generate intense pressure waves in the tissue, leading to both mechanical shearing and thermal denaturation of the adjacent tissue. Ablation with these lasers requires sufficient energy to vaporize water in the volume of tissue being removed. The conversion of water to steam results in a massive increase in the volume of the irradiated matter. However, the water vapor and tissue components are confined by the surrounding tissue. As more water is converted to vapor, and the pressure and temperature rise, a small scale explosion occurs. Using stop frame photography this process can be visualized (Fig. 2).

Photochemical Processes

A second form of tissue ablation results from irradiation of tissue with short (nanosecond) pulse duration ultraviolet laser energy. Below 320 nanometers ultraviolet photons contain sufficient energy per photon (3.6 eV) to break molecular bonds. This electronic process is more efficient than thermal processes as the laser energy is employed directly in bond breaking without a thermal intermediate. The primary chromophore (energy absorbing material) is protein or lipid not water. Thus, pulsed ultraviolet light can lead to direct electronic bond breaking of organic material and does not require vaporization of water for tissue ablation. As large molecules are converted to small molecules they are ejected from the surface of the material, removing much of the energy used to break the chemical bonds [14]. Since the pulse duration is less than 500 nanoseconds, there is little time for radiative or conductive heat transfer to the adjacent tissue. Thus, the input energy is not deposited in the adjacent tissue.

In order for the process to be effective, the tissue must be a strong absorber of the laser wavelength. Atherosclerotic tissue, although highly heterogeneous, is composed primarily of water and organic compounds with inorganic salts. The atherosclerotic proteins and lipids strongly absorb ultraviolet light and serve as the primary chromophore. Photochemical change can occur as a result of direct excitation of electronic bonds by the laser energy and is one of the proposed mechanisms of action of pulsed, ultraviolet lasers. Electronic excitation of tissue molecules by laser light is not 100% efficient; therefore, heat is also generated during this process. While the exact nature of this process remains the subject of intense debate, ablation produced by pulsed ultraviolet light at levels above threshhold is precise, controllable, and predictable (Fig. 3).

Two potential mechanisms have been proposed to explain the precise ablation of tissue with minimal thermal damage produced by pulsed ultraviolet laser irradiation of tissue. At shorter wavelengths, tissue components, proteins, and lipids absorb photons and become electronically excited. This "photoexcitation" leads to rupture of molecular bonds and formation of molecular fragments. These molecular fragments then undergo a process known as photochemical desorption and are ejected from the irradiated surface in less than 200 nanoseconds. The ejected fragments carry with them much of the energy that was initially deposited within the tissue to generate the fragments. This electronic excitation occurs before conversion to heat or thermal diffusion occurs.

A second possible mechanism to explain this phenomenon is very high-speed, localized absorption, which leads to formation of a very small area

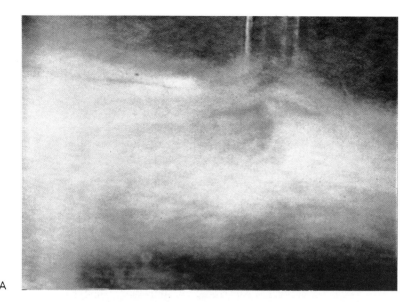

A

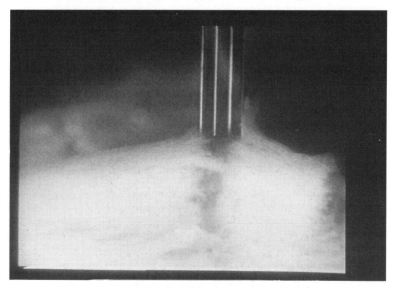

B

Figure 2. Holmium:YAG ablation of atherosclerotic tissue. This sequence of images demonstrates the impact of shock waves on tissue ablation. The Holmium:YAG laser was delivered to human atherosclerotic aortic tissue through a 0.4 mm low-OH silica fiber. The fiber spot size at the tissue was 0.5 mm at an energy density of $700\,mj/mm^2$. Figure 2A illustrates the effect of the blast wave on the intimal surface. Note the upward and outward motion of the debris and tissue edges. The haziness of the image is due to the rapid motion of the tissue. Figure 2B shows the generation of dissection planes within the tissue. The combination of intense shock waves, gas bubble generation and ejection of large particulate debris limits the applicability of this laser for laser angioplasty.

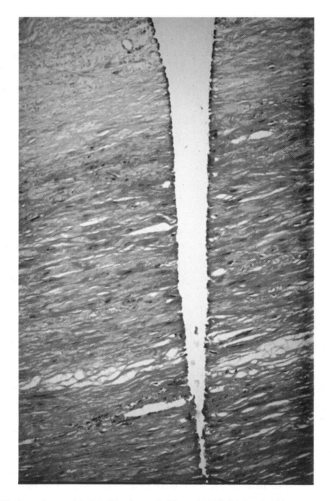

Figure 3. Excimer laser ablation histology. In June 1983 initial experiments revealed that the 308 nanometer excimer laser could ablate tissue with great precision and minimal thermal damage. This histologic section of human atherosclerotic aorta received 96 pulses of 308 nm laser radiation at an energy density of 30 mj/mm². Note the lack of carbonization and lateral thermal injury. Compared to the histology obtained from continuous wave lasers this was a dramatic reduction in tissue injury.

of vaporized photoproducts. These products expand rapidly away from the tissue surface, again carrying away the incident energy. By either mechanism the result is the removal of tissue with minimal thermal damage to adjacent structures. Based on these theoretical considerations, pulsed ultraviolet light appears to be the optimal energy source for laser angioplasty [15].

Photoacoustic Processes

The deposition of large numbers of photons in a short period of time produces a very intense local alteration in the electric field which surrounds all matter. This sudden rise in electrical energy disrupts the outer electronic configuration of molecules. These excited electrons produce a plasma. These plasmas can be produced through a variety of mechanisms. The most common of these is dielectric breakdown, in which large numbers of electrons are released as the conductivity of the material is altered due to the intense electric field generated by the absorption of laser light. This energy is then transferred to the surrounding tissue, producing a small area of vaporized material. The sudden expansion of the vaporized material generates an intense shock wave. As the shock wave expands radially outward, tissue disruption and ejection of material may result. This mechanism is employed in the treatment of thickened posterior capsule membranes which occur after cataract operations.

Typically, two infrared beams of subthreshhold energies are focused to the spot on the posterior capsule of the lens where membrane disruption is desired. While each beam is insufficient to destroy the tissue, the two beams together produce a photoplasma which disrupts the tissue [16]. The high peak powers and short pulse durations required for this process to occur tend to destroy the fiber optics as well as the tissue. Thus, this mechanism is not readily adaptable to fiber optic transmission. Alternatively, longer pulses can be transmitted through fibers and deposited in an area where intense absorption occurs. The deposition of green light at pulse durations of 1–50 microseconds produces an intense shock wave from the rapid vaporization of the hemoglobin and adjacent water. This mechanism does not work well in heterogeneous tissue such as atheroma due to the variations in elasticity and absorption (Fig. 4). Therefore, application of photoacoustic ablation mechanisms to atherosclerotic tissue produces variable results.

During tissue ablation, these three ablation processes, photothermal, photoacoustic, and photochemical, can occur simultaneously. However, the desired outcome can be achieved by selection of the appropriate wavelength and energy delivery parameters. Unless the appropriate parameters are selected, the desired process may be accompanied by other, less desirable ablation pathways. For pulsed ultraviolet ablation of tissue to occur through a photochemical mechanism there must be sufficient energy per photon and sufficient numbers of photons to break molecular bonds [17]. This occurs only above a certain threshhold level which is a unique combination of both the laser wavelength and the tissue under irradiation [18] (Fig. 5). If the light irradiating the tissue is at subthreshhold levels, insufficient chemical intermediates are formed for the photochemical processes to occur and the light is converted to heat. If too much energy is employed, dieiectric breakdown occurs and a photoacoustic mechanism predominates. Thus, the same

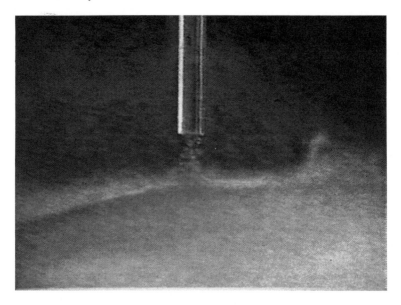

Figure 4. Pulsed dye laser irradiation. This image demonstrates the scatter of 480 nm laser light through tissue. This human atherosclerotic cadaveric aorta was irradiated at 480 nm via a 200 micron diameter silica fiber at 65 mj/mm^2. While this energy is more than sufficient to shatter most kidney stones and gallstones, it had little effect on the aorta. When the tissue is irradiated in blood (not shown) the blood absorbs the energy producing a shock wave which tears apart the tissue. However, in saline only minimal ablation occurs. Tissue that is relatively unpigmented is only minimally affected at this wavelength. Tissue which is yellow absorbs this wavelength and the resulting shock wave causes ejection of the irradiated material. However, due to the great variation in coloration of human atheroma, this laser is inappropriate for laser angioplasty.

laser, if operated in a different mode, can produce considerably different tissue effects even though the wavelength is the same.

Based on early observations that continuous-wave lasers produce significant thermal damage during ablation of atherosclerotic material, our group began to investigate the possibility of pulsed ultraviolet laser ablation of tissue in 1983. Thus we began our search for a laser source which produced pulsed ultraviolet light that could be transmitted through fiber optics [19, 20]. In addition, ablation had to proceed in a relatively uniform fashion in all types of atheroma. Concommitant with our laser studies, our ability to view the lumen of coronary arteries in patients demonstrated the need for a laser wavelength which would uniformly ablate the broad range of atherosclerotic tissue [21].

At 308 nm each photon has 3.8 eV; thus, this wavelength is the shortest which can produce direct photochemical excitation and still be transmitted at sufficient intensity through fiberoptics. Transmission of this wavelength through fiber optics requires pulse stretching of the laser. Research by Litvack et al [22, 23] has demonstrated that over the range of 10–500 nano-

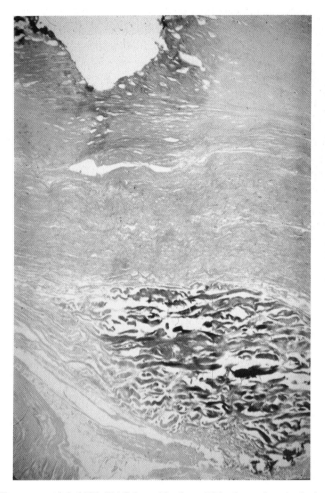

Figure 5. Frequency tripled Nd: YAG laser histology. This photomicrograph shows the results of irradiation of human cadaveric aorta at 353 nm at 7 nanoseconds at 45 mj/mm². Note that the crater walls show evidence of vacuolization and coagulation injury. Thus, energy is absorbed and converted to heat which produces the resulting observed damage. Thus, the near UV wavelengths can ablate tissue but do not entirely eliminate thermal damage when delivered in a pulsed mode.

seconds, energy density is the key parameter in determining ablation thresholds. In contrast, fiber optic damage occurs as peak powers are increased (as pulse duration is decreased). Thus, a long pulse (200 nanoseconds) of 100 millijoules can be easily transmitted through a multifiber catheter, while a short pulse (60 nanoseconds or less) at the same energy invariably leads to fiber destruction within a few pulses. Stretching the pulse decreases the shock wave during ablation since the ejection of material and escape of gases occurs over a longer time period. However, as the pulse duration increases, poor beam quality and high repetition rates may lead to thermal injury of the tissue. Optimal pulse durations for ablation of tissue with minimal thermal damage and shock waves appear to be between 200–350 nanoseconds.

308 nm light is strongly absorbed by most vascular and atherosclerotic tissues. Depth of penetration ranges from 10 microns for blood to 30 microns for lipoid atheroma. As calcification increases the energy threshhold rises. At 308 nm ablation threshholds for noncalcified tissue are between 18–25 millijoules/mm^2. For moderately calcified atheroma the threshhold rises to 35 millijoules/mm^2, and for densely calcified tissue, such as calcified heart valves, the ablation threshold can exceed 60 millijoules/mm^2. In densely calcified tissues, dead space from the cladding of the fiber optics may often limit the ability to advance the fiber. In clinical practice this is potentially a serious problem. To avoid this problem, careful attention must be paid to the fiber optic design of the delivery system.

Ablation at 308 nm proceeds with minimal transfer of heat into the adjacent tissue. High-speed filming, histologic and thermographic studies have all demonstrated that tissue adjacent to areas ablated by an excimer laser suffer minimal, if any, thermal trauma. When properly operating, i.e., with uniform beam quality and minimal variation of energy from pulse to pulse, ablation occurs uniformly across the area irradiated by the laser beam. If the beam is irregular an irregular crater will form. If the delivery system injects energy into the tissue at subthreshhold levels, this energy is converted to heat. Thus, the challenge for system engineers is to produce a relatively uniform energy output across the surface of the catheter while maintaining flexibility and trackability of the angioplasty system. This complex engineering problem requires multiple iterative design sequences.

Excimer Lasers

Excimer lasers consist of a family of gas lasers in which the lasing action is produced by a chemical reaction. The chemical reaction is induced by transmitting a high voltage electrical discharge through a gas mixture [24]. The gas mixture is primarily composed of an inert gas such as helium or neon into which a few per cent of another inert gas such as argon, xenon or krypton and trace amounts (0.1–0.5%) of a halogen such as chlorine or fluorine are added. The excimer gas laser emits pulsed light directly in the ultraviolet region of the spectrum. These lasers operate only in the pulsed mode. The word "excimer" is derived from the initial description of these lasers as emitting from an excited state dimer molecule. While this characterization proved to be a simplification of the actual physical process, the name "excimer" was used to describe this class of lasers.

The XeCl excimer laser can be made to operate in the so-called "long

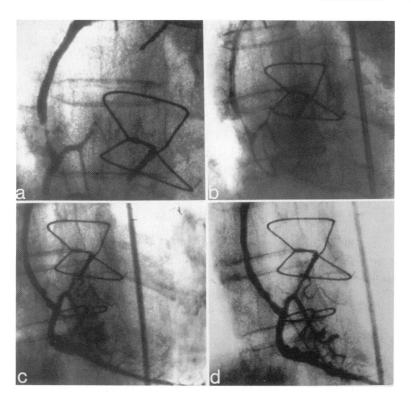

Figure 6. Excimer Laser Angioplasty of a Sapheneous vein graft in the first clinical trial. This four panel angiographic sequence shows the iniitial angiogram (a), the wire across the lesion (b), the results of excimer laser angioplasty in the saphenous vein graph (c), and the final result after adjunctive balloon angioplasty (d). This 85 year old female is still alive as of 11/91 with no evidence of restenosis.

pulse" mode. Typical commercially available excimer lasers for industrial applications operate between 7–40 nanoseconds. For ablation of biologic tissue approximately 35–70 millijoules of energy per pulse are required to ablate tissue. The power produced by such a pulse in units of energy per time is enormous and is calculated in the megawatt range. These high peak power pulses cause destruction of the fiber optics with corresponding loss of transmission of the laser light. When short pulse excimer laser designs are used for clinical applications they do not have sufficient reliability and predictability to produce optimal results. Recent results reported by Karsch et al using a XeCl excimer laser with 60 or 110 nanosecond pulse durations showed significant loss of energy transmission during the procedure. However, the XeCl excimer laser can be operated at 200–300 nanoseconds pulses producing a significant (fivefold) reduction in the peak power. This stretching of the pulse permits reliable fiber optic transmission.

Critical to the development of clinical systems for excimer laser angioplasty is the iterative design process. Experiments by Laudenslager [25] and Goldenberg [26] have demonstrated that the transmission of pulsed ultraviolet light through fiber optics is a function of peak power, spatial and temporal uniformity of the beam, and the construction of the fiber optics themselves. Having a long pulse excimer laser is not sufficient to achieve fiber optic transmission. The laser must have a relatively uniform beam profile with an output of sufficient size to power large diameter (3 mm or greater) fiber optic arrays. If the laser is underpowered, there will be insufficient energy to ablate with large diameter catheters. When only small catheters can be employed, the laser must be used primarily as an adjunctive hole-drilling device.

Our laboratory investigations have defined the optimal laser system given current fiber optic technology [27]. The laser, a 308 nanometer excimer laser, is designed to emit pulsed ultraviolet light at a pulse duration of 225 nanoseconds at energy levels of 250–300 millijoules/pulse. These requirements permit uniform transmission of the laser pulse through a multifiber concentric over-the-wire catheter. The catheters are designed to deliver 50–70 millijoules/mm^2 in contact with the tissue. Given the losses in the system from both fiber optics and coupler, an energy pulse from the laser must be sufficient to deliver this fluence through the catheter. The high energy output of the laser accounts for these energy losses which occur in the optical train and optical coupler and losses which occur during transmission through the fiber optics. Therefore, the clinical unit was designed specifically to meet these requirements.

References

1. Choy D S J, Stertzer S H, Myler R K, Marco J, Fournial G (1984) Human coronary laser recanalization. *Clinical Cardiology* 7:377–381
2. Ginsburg R, Wechsler L, Mitchell R S, Profitt D (1985) Percutaneous transluminal laser angioplasty for the treatment of peripheral vascular disease. *Radiology* 156:619–624
3. Abela G S, Fenech A, Crea F, Conti C R (1985) "Hot Tip": another method of laser vascular recanalization. *Lasers Surg Med* 5:327–335
4. Cumberland D C, Sanborn T A, Taylor D I, Moore D J, et al (1986) Percutaneous thermal laser angioplasty: initial clinical results with a laser probe in total peripheral artery occlusions. *Lancet* 1457–1459
5. Leon M B, Provosti L G, Smith P D, et al (1987) In-vivo laser induced fluorescence plaque detection: preliminary results in patients. *Circulation* 76(Suppl IV):IV 408
6. Forrester J S, Litvack F, Grundfest W S (1986) Laser angioplasty and cardiovascular disease. *Am J Cardiol* 57:990–992
7. Litvack F, Grundfest W S, Adler L, Hickey A, et al (1989) Percutaneous excimer laser angioplasty of the lower extremities: Results of an initial clinical trial *Radiology* 172:331–335
8. Litvack F, Grundfest W S, Eigler N, Tsoi D, Goldenberg T, Laudenslager J (1989) Percutaneous excimer laser coronary angioplasty. *Lancet* 2:102–103
9. Grundfest W S, Litvack F, Doyle L, et al (1986) Comparison of in vitro and in vivo thermal effects of argon and excimer lasers for laser angioplasty. *Circulation* 74(suppl II):II-204

10. Litvack F, Doyle L, Grundfest W S, et al (1986) In vivo excimer laser ablation: acute and chronic effects on canine aorta, abstracted. *Circulation* 74(suppl II):II-360
11. Srinivasan R (1986) Ablation of polymers and biological tissues by ultraviolet lasers. *Science* 234:559-565
12. Anderson R R, Parrish J A (1983) Selective photothermolysis: precise microsurgery by selective absorption of pulsed radiation. *Science* 220:524-527
13. Hu C, Barnes F S (1970) The thermal-chemical damage in biological material under laser irradiation. *IEEE Trans Biomed Eng* 17:220-231
14. Boulnais J L (1986) Photo physical processes in recent medical laser developments: a review. *Lasers Med Sci* 1:47-66
15. Grundfest W S, Litvack F, Morgenstern L, Forrester J S, Goldenberg T, Swan H J C, Fishbein M, McDermid I S, Rider D M, Pacala T J, Laudenslager J B (1984) Effect of excimer laser irradiation on human atherosclerotic aorta: amelioration of laser-induced thermal damage. *IEEE-CLEO Technical Digest* 248-249
16. Prince M R, Deutsch T F, Mathews-Roth M M, et al (1986) Preferential light absorption in atheromas in vitro: Implications for laser angioplasty. *J Clin Invest* 78:295-302
17. Garrison B J, Srinivasan R (1984) Microscopic model for the ablative photodecomposition of polymers by far ultraviolet radiation (193 nm). *Appl Phys Lett* 44:849-851
18. Srinivasan R, Braren B, Dreyfus R W, Hadel L, Seeger D E (1986) Mechanism of the ultraviolet laser ablation of PMMA at 193 and 248 nm: *Optic Soc Am* (B) 3:785-791
19. Grundfest W S, Litvack F, Forrester J S, Goldenberg T, Swan H J C, Morgenstern L, Fishbein M, McDermid I S, Rider D M, Pacala T J, Laudenslager J B (1985) Laser ablation of human atherosclerotic plaque without adjacent tissue injury. *J Am Coll Cardiol* 5(4):929-933
20. Grundfest W S, Litvack F, Goldenberg T, Sherman T, Morgenstern L, Carroll R, Fishbein M, Forrester J, Margitan J, McDermid S, Pascala T J, Rider D M, Laudenslauger J B (1985) Pulsed ultraviolet lasers and the potential for safe laser angioplasty. *Am J Surg* 150:220-226
21. Forrester J S, Litvack F, Grundfest W S (1987) A perspective of coronary disease seen through the arteries of living man. *Circulation* 75:505-513
22. Litvack F, Grundfest W S, Goldenberg T, Laudenslager J, Pacala T, Segalowitz J, Forrester J (1988) Pulsed laser angioplasty: wavelength power and energy dependencies relevant to clinical application. *Lasers in Surgery and Medicine* 8(1):60-65
23. Grundfest W S, Litvack F, Hickey A, Doyle L, Glick D, Treiman R, Lee M, Chaux A, Cohen L, Foran R, Levin P, Cossman D, Carrol R, Morgenstern L, Forrester J (1987) The current status of angioscopy and laser angioplasty. *J. Vasc Surg* 5(4):666-673
24. Laudenslager J B, Pacala T J, Wittig C (1976) Electric discharge pumped nitrogen ion laser. *Appl Phys Lett* 29:580-582
25. Grundfest W S, Litvack F, Goldenberg T, Doyle L, Pacalla T, Laudenslager J (1986) Laser ablation and fiber optic damage thresholds for laser angioplasty. ILS-2, APS/OSA International Laser Science Conference Technical Digest, Paper FE1 Pg 66
26. Laudenslager J B (1988) Excimer lasers adapt to angioplasty. In: *Laser Focus World*, 60-70
27. Litvack F, Grundfest W S, Goldenberg T, Laudenslager J, Pacala T, Segalowitz J, Forrester J (1988) Pulsed laser angioplasty: wavelength power and energy dependencies relevant to clinical application. *Lasers in Surgery and Medicine* 8(1):60-65

16. Improved Luminal Dimensions and Local Pharmacological Therapy with Laser Balloon Angioplasty for Potential Mitigation of Angioplasty Restenosis

J. RICHARD SPEARS

Pathogenetic Mechanisms of Restenosis and the Potential Role of LBA

As shown in Fig. 1, restenosis lesions very likely consist of one or a combination of 4 different components. Smooth muscle cell and/or fibroblast cell proliferation has received the greatest attention in view of the cellular nature of restenosis lesions found histologically and the multiple potential inciting pathways for this response [1]. However, organization and encapsulation of thrombi can also result in a lesion with a similar histologic appearance. The majority of restenosis lesions examined histologically by Nobuyoshi et al [2] at 1 month after PTCA demonstrated the presence of thrombus, unlike lesions examined at later intervals, but whether the mass effect of thrombus following its organization, its encapsulation, and its potential for stimulating cellular proliferation contributed to late restenosis lesions can only be surmised. A variable amount of extracellular matrix also contributes to restenosis lesions, and the possibility exists that, if collagen is deposited along with glycosaminoglycans before the endothelial lining layer has regenerated, additional platelet adhesion and activation may occur at the site of exposed collagen, thereby potentially renewing the process of restenosis. Many interacting pathogenetic sequences are possible, and the schematic figure, despite its complexity, is undoubtedly incomplete, but it is likely that the 4 different basic causes listed (presence of thrombus; inflammation; endothelial cell loss; and lumen geometry) contribute to restenosis lesions to varying degrees in different patients.

Lesion growth is superimposed on a lumen which may be significantly compromised acutely after angioplasty. Very likely, in order to significantly reduce the incidence of PTCA restenosis, it will be necessary to improve the acute luminal dimensions as well as to mitigate adverse biologic reactivity to arterial injury. In this regard, the preliminary long-term encouraging results of single stent implantation in coronary arteries suggests that the combination of excellent acute luminal geometry and aggressive anticoagulation may be an effective approach [3].

P.W. Serruys, B.H. Strauss and S.B. King III (eds), Restenosis after Intervention with New Mechanical Devices, 347–357.

348   *J.R. Spears*

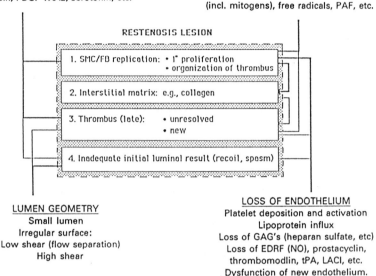

Figure 1. Potential pathogenetic mechanisms of restenosis: In addition to improved luminal morphology compared to that achieved with PTCA, local pharmocologic therapy with LBA could, in theory, be used to reduce the thrombogenicity of both thrombus and the mechanically-injured surface and to reduce inflammatory cell responses.

During laser balloon angioplasty (LBA), heat from a cw Nd: YAG laser (1.06 μm) and pressure are applied simultaneously to the arterial wall during balloon inflation in an attempt to: 1.) reduce arterial recoil, both active and passive; 2.) fuse separated tissue layers together; 3.) and dessicate and re-model thrombus [4]. Once an angioplasty balloon has been successfully expanded at the site of a lesion, essentially no other tissue effect would be required to ensure an adequate acute luminal result. In addition, we have recently demonstrated the feasibility of using LBA to induce adherence of a drug/ carrier preparation to the luminal surface and to deeper layers of the arterial wall, so that specific adverse biologic responses to angioplasty injury can potentially be mitigated [5]. As discussed below, it appears quite likely that the same laser dose can be used simultaneously for all 3 luminal geometric effects and for local drug application, thereby simplifying the procedure.

A series of in vitro studies of the laser dosimetry and tissue temperature history requirements for effective thermal fusion of separated intima-media layers of human postmortem atherosclerotic aortic sections were performed in my laboratory prior to experimental in-vivo studies. Although these studies are reviewed in depth elsewhere (see references in 4) a few observations are nonetheless noteworthy. The 1.06 μm wavelength of a cw Nd: YAG laser appears to be ideal in terms of the degree of effective tissue penetration, approximately 2 mm, through neointima in order to seal dissections to this depth; relatively strong scattering, including backscattering, and reflection at the luminal surface across the relatively transparent balloon, result in an "integrating sphere" effect [6] which helps to provide a uniform power density within the cylindrical sleeve of irradiated tissue; and the relatively strong absorption by thrombus compared to the arterial wall results in the selective dessication of the latter when a dose is delivered which is adequate to fuse tissue layers together. An important finding was that a minimum peak temperature of 80 °C, for a minimum duration of 10 seconds, was necessary to thermally bond separated layers of arterial tissue. Higher temperatures up to the threshold level of 180 °C are required for vaporization of the non-aqueous components of soft tissue and longer exposure durations produce stronger tissue "welds," but peak temperatures <130 °C and exposure durations <30 sec have been utilized clinically for several reasons. At excessively high temperatures, homogenization of structural detail at the light microscopic level is found, consistent with destruction of connective tissue components. In addition, since peak tissue temperature responses to a given laser dose may vary by 10–20 °C, we felt that a wide margin of safety should be employed to avoid inadvertant tissue vaporization.

The mechanism of thermally-induced tissue fusion very likely involves, at least in part, establishment of non-covalent bonds between interdigitating fibrillar substructures of juxtaposed collagen fibers [7], after transformation of the tertiary structure of collagen from a triple helix to a random coil. Reduction of arterial recoil with heat may also result from reshaping the tertiary structure of connective tissue proteins, and it may not be surprising, therefore, that the laser dosimetry required to reduce arterial recoil in vivo or to reshape human postmortem atherosclerotic aortas appears to be similar to that required to effect tissue fusion. It should be noted, however, that arterial recoil is a complex phenomenon which incorporates vasomotor tone along with passive visco-elastic properties of the arterial wall. The laser dose which is sufficient to destroy the viability of smooth muscle cells appears to be lower than that required to fuse tissues, but it is the author's opinion that passive recoil is by far the more important component of the acute recoil noted in most arteries subjected to balloon angioplasty.

The improvement in luminal diameter provided by LBA compared to conventional balloon angioplasty with a balloon of identical dimensions (3.0 × 20 mm) is on the order of 0.2 to 0.3 mm for normal arteries in experimental animal models [8, 9] and for atherosclerotic lesions in the clinical setting of successful PTCA (17), with "success" defined as a residual diameter stenosis of <50% immediately after PTCA. The improvement provided by LBA in the clinical setting of either initially unsuccessful PTCA [4], defined as a residual stenosis of >50%, with or without acute closure, has been on the order of 1.5 mm. Some of this marked improvement has possibly been related to a reduction of prominent recoil, but the bulk of the improvement in these cases very likely has resulted primarily from either sealing dissections or dessication/remodelling of thrombus.

Although Motamedi and colleagues in our laboratory have found that the scattering coefficient at 1.06 μm for thrombus is about one-half that of the arterial wall in vitro, the absorption coefficient of thrombus is many times greater than that of the arterial wall. It is not surprising, therefore, that the temperature response of thrombus is greater than that of the arterial wall for a given laser dose experimentally and in a mathematical model of LBA developed by Cheong and Welch [6]. As a result, when thrombus is compressed between the surface of the balloon and the tissue luminal surface and is exposed to a laser dose sufficient to fuse separated tissue layers, the thrombus is both dehydrated and remodelled into a thin non-obstructive film which is adherent to the luminal surface in a canine model of thrombotic occlusion (unpublished observation).

Preliminary clinical results of the application of LBA for treatment of unsuccessful PTCA, without acute closure [10], suggest that 98% of these patients have an adequate post LBA acute angiographic luminal diameter, while the in-hospital success rate for LBA reversal of PTCA-induced acute closure is on the order of 80%. Thus, if LBA were applied electively to the same population of patients currently treated with PTCA, it is likely that >95% of patients would have <50% diameter stenosis acutely, since acute closure is relatively uncommon and would be treatable with LBA in most patients.

Refinements in LBA catheter technology and laser dosimetry could further improve the success rate of treatment of PTCA-induced acute closure. For example, both the laser power and exposure duration could be increased substantially beyond currently used levels without risk of adverse acute reactions, and the efficacy of sealing a thick-walled dissection, reducing arterial recoil, and dessicating thrombus would be improved accordingly. The pattern of laser radiation emitted from the balloon currently has a roughly 30% variation in power density in both axial and azimuthal directions over a 15–17 mm length of the 20 mm balloon, which is considerably improved compared to the first LBA catheters available, but a truly cylindrically uniform pattern of emitted radiation is an eventual technological goal which may improve the efficacy of the procedure.

The mean residual diameter stenosis (by computer analysis) following LBA applied electively in over 150 patients is approximately 25%, which is statistically significantly improved over the mean value of 35% found after initial successful PTCA. In order to greatly reduce restenosis rates, however, it may be necessary to reduce the mean residual stenosis to closer to zero as suggested by Kuntz et al [11] in a clinical study of the chronic loss of angiographic luminal diameter after angioplasty with 3 different new devices (directional atherectomy, stent, and LBA), since the magnitude of the loss appeared to be independent of the type of device used.

By computerized analysis of cineangiograms [12], the mean minimum

Table 1. Incidence of restenosis (%) (by 6 month angiographic follow up).

	Min. Diam <1.5 mm	Min. Diam <1.0 mm	% Stenosis >50%	% Stenosis >70%
Elective LBA				
Successful PTCA	44 (89)	30 (89)	43 (89)	26 (89)
Failed PTCA	56 (27)	41 (27)	59 (27)	37 (27)
Emergent LBA				
Acute PTCA Closure	64 (33)	48 (33)	64 (33)	42 (33)

Number in parenthesis = no. of patients

diameter of patients having initially successful PTCA followed by LBA (2.3 mm, n = 151) is acutely greater than LBA after unsuccessful PTCA (2.0 mm, n = 49) in patients without acute closure. In patients with LBA treatment of acute closure, the immediate mean post-LBA result is lower still (1.9 mm, n = 85). The long-term mean minimum luminal diameters for each group are consistent with the acute results, so that the successful PTCA/LBA group has at follow-up a mean minimum luminal diameter of 1.4–1.5 mm (n = 84), which is not statistically different (p > 0.05) from that of a small PTCA control group, while the unsuccessful PTCA/LBA and PTCA acute closure groups have minimum luminal diameters of 0.1 to 0.4 mm less, respectively, than that of the successful PTCA/LBA group. Thus, the acute luminal result following LBA depends greatly on the degree of difficulty encountered during initial PTCA, and the restenosis rates will vary accordingly (Table 1). It should be emphasized that the restenosis rate following successful PTCA/LBA is not statistically different from that of the small PTCA group despite the greater frequency of difficult lesions (type B and C) treated in the former group. Moreover, the mean minimum luminal diameter of this group at long-term angiographic follow-up is nearly identical to that found by Nobuyoshi et al 3 months after PTCA. The relatively high restenosis rate of the unsuccessful PTCA/LBA group is similar to that reported for PTCA acute closure successfully reversed with a prolonged balloon inflation. The somewhat still higher restenosis rate of patients treated with LBA for PTCA-induced acute closure should not be surprising, since failure of a prolonged balloon inflation to reverse poor angiographic flow or clinical ischemia has been a prerequisite for entry into the trial, and these cases are more difficult, therefore, than the group of patients successfully treated with a prolonged balloon inflation. The higher incidence of restenosis as a function of increasing laser doses noted in a subset of LBA patients by Plokker elsewhere in this book suggests, in light of the above data, that the more difficult lesions causing acute closure after initial PTCA required more laser exposures and would be expected to have a higher incidence of re-stenosis. In fact, when the long-term angiographic results of a prospective, randomized trial of 3 different laser doses applied electively after successful PTCA were compared, no difference in mean luminal diameter or in the incidence of restenosis between groups was found. However, with the use of relatively high laser doses in a normal rabbit iliac artery model (but not in a normal dog coronary artery model) and, clinically, with high doses delivered from the first generation LBA catheter which had a "hot spot" adjacent to the relatively nonuniform diffusing tip, restenosis was more problematic. Additional studies will be required to formally define the relationship between laser dose and restenosis. The possibility also exists that the effect of laser dose on restenosis may depend at least in part on the type of lesion treated, particularly thrombotic vs thrombus-free lesions.

Two different approaches could be taken to further improve the acute luminal results of LBA. Firstly, the use of a LBA balloon which is oversized (e.g., 20%) relative to the diameter of adjacent reference segments might improve luminal dimensions without incurring a substantial risk of acute closure as is the case with PTCA. Application of laser/thermal energy during the first inflation, or at least within the first several minutes of the first inflation, might also prove more effective in terms of prevention of a dissection compared to the current use of LBA to treat the dissection only after it has propagated. Secondly, the use of LBA, including with an oversized balloon, could be employed after an atherectomy procedure.

The achievement of a minimal residual stenosis will be insufficient alone, of course, to ensure a successful long-term result. It will also be necessary to mitigate adverse biologic reactivity. In this regard, LBA could be helpful in two ways: 1) potential thermal reduction of luminal surface thrombogenicity and, probably more importantly, 2) thermal induction of semi-permanent adherence of a potentially useful drug/carrier preparation to the luminal surface and to deeper layers of the arterial wall [5].

Borst et al [14] recently demonstrated in an in vitro preparation of a deendothelialized human umbilical artery that platelet deposition is markedly reduced, acutely, by laser energy exposure when the luminal surface is heated to approximately 100 °C. Experimentally in vivo, Abela likewise demonstrated a reduction in acute platelet deposition following luminal surface heating with a laserprobe to approximately 80 °C [15]. Scanning electron microscopy studies by Sinclair et al [16] also suggested that platelet adhesion to the luminal surface of canine coronary arteries, shortly after balloon angioplasty, was reduced by similar temperatures achieved during LBA. We have recently found that when thrombus is heated to approximately 100 °C during cw Nd: YAG laser exposure, its in vitro thrombogenicity is reduced as determined by measurement of thrombin-antithrombin III levels in non-anticoagulated blood in contact with the thrombus (unpublished observation). The potentially beneficial effect may result from thermal denaturation of thrombin, which appears to be markedly inhibited by exposure to 80 °C for 20 sec. Whether other potentially thrombogenic proteins in the arterial wall, such as collagen type I, thromboplastin, etc, will demonstate a similar effect to heat remains to be studied. However, Gentry et al [17] noted a reduction in platelet adhesion to burro aortic collagen type I after heating to 55 °C.

Although it may be possible to reduce the thrombogenicity of the arterial wall and thrombus with an appropriate level of thermal exposure, the possibility exists that increased inflammatory responses associated with LBA, compared to conventional balloon angioplasty, may counteract this potentially useful effect. For example, when peak temperatures of <120 °C within tissue adjacent to an LBA balloon were achieved in the normal rabbit iliac artery, we found that, unlike the response to peak temperatures of 100–110 °C, excessive inflammation and fibrosis of perivascular tissue produced moderately severe strictures on 1 month follow-up angiographic and histologic examinations [8]. In contrast, an even greater degree of thermal injury from 7 to 10 LBA doses in the dog circumflex artery failed to produce any evidence of chronic stricture formation, including in 4 animals examined 1 year after treatment [9]. The fact that inflammatory responses to laser/ thermal anastomosis of arteries and other soft tissues are less prominent experimentally than those associated with conventional suture technique suggests that an appropriate level of thermal injury to the arterial wall may not be problematic [18], but a great deal of experimental work remains to define the relationshlp between tissue temperature history and inflammatory cell responses.

Local application of a suitable drug to the luminal surface and to deeper layers of the arterial wall during or after an angioplasty procedure would, in theory, be attractive to reduce the thrombogenicity and inflammatory cell responses to injury. Many potentially useful drugs, when given systemically in large doses, are toxic, and some drugs cannot be given orally. Wolinsky et al [19] suggested the use of a perforated balloon to delivery an agent, such as heparin, locally during balloon inflation. Such an approach is limited, however, in that persistence of the drug in tissue is relatively brief.

The author devised a method using LBA wherein the heat generated during laser exposure would induce adherence of a drug/carrier combination to the arterial wall in one of two ways [5]. A suspension of the drug/carrier preparation is injected into the lumen proximal to the site of a lesion during balloon inflation, so that the preparation is physically trapped by pressure from the inflated balloon. Application of thermal energy from the LBA catheter would then be used to induce adherence of the carrier and/drug to the arterial wall (Fig. 2). Since LBA with cw Nd: YAG laser radiation obliterates vasa vasorum and perivascular capillaries in addition to bonding separated tissue layers, the drug/carrier would become entrapped within deeper layers of the arterial wall and adjacent tissues. The use of a water-insoluble carrier would help provide a semi-permanent coating of the drug at the luminal surface, and the diffusion of the preparation from deeper tissue layers would be expected to be relatively slow. In an alternate or complementary approach, a sleeve of a drug/carrier would be transferred

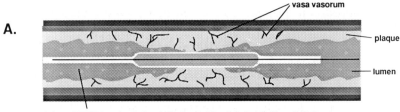

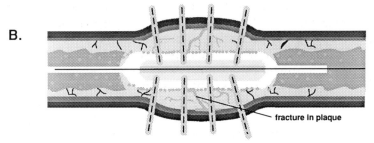

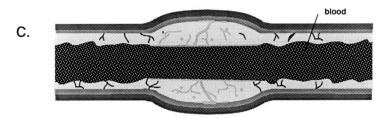

Figure 2. LBA application of bioprotective materials (BPM = drug plus carrier). Heat generated during LBA can be used to induce adherence of a BPM, such as albumin microspheres fabricated from heparin/albumin conjugates, at the luminal surface and within deeper layers of the arterial wall.

from the surface of the balloon to the luminal surface, and thermal energy would be used to induce semi-permanent adherence of the sleeve of material.

It should be apparent that either of the above approaches would be applicable as an adjunct to not only balloon angioplasty, but also to virtually any other angioplasty procedure. For example, LBA with local application of a drug/carrier could be performed after mechanical or laser atherectomy, so that the residual stenosis would be minimal and a potentially useful drug at the luminal surface and within the arterial wall could mitigate adverse biologic reactivity to angioplasty injury. In the case of stents, transfer of a sleeve of a drug/carrier after stent deployment could theoretically be used to fill in recesses between struts and the luminal surface, thereby potentially reducing local separated flow patterns which would be expected to enhance thrombus formation. The use of an anticoagulant such as heparin or hirudin within the transferred sleeve of material would probably be useful for virtually any type of angioplasty procedure, and in the case of stents, the combination of a smooth luminal surface and the presence of an anticoagulant might obviate the need for aggressive anticoagulation after the procedure.

The results of preliminary experimental studies in our laboratory demonstrate that, among a large number of potential candidate drug carriers, albumin microspheres, red blood cells, and starch preparations show the most promise in terms of thermal inducibility of adherence to the arterial tissue luminal surface and biocompatibility. Although albumin in solution can be thermally precipitated onto the luminal surface of mechanically injured porcine aortas, adherence of the precipitate is weak. On the other hand, the adherence of albumin microspheres to the luminal surface after heating to 90–100 °C for 20–30 seconds is quite adequate. In fact, when albumin microspheres were applied during LBA in vivo in canine peripheral arteries, minimal loss was found 24 hours after re-establishment of blood flow as noted by the use of a flourescent label (FITC), and we have noted in vivo persistence for at least one week in additional unpublished studies. The degree of thermal or chemical cross-linking achieved during preparation of the microspheres determines the rate of biodegradation, the half-life of which can be varied from minutes to many months in other applications of such preparations [20].

Albumin per se has been shown to be relatively non-thrombogenic when coated onto surfaces [21]. Hennick et al [22] have recently demonstrated that conjugates of heparin and albumin can be used to further render the surface of prosthetic vascular grafts non-thrombogenic in experimental studies. Heparin has also been shown, of course, to inhibit smooth muscle cell proliferation. Therefore, we prepared albumin microspheres with heparin covalently linked to albumin with 1-ethyl-3-(dimethylaminopropyl)carbodiimide by sonicating the conjugates in aqueous solution along with additional free heparin at elevated temperatures at an oil-water interface. The resultant preparation has heparin both physically entrapped within the matrix of the microsphere as well as chemically bound at the surface and within the microspheres. Heparin activity does not appear to be affected by this technique, including the use of prolonged heating of the oil/water emulsion at 150 °C, nor is it affected by exposure to temperatures generated during LBA at clinical used laser doses. Thus, we found that the surfaces of a variety of materials coated with this preparation in vitro, including thrombus, mechanically-injured porcine aorta, and glass slides, appear to have a resultant marked reduction of their thrombogenicity. Preliminary experimental in vivo studies with 1 hour to 24 hours after application of this preparation to the mechanically injured luminal surface have shown no thrombus formation at the site of the preparation, unlike control adjacent segments, which is consistent with the probable in vivo activity of the locally applied heparin.

Albumin microspheres fabricated with heparin/albumin conjugates may represent a highly useful preparation to be applied during LBA. However, we anticipate a delay of several years before a fully developed and pharmacologically characterized preparation would gain experimental clinical approval. Our recent efforts have therefore been devoted to testing the potential utility of red blood cells as drug carriers. Many groups of investigators have shown, by either electroporation or by resealing after hemolysis, that various drugs can be entrapped within red blood cells. Preliminary studies in our laboratory demonstrate that, very likely, heparin can be both bound to and entrapped within the red cell. Application of laser/thermal energy during LBA in vitro and experimentally in vivo has resulted in at least semi-permanent adherence of the red cell membrane to mechanically injured arterial tissues, and various thrombogenic surfaces coated with heparinized red cells acutely are rendered non-thrombogenic. Given the ease with which heparinized red cells can be prepared, one such preparation (albeit with a relatively low heparin concentration) has already been applied clinically at our institution during LBA treatment of PTCA-induced acute closure. A great deal of work will be required, of course, to optimize this type of preparation and to characterize the pharmacokinetics of heparin persistence and activity at both the luminal surface and within deeper layers of the arterial wall.

In summary, it should be possible with LBA to address 3 of the 4 major pathogenetic processes shown in Fig. 1. One would anticipate that, if an appropriate concentration and persistence of drugs with anticoagulant, anti-proliferative, and anti-inflammatory activities can be achieved within the arterial wall as well as at the luminal surface following any type of angioplasty procedure, the incidence of restenosis would be reduced. Loss of endothelial cells could not be directly addressed with this approach, but it is possible that inhibition of the other pathogenetic pathways of restenosis would allow regrowth of the endothelial lining layer in an unimpeded manner.

Acknowledgements

This work was supported in part by grants from the NHLBI (HL 37349), Bethesda, MD and C.R. Bard, Inc., Billerica, MA.

References

1. Ross R (1986) The pathogenenis of atherosclerosis – an update. *N Engl J Med* 314:488–500
2. Nobuyoshi M, Kimura T, Ohishi H, Horiuchi H, Nosaka H, Hamasaki N, Yokoi H,

Kim K (1991) Restenosis after percutaneous transluminal coronary angioplasty: pathologic observations in 20 patients. *J Am Coll Cardiol* 17:433–9

3. Schatz R A, Baim D S, Leon M, Ellis S G, Goldberg S, Hirshfeld J W, Cleman M W, Walker C, Stagg J et al (1991) Clinical experience with the Palmaz-Schatz coronary stent. Initial results of a multicenter study. *Circulation* 83:148–61

4. Spears J R, Reyes V P, Wynne J, Fromm B S, Sinofsky E L, Andrus S, Sinclair I N, Hopkins B E, Schwartz L, Aldridge H E, Plokker H W T, Mast E G, Rickards A, Knudtson M L, Sigwart L, Dear W E, Ferguson J J, Angelini P, Leatherman L L, Salan R D, Jenkins R D, Douglas J S, King III S B (1990) Percutaneous coronary laser balloon angioplasty: Initial results of a multicenter experience. *JACC* 16:293–303

5. Spears J R, Kundu S K, McMath L P (1991) Laser balloon angioplasty: Potential for reduction of thrombogenicity of the impaired arterial wall and for local application of bioprotective materials. *JACC* (in press)

6. Cheong W F, Welch A J. A model for optical and thermal analysis of laser balloon angioplasty. *IEEE Trans Biomed Eng* 36:1233–43, 1989

7. Schober R, Ulrich F, Sander T, Durseken H, Hessel S (1986) Laser-induced alteration of collagen substructure allows microsurgical tissue welding. *Science* 232:1421–1422

8. Jenkins R D, Sinclair I N, Leonard B M, Sandor T, Schoen F J, Spears J R (1989) Laser balloon angioplasty vs balloon angioplasty in normal rabbit iliac arteries. *Lasers Surg Med* 9:237–47

9. Spears J R, Sinclair I N, Jenkins R D (1990) Laser balloon angioplasty: experimental in vivo and in vitro studies. In: Abela G (ed) *Lasers in Cardiovascular Medicine & Surgery.* Norwell, MA: Kluwer, 167–88

10. Reyes V P, Plokker H W M, Leatherman L L, Dear W E, Sinclair I N, Douglas J S, King III S B, Safian R D, Jenkins R D, Rickards A, Sigwart U, Pichard A, Morice M C, Spears J R, and the LBA Study Group (1990) Laser balloon angioplasty effectively treats unsuccessful PTCA (abstr). *Circulation* 82:III–71 (Suppl III)

11. Kunze R E, Sehmidt A, Levine M J, Reis G J, Safian R D, Baim D S (1990) Importance of post-procedure luminal diameter on restenosis following new corony intervenions. Suppl III, *Circulation* 82:314

12. Spears J R, Sandor T, Als A V et al (1983) Computerised image analysis for quantitative measurment of vessel diameter from cineangiograms. *Circulation* 68:453–61

13. Ba'albaki A H, Weintraub W S, Tao X, Ghzal Z M B, Liberman H A, Douglas J S, King III S B (1990) Restenosis after acute closure and successful reopening: implications for new devices. Suppl III, *Cirulation* 82:314

14. Borst C, Bos A N, Zwaga J J, Rienks R, de Groot, Sixma J J (1990) Loss of blood platelet adhesion after heating native and cultured subendothelium to 100 °C. *Cardiovasc Res* 24:665–8

15. Abela G S, Tomaru T, Mansour M, et al (1990) Reduced platelet deposition with laser compared to balloon angioplsty (abstr). *J Am Coll Cardiol* (suppl A); 245A

16. Sinclair I N, Robertsom T A Papamitiou J M (1989) Thrombogenic potential of dog coronary artery after laser balloon angioplaty (abstr). *Circulation* 80 (suppl II): II–24

17. Gentry P A, Schneider M D, Miller J K (1981) Plasma clot-promoting effect of collagen in relation collagen-platelet interaction. *Am J Vet Res* 42:708–15

18. White R A, Kopchok G, Donayre C, Abergel R P, et al (1986) Comparison of laser-welded and sutured arteriotomies. *Arch Sug* 121:1133

19. Wolinsky H, Thung S N (1990) Use of a perforated balloon atheter to deliver concentrated heparin in the wall of the normal canine artery. *J Am Coll Cardiol* 15:475–81

20. Yapel A F Jr. Albumin microspheres: heat and chemical stabilization. In Ref 76:3–18

21. Chang T M S (1974) Platelet-surface interaction: effect of albumin coating or heparin complexing on thrombogenic surfaces. *Can J Physiol Pharmacol* 52:275–85

22. Hennink W E, Kim S W, Feijen J (1984) Inhibition of surface induced coagulation by preadsorption of albumin-heparin conjugates *J Biomed Mater Res* 18:911–26

17. Laser Balloon Angioplasty: European Experience

H.W. THIJS PLOKKER and E. GIJS MAST

Introduction

Andreas Grüntzig performed the first percutaneous coronary angioplasty in a patient in 1977 [1]. After more than a decade of percutaneous transluminal coronary angioplasty (PTCA) as Grüntzig baptized his technique, the worldwide growth of the number of procedures demonstrates the faith that cardiologists have in this technique. It has been proven that it can successfully and predictably induce regression of coronary artery disease. Thus, symptoms can be relieved and the need for coronary artery bypass surgery (CABG) can be postponed or even eliminated because late recurrences after successful PTCA are extremely rare. However, the limitations of PTCA have also become clear. Its Achilles heel remains the problem of restenosis within the first six months after a successful procedure. The restenosis rate has been reported to range between 17 and 40% [2–9]. The other limitations of PTCA, such as the limited range of indications, and the risk of abrupt closure remain outside the scope of this contribution.

To overcome these limitations many efforts have been made to develop new pharmacologic and mechanical intervention techniques, with a strong emphasis on tools to reduce the recurrence rate after successful PTCA. Namely, only if this restenosis rate can predictably be reduced, one may expect true replacement of CABG by PTCA. Among all new developments the laser systems have particular appeal. If lasers can create holes in concrete walls, they should easily be able to remove plaque and cross previously impenetrable occlusions. Today, this perspective of what the laser systems can achieve has been blurred by high hopes, confusing claims, and short term disappointments.

A novel use of laser energy has been pioneered by Richard Spears [10–16]. He proposed that diffuse energy-scattering of ND:YAG laser could be used to improve the results of conventional angioplasty. The primary goal of Laser Balloon Angioplasty (LBA) is to reduce restenosis, and not to remove plaque. The combination of heat (90–120° Celcius) and the pressure

P.W. Serruys, B.H. Strauss and S.B. King III (eds), Restenosis after Intervention with New Mechanical Devices, 359–372.
© 1992 Kluwer Academic Publishers. Printed in the Netherlands.

from the inflated balloon would leave the smoothest and largest possible lumen after PTCA.

It also might reduce the potential for elastic recoil that immediately follows deflation after conventional balloon angioplasty. Furthermore it has been demonstrated (in vitro) that the LBA system also can seal or weld loose flaps back to the wall in the event of major intimal dissections following balloon inflation [11, 13, 14, 16]. It also has been demonstrated in canine experiments that thrombus can be removed by desiccation, which would eliminate another cause for (acute) closure following conventional PTCA [17]. Finally, subendothelial proteins can be denatured thermally which in theory may prevent a thrombogenic subendothelial surface.

On this basis our group at the St. Antonius Hospital joined the USCI laser balloon angioplasty project in September 1988. Within a few weeks, the groups at the National Heart Hospital in London (A.F. Rickards) and at the University Hospital in Lausanne (U. Sigwart) followed. One year later (June 1989) the Centre Cardiologique du Nord in Paris (Madame Maurice) was the fourth European centre to join the group of LBA investigators. Today, 111 patients have been included in the European LBA experiment. It is the purpose of this chapter to provide an overview of the results of LBA on restenosis rates.

Methods

Study Purpose. The purpose of the Laser Balloon Angioplasty Study was to determine the safety and efficacy of the LBA catheter in reducing the incidence of restenosis of coronary artery lesions dilated during routine PTCA. Coronary vessel patency was assessed by angiography and clinical evaluation for both treatment and control groups at 6 months after the therapeutic procedure. An initial group of non randomized patients was first treated with LBA in order to gain experience with the device and the technical procedure [18]. After the initial pilot study, the LBA system was used in a prospective randomized trial comparing three different laser doses (maximal energy 25, 20 and 15 Watts respectively) with a 0 Watt (=PTCA only) group (see Table 1).

The study was conducted under IDE regulations and conditions of the Institutional Review Boards and the FDA. Informed consent was obtained. All cineangiogram films were submitted to the Laser Lab of Wayne State University in Detroit for quantitative analysis. All LBA catheters were returned to USCI for engineering analysis. The USCI safety and data monitoring committee recorded all medical complications, and anticipated adverse device defects.

Pre entry patient selection criteria are given in Table 2.

Table 1. Study design of randomized and acute LBA protocols.

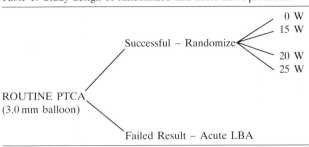

Method

Each patient was treated initially with conventional PTCA until an optimal angiographic result was achieved. Since we were initially limited to 3.0 mm laser balloons, only lesions treated with a 3.0 mm angioplasty balloon were included in the series. If a balloon larger than 3.0 mm in diameter was used as the final balloon during PTCA, the patient was excluded from the series.

All lesions were first crossed with an 0.014 inch ACS high torque floppy (exchange) guidewire and a 3.0 mm USCI Simplus or USCI Mini balloon was advanced through a standard 8F Judkins guiding catheter. The standard balloon was inflated in the stenotic segment at least three times to a maximal 10 atmospheres for at least 60 seconds per inflation. The balloon catheter was then withdrawn and if a satisfactory angiographic result (defined as an estimated residual stenosis of less than 30%) was not achieved the balloon catheter was readvanced across the lesion for at least one additional inflation.

In the LBA system a 15–50 Watt ND:YAG air cooled laser delivery

Table 2. Pre entry patient selection criteria.

Inclusion:
1) Written informed consent
2) Acceptable candidate for CABG
3) Clinically stable prior to PTCA
4) Only one lesion of > 50% in the vessel to be treated with PTCA/LBA

Exclusion
1) Totally obstructed coronary arteries
2) Left main coronary disease
3) Prinzmetal coronary artery spasm
4) Mid vein graft lesions
5) Ostium left main, ostium LAD, ostium RCA, ostium LCX lesions
6) Bifurcation lesions involving the origin of vessels
7) Unstable angina with documented ST-elevations at rest
8) Patients with poor left ventricular function or those at high risk of death due to cardiac or other causes
9) Patients previously treated with LBA

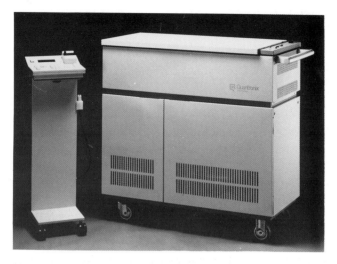

Figure 1. The 15–50 Watt ND:YAG air cooled laser system. Only the console (on the left) is positioned in the cathlab.

system (Quantronic Inc., Smith Town, N.Y.) (see Fig. 1) is used to deliver laser radiation at 1064 nanometer into the fiber optic system. Standard fiber optic connectors allow rapid coupling of the fiber optic within the catheter to another fiber optic coupled to the laser source.

The mechanical function of the Spears/USCI balloon catheter (see Fig. 2) is similar to that of a conventional balloon catheter in terms of balloon size, shape, and balloon material (polyethylene terephthalate).

The flexibility and trackability of these LBA balloons is somewhat diminished as compared to the standard balloons, probably because of the extra channel which carries the 100 micron silica fiber. This fiber ends as a helical

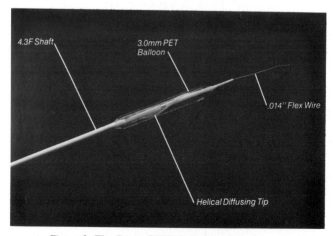

Figure 2. The Spears/USCI balloon catheter.

Table 3. Four laser dosage groups of the randomized LBA trial.

-0 W 40 sec	(0 W)
-15 W 5 sec $+ 11$ W 5 sec $+ 8$ W 10 sec $+ 0$ W 20 sec	(15 W)
-20 W 5 sec $+ 13$ W 5 sec $+ 11$ W 10 sec $+ 0$ W 20 sec	(20 W)
-25 W 5 sec $+ 15$ W 5 sec $+ 12$ W 10 sec $+ 0$ W 20 sec	(25 W)

diffusing tip, wrapped around the distal shaft, within the balloon in its 1.0 cm. long mid portion. Prior to use, power output from both the laser and the fiber optic coupled to the laser was calibrated to ensure delivery of a programmed twenty seconds step-wise decremental dose. The laser dosages are further specified in Table 3.

Prior to use, the balloon is filled with metrimazide and deuterium oxide because this has a very low absorption of 1064 nm radiation. Unfortunately it makes the balloon filling rather expensive. Immediately before clinical use, the pattern of radiation provided by the diffusing tip is visually assessed with the use of a red helium-neon laser reference beam.

In addition, a 35 Watt $\times$ 3 seconds exposure is performed in a reservoir of sterile sodium chloride solution to ensure the functional integrity of the system.

Once the system has been tested the laser balloon catheter is then advanced over the exchange wire, carefully avoiding damage while entering the Y-connector, and advanced across the previously dilated lesion. Because of the reported severe burning pain experienced during laser irradiation in the initial patients, all our patients were given intravenous analgesics. In order to prevent coagulation of blood at the proximal side of the balloon or at the distal side, 10 to 20 cc of 37 °C saline were injected both through the guiding catheter and through the guidewire lumen along the guidewire which was left in place during the procedure. Balloon inflation is maintained for another 30 seconds after the termination of laser exposure to ensure return of wall temperatures to baseline before balloon deflation. The LBA balloon catheter is then removed. When the result after LBA was considered to be suboptimal, one or two additional identical laser doses could be given.

LBA Patients

To date 111 patients have been included in the European LBA experience, 68 from the St. Antonius Hospital, 21 from the Centre Cardiologique du Nord, 10 from the National Heart Hospital and 7 from the University Hospital in Lausanne. However, 27 of those are included in the so called acute protocol, where LBA is used as a bail-out device for abrupt vessel closure after initially successful PTCA. Although control angiography has been performed in most of the "bail-out" patients, they are not included in the

Table 4. Clinical characteristics of the randomized LBA patients.

Mean age		56
Male sex		75%
Angina class	I	2%
	II	35%
	III	46%
	IV	17%
Previous AMI		23%
Previous PTCA		6%
Previous CABG		2%
Single VD		88%
Double VD		12%

restenosis study. Of the 111 European patients, 27 were treated in the bail-out protocol leaving 84 in the restenosis trial. Within this group of 84, 16 patients were randomized to the PTCA only (or 0 Watt) group, leaving 68 European patients to be treated with ND:YAG laser via the LBA balloon.

In the St.Antonius Hospital all patients were given 10.000 units heparin intravenously immediately prior to the procedure and heparin was continued after the procedure until adequate anticoagulation was taken over by oral coumadin. The patients were discharged two days after LBA and maintained on acetyl-salicylic acid 100 mg daily and coumadin for the first six months after the procedure.

From January 19th, 1989 to December 22nd, 1990 in the St. Antonius Hospital 48 patients were entered in the prospective randomized restenosis trial, divided over four laser energy doses-subgroups, following the first 7 patients in that pilot study. The baseline clinical and angiographical characteristics of the Dutch LBA patients are given in Tables 4 and 5. The clinical and angiographical data indicate that this group of patients is similar to the average PTCA patient population.

The laser dosages given to these patients are specified in Table 3.

Table 5. Angiographic characteristics of the randomized LBA patients. Type A and B according to the ACC/AHA task force.

	No.	Type A	Type B
RCA	14	8	6
LAD	27	10	17
LCX	7	2	5

AMI = Acute myocardial infarction.
PTCA = Percutaneous Transluminal Coronary Angioplasty.
CABG = Coronary Artery Bypass Grafting.
VD = Vessel Disease.

Results

Acute Results. There were few complications during the procedures. In two patients the LBA dosage was incomplete, because the laser was automatically switched off after only 10 seconds of laser exposure, due to a technical problem.

In one (Swiss) patient the result immediately after LBA was unsuccessful with acute vessel closure, and a stent was (successfully) implanted. In one of the early Dutch patients, a small thrombus in a sidebranch distal to the laser site in the right coronary artery was noted without any clinical consequences.

The vessel wall contour after successful LBA usually appeared much smoother than after the preceeding PTCA (see Figs 3–10).

Follow-up Results

The clinical and angiographical follow up data of the Dutch LBA patient groups are summarized in Table 6. During clinical follow up, which was completed in all 48 patients, 30 patients remained free of angina. Fourteen had recurrence of angina class II, and one class IV according to the Canadian Cardiovascular Society. There were no myocardial infarctions. One patient died due to a ruptured abdominal aneurysm. Angiographic follow up was obtained in 42/48 of the patients (84%). In our study, restenosis was defined as a stenosis ≥50%, as measured by electronic calipers. It is interesting to

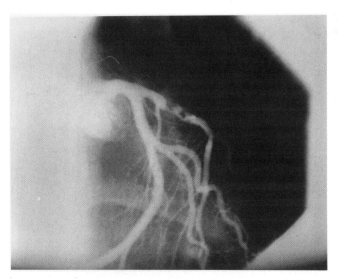

Figure 3. Stenosis in the left anterior descending artery (LAD) in right anterior oblique projection (RAO) pre-PTCA.

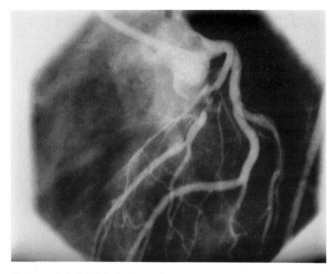

Figure 4. Stenosis in LAD in left anterior oblique projection (LAO) pre-PTCA.

note that of the 29 asymptomatic LBA treated patients, 11 did have a recurrence. Asymptomatic recurrences, and especially asymptomatic occlusions are known to occur in 2 to 30% [6, 19–23]. In this group of LBA patients, the asymptomatic recurrence rate of 38% seems to be extremely high. Restenosis ≥50% was seen in 2 patients in the 0 W (=PTCA only) group of 9 patients, which indicates a restenosis rate of 22% in this group. The restenosis rate was 45% in the 15 W group, 73% in the 20 W group and

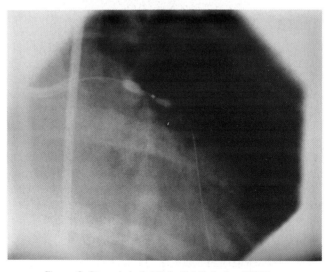

Figure 5. Stenosis in LAD in RAO during PTCA.

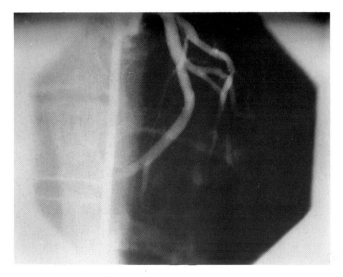

Figure 6. LAD in RAO following PTCA. Note slight haziness at the dilated site.

73% in the 25 W group (see Table 7). Reintervention due to restenosis was required in 11 patients (PTCA, n = 9; CABG, n = 2).

Although they were not part of this study, thirteen patients in our institution underwent LBA to prevent emergency CABG after abrupt closure. Nine of the patients were restudied angiographically and 7 of those had a recurrence (77%).

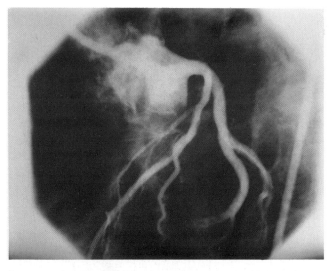

Figure 7. LAD in LAO following PTCA. Although the result looks excellent, some haziness and vagueness of the vessel wall contours at the PTCA-site can be noticed.

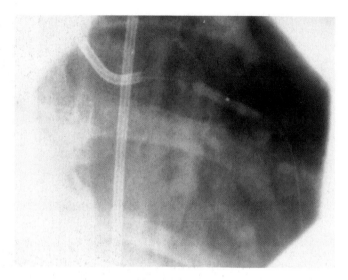

Figure 8. LAD in RAO during LBA.

Conclusions

Our results show that the laser balloon angioplasty is easy to use, with a very low complication rate. Its immediate effect results in smooth vessel wall contours and it can successfully restore patency after abrupt reclosure following initially successful PTCA. The ability to "weld" dissections that are usually the main cause of acute occlusions following initially successful

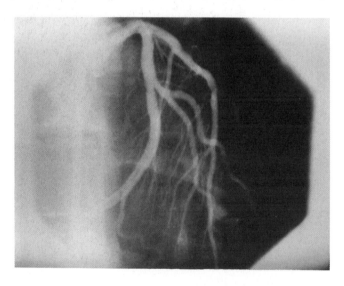

Figure 9. LAD in RAO following LBA.

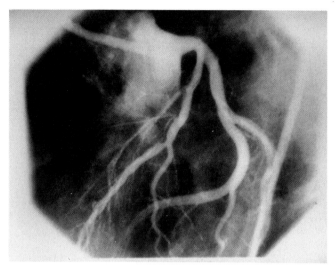

Figure 10. LAD in LAO following LBA. As compared to Fig. 7 the much smoother contours of the vessel wall at the dilated site can be noticed.

PTCA, and the ability to dissecate acute thrombus make it a useful but expensive system to "bail one out" of acute PTCA related problems. It remains to be seen whether cheaper devices which can combine pressure and heat will be as effective.

However, it appears from our data that with the present system and dosages, LBA seems to increase the incidence of restenosis. This recurrence seems at be directly related to the amount of laser energy used (see Table 8). If the total number of joules given is lower than 600, the restenosis rate is 58%, and if more than 600 joules have been delivered, the restenosis rate is as high as 80%.

Due to the relatively large proportion of patients remaining symptomfree after PTCA followed by LBA, we initially had hopes that this system would indeed reduce the recurrence rate after successful PTCA. The reason why such a high proportion of patients with a recurrence remain symptomfree remains to be explained.

Given the present high recurrence rate, the LBA program to reduce restenosis after initially successful PTCA has been stopped in Europe, and only the "acute protocol" is being pursued at this moment.

Perhaps in the near future, with reduced amounts of laser energy and lower temperatures, the Spears-concept to reduce restenosis rates will be retested.

Table 6. Clinical and angiographic follow-up data of the Dutch LBA patient groups.

Sex	Laser Dose	Lesion	Result	Restenosis (%)	Angina	Remarks
PILOT PHASE						
M	30W	CX	Success	80%	APII	Re-PTCA
M	30W	CX	Success	30%	Asymp	
M	30W	LAD	Success	60%	Asymp	Conservative
F	25W	CX	Success	20%	Asymp	
F	25W	RCA	Success	NA	Asymp	
M	25W	LAD	Success	85%	Asymp	Re-PTCA
M	25W	LAD	Success	13%	Asymp	
RANDOMIZED 25W						
F	25W	LAD	Success	15%	Asymp	
F	25W	LAD	Success	85%	APII	CABG
M	25W	RCA	Success	75%	APII	Re-PTCA
M	25W	LAD	Success	100%	APII	Re-PTCA
M	25W	RCA	Success	95%	Asymp	CABG
F	25W	CX	Success	99%	APIV	Re-PTCA
M	25W	RCA	Success	25%	Asymp	
M	25W	LAD	Success	85%	APII	Re-PTCA
F	25W	LAD	Success	70%	APII	Conservative
M	25W	RCA	Success	90%	Asymp	Conservative
M	25W	RCA	Success	15%	Asymp	
RANDOMIZED 20W						
M	20W	LAD	Success	NA	NA	Deceased Non LBA related
M	20W	CX	Success	67%	Asymp	Conservative
M	20W	LAD	Success	30%	Asymp	
M	20W	LAD	Success	90%	APII	Re-PTCA
M	20W	LAD	Success	55%	APII	Conservative
M	20W	LAD	Success	60%	APII	Re-PTCA
F	20W	RCA	Success	5%	Asymp	
M	20W	RCA	Success	70%	APII	Re-PTCA
M	20W	RCA	Success	30%	Asymp	
M	20W	LAD	Success	60%	Asymp	Conservative
M	20W	RCA	Success	100%	APII	Conservative
M	20W	LAD	Success	80%	APII	Re-PTCA
RANDOMIZED 15W						
M	15W	LAD	Success	10%	Asymp	
M	15W	LAD	Success	0%	Asymp	
F	15W	CX	Success	10%	Asymp	
M	15W	LAD	Success	55%	Asymp	Conservative
F	15W	CX	Success	100%	Asymp	Conservative
F	15W	LAD	Success	NA	Asymp	
M	15W	RCA	Success	100%	Asymp	Conservative
F	15W	LAD	Success	55%	Asymp	Conservative
M	15W	LAD	Success	85%	Asymp	Re-PTCA
F	15W	LAD	Success	45%	Asymp	
M	15W	CX	Success	30%	Asymp	

Table 6. (Continued)

Sex	Laser Dose	Lesion	Result	Restenosis (%)	Angina	Remarks
M	15W	1st septal	Success	NA	Asymp	
M	15W	CX	Success	30%	Asymp	
RANDOMIZED PTCA ONLY						
M	PTCA	LAD	Success	53%	APII	Conservative
M	PTCA	LAD	Success	45%	Asymp	
M	PTCA	RCA	Success	NA	Asymp	
F	PTCA	LAD	Success	0%	Asymp	
M	PTCA	LAD	Success	60%	APII	Conservative
M	PTCA	LAD	Success	45%	Asymp	
M	PTCA	RCA	Success	35%	Asymp	
M	PTCA	CX	Success	10%	Asymp	
M	PTCA	RCA	Success	20%	Asymp	
F	PTCA	LAD	Success	NA	Asymp	
M	PTCA	LAD	Success	25%	Asymp	
M	PTCA	RCA	Success	NA	Asymp	

Abbreviations: APII = Angina pectoris class II according to the Canadian Cardiovascular Society. Asymp = Asymptomatic.

Table 7. Angiographic Follow-up of the Randomized LBA Patients. Restenosis Rate Per LBA Dosage Group.

	No.	Restenosis >50%
0 W (= PTCA only)	9	2 = 22%
15 W protocol	11	5 = 45%
20 W protocol	11	8 = 73%
25 W protocol	11	8 = 73%

Table 8. Angiographic Follow-up of the Randomized LBA Patients. Restenosis Rate Per Total Amount of Laser Energy.

Total Joules		Restenosis 75%
0 J = PTCA only		2/9 = 22%
< 600 J		15/26 = 58%
600–1200 J	6/7 = 80%	
	p = 0.036	

References

1. Gruentzig A R, Senning A, Seigenthaler W E (1979) Nonoperative dilatation of coronary-artery stenosis: percutaneous transluminal coronary angioplasty. *N Engl J Med* 301:61–8.
2. Kaltenbach M, Kober G, Schmidt-Moritz A, Scherer D (1983) Rezidivhaufigkeit nach erfolgreicher transluminaler Koronar-angioplastie. *Dtsch Med Wochenschr* 108:1387–90.
3. Kaltenbach M, Kober G, Scherer D, Vallbracht C (1985) Recurrence rate after successful coronary angioplasty. *Eur Heart J* 6:276–81.
4. Dangiosse V, Val P G, David P R et al (1982) Recurrence of stenosis after successful percutaneous transluminal coronary angioplasty (PTCA) [abstract]. *Circulation* 6(suppl II):331.
5. Jutzy K R, Berte L E, Alderman E L, Ratts J, Simpson J B (1982) Coronary restenosis

Table 1. Characteristics of current clinical cardiovascular lasers: 1991.

Laser Characters	Excimer	Pulsed Dye	Argon	Nd:YAG
Spectral region	Ultraviolet	Visible	Visible	Near infrared
Wavelength (nm)	308	480	488,514	1,060
Temporal mode	Pulsed (P)	P	Continous wave (CW)	P, CW
Delivery system	Single & multiple fiberoptics	Single fiberoptic, spectroscopic recognition	Single & multiple fiberoptics, metal cap, sapphire tip, lensed tip	Single fiberoptic metal cap, sapphire tip, rotational catheter

laser catheters. The early experience with these systems is just now being published [7–14] and six month angiographic follow-up has only been reported in a small number of patients [12–14]. While not yet published as of this writing, preliminary results from two separate registries indicate that at least one laser, the excimer laser, used either alone or in combination with conventional balloon angioplasty may have a benefit in the treatment of long lesions, greater than 20 mm, by increasing the success rate and decreasing the complications rate in these complex lesions. Other laser systems besides the excimer laser are also under investigation. While some approaches have already been discarded due to the lack of safety or efficacy in initial clinical trials [3, 4], the present review will attempt to present a current perspective on this rapidly changing field.

Current Cardiovascular Laser Technology

The current laser systems in clinical use or under investigation in either the peripheral or coronary circulation are summarized along with several of their laser characteristics in Table 1. In the cardiovascular system, different laser wavelengths may be required for different desired effects. For example, the 308 nm wavelength excimer laser which is readily absorbed by atherosclerotic tissue may be ideal for tissue ablation. On the other hand, the less readily absorbed Nd:YAG laser wavelength may be more appropriate for sealing or welding intimal flaps and dissections as in laser balloon angioplasty. Furthermore, the temporal mode (pulsed versus continuous wave) also appears to be an important laser parameter, particularly in smaller coronary arteries. Based on the initial clinical experience [7–14] and comparative studies in pig coronary arteries [15], pulsed excimer lasers appear safer than thermal laser angioplasty performed with a continuous wave laser [3, 4]. Whether smaller solid state pulsed lasers (holmium, erbium, etc) which are less expensive and require less maintenance will be superior to the excimer laser remains to be determined. However, compared to the excimer wavelength these near infrared lasers are less readily absorbed by atherosclerotic tissue and are more readily absorbed by water. Absorption by water can lead to "steam" production (O_2, H_2 and CO_2 gases) and significant disruption of arterial cells which may not be a desired effect. Additional experimental and clinical trials are obviously required to determine the ideal laser source for coronary laser angioplasty. For a more detailed review of laser physics and the fundamental aspects of lasers for cardiovascular use, the reader is referred to several recent textbooks on the subject [16–18].

Laser Catheter Design

The desired laser effect (recanalization, treatment of abrupt closure, or ablation) has a great deal to do with how the various lasers catheters are designed. Early cardiovascular laser catheters with modified tips (metal, sapphire, lens) were initially developed as recanalizaton devices for peripheral angioplasty when conventional attempts with a balloon or guidewire failed [1, 2, 5, 6, 19]. However, the application of these argon or Nd:YAG continuous wave laser systems in coronary arteries was limited by the thermal damage to the arterial wall mentioned above as well as the difficulty recanalizing coronary occlusions with the devices using angiographic and fluoroscopic guidance alone. The laser balloon catheter represents an entirely different concept of using low level Nd:YAG laser energy after balloon dilation to seal intimal dissection as a treatment for abrupt closure. Initial experience with this system was recently presented [6] and, therefore, will not be discussed further. Thus, the remainder of this review will discuss the over-the-wire ablative excimer laser angioplasty systems.

Besides the various laser parameters such as wavelength, pulse duration, etc, the actual catheter delivery system for intracoronary laser angioplasty may be one of the most important features in determining whether laser angioplasty will become a useful coronary therapeutic modality. Certain concepts such as a central lumen for guidewire passage have reduced but not eliminated the risk of vessel perforation. The packaging of multiple flexible fiberoptics into a single catheter has enabled investigators to create larger laser recanalized channels. At present, there are three percutaneous coronary excimer laser angioplasty systems under investigation (Advanced Interventional Systems, Spectranetics, and Technolas). While at present, different systems may have separate advantages in terms of individual laser generators or catheters, these laser delivery systems are undergoing such rapid modifications and adjustments that it is not possible to catalogue or compare different laser catheter designs and manufactures as has been done with balloon catheters. Many issues such as the optimum catheter flexibility, trackability, and tip geometry as well as the least amount of catheter "dead space" (nonfiber components) remain to be determined. However, the early experi-

residual lesion of less than 50% to be adequate such that no further balloon angioplasty is performed. This latter approach may lead to a higher incidence of angiographic restenosis.

In the majority of cases, systemic heparinization is maintained overnight and sheaths are removed the following morning. Discharge medications include aspirin (325 mg/day) and other cardiac medications as prescribed by the referring physician. Systemic anticoagulation with coumadin has not been a part of this protocol.

Procedural Definitions. Successful excimer laser angioplasty or laser recanalization is defined as passage of the laser catheter through the stenosis and a greater than 20% improvement of the luminal diameter stenosis (visual estimate) without perforation. Procedural success is defined as less that 50% residual stenosis without major complications of myocardial infarction (CPK > 200mg/dl), emergency bypass surgery, or death.

Initial Multicenter Results

The initial clinical experience of percutaneous coronary excimer laser assisted balloon angioplasty with the Spectranetics excimer laser catheter was recently published [13–14] and is briefly summarized as follows.

Acute Angiographic Results. The clinical and angiographic variables for this series are summarized in Table 2. Based on an intention to treat analysis, the excimer laser catheter was able to traverse the lesion and reduce the percent diameter stenosis by at least 20% in 138 of 158 (87%) coronary artery stenoses. Laser failure was attributed to the following: inability to cross the lesion [n = 15, due to vessel tortuosity (n = 5), low energy fluence (n = 4), calcified lesion (n = 3), and large device profile or catheter dead space between the fibers (n = 3)]; vessel perforation (n = 3); laser generator failure (n = 1); or radiographic failure (n = 1).

In this early feasibility study with small 1.5 and 1.75 mm diameter catheters, excimer laser angioplasty was able to reduce the residual stenosis to less than 50% in 77 of 158 (49%) lesions; however, due to protocol design to obtain the largest lumen and the greatest reduction in the stenosis only 9 of 158 (5.7%) lesions were treated with excimer laser angioplasty alone. An angiographic example of a patient treated with "stand alone" excimer laser angioplasty that resulted in a smoother lumen with less dissection than on a prior attempt with ballon angioplasty is shown in Fig. 1 along with a nine month follow-up angiogram which demonstrates no restenosis. Overall, laser-assisted balloon angioplasty was successful (residual stenosis less than 50% without major complication) in 129 of 141 (91%) patients.

Complications. Laser perforation is the most feared complication of coronary

Table 2. Clinical and angiographic variables.

Clinical variables: (141 pts)	
Age (yr)	
Mean	60
Range	32–84
Sex	
Male	98 (69%)
Female	43 (31%)
Angina	
Stable	78 (55%)
Unstable	63 (45%)
Functional class (CCS)	
I	4 (3%)
II	16 (11%)
III	47 (33%)
IV	74 (53%)
Angiographic variables: (158 stenoses)	
Vessel treated	
LAD	95 (60%)
RCA	29 (18%)
LCX	26 (16%)
SVG	8 (5%)
Repeat angioplasty	30 (19%)
Multivessel angioplasty	15 (11%)
Severity of stenosis prior to treatment (mean + standard error)	87 + 09

CCS = Canadian Cardiovascular Society.

laser angioplasty. However, with the over-the-wire approach, this occurred in only 3 (1.9%) attempts. Two of these cases required emergency bypass surgery while one was successfully treated with prolonged balloon inflation [20]. One diseased small diagonal vessel became occluded after five passes of the excimer laser catheter and could not be recanalized with a guidewire; this resulted in a small non-Q wave myocardial infarction (peak CPK 381 mg/dl). These four immediate laser related complications occurred during a modification of the catheter tip design. This design was abandoned after these four cases and no further laser perforations occurred in subsequent cases. Single episodes of vessel spasm or intraluminal filling defects seen after excimer laser angioplasty were not angina producing and were successfully treated with intracoronary nitroglycerin and balloon dilation. A summary of these complications is presented in Table 3.

While it is difficult to separate and attribute complications to either the laser or balloon angioplasty procedure when the catheters were used sequentially, those observed after balloon dilatation were also low (Table 3). Except for the above mentioned complications seen after laser attempts, the use of

rate, pulse duration) and operator techniques (number of passes, rate of advancement through the lesion, etc). These questions are just now being addressed. Currently, larger 2.0 mm laser catheters are being evaluated that are capable of producing larger channels to obviate the requirement for follow-up balloon angioplasty [22]. These improved catheters will allow for more independent analysis of excimer laser angioplasty alone. Whether there will be a benefit of "debulking" a lesion with excimer laser-assisted balloon angioplasty will require a randomized trial comparing acute and follow-up results to balloon angioplasty alone. Preliminary quantitative angiographic analysis suggest that if the laser is able to reduce the lesion to less than 30% residual stenosis then the incidence of restenosis is reduced [23].

Better Angioplasty? Figure 1 is a representative angiographic example of an observation made numerous times in this study; that is, the angiographic result after excimer laser angioplasty appears to result in less vessel dissection then that often seen after conventional balloon angioplasty. While it is difficult to prove that excimer laser angioplasty results in a smoother lumen than balloon dilation using angiography alone, it will be interesting to analyze the incidence of complications as more cases are performed by excimer laser angioplasty alone without subsequent balloon angioplasty. Intraluminal ultrasound may be able to determine whether this impression of a "smoother" channel does exist after excimer laser recanalization as compared to the fractures and dissections of balloon dilation.

Future Directions. The feasibility of excimer laser angioplasty and excimer laser-assisted balloon angioplasty has been demonstrated in several clinical registries. There is some preliminary data that this technique may have its initial application in improving the success rate and reducing complications for angioplasty of long diffuse stenoses greater than 20 mm. There are still many questions regarding the optimal operator techniques as well as the actual laser catheters which will require significant evaluation and modifications in the near future. Catheter related issues will center on such aspects as flexibility, trackability, profile, and maximal ablative potential. There is also a need to create larger laser channels safely. Whether the latter will require larger sized catheters or can be accomplished by positioning the catheter to one side of the vessel or another as in directional atherectomy remains to be determined. Hopefully, there will be answers to these questions with greater clinical experience.

References

1. Cumberland D C, Sanborn T A, Tayler D I, et al (1986) Percutaneous laser thermal angioplasty: initial clinical results with a laser probe in total peripheral artery occlusions. *Lancet* 2:1457–9

2. Sanborn T A, Cumberland D C, Greenfield A J, Welsh C L, Guben J K (1988) Percutaneous laser thermal angioplasty: initial results and 1–year follow-up in 129 femoropopliteal lesions. *Radiology* 168:121–5

3. Sanborn T A, Faxon D P, Kellett M A, Ryan T J (1986) Percutaneous coronary laser thermal angioplasty. *J Am Coll Cardiol* 8:1437–40

4. Cumberland D C, Starkey I R, Oakley G D G, et al (1986) Percutaneous laser-assisted coronary angioplasty. *Lancet* ii:214

5. Nordstrom L A, Castaneda-Zuniga W R, Young E G, Von Seggern K B (1988) Direct argon laser exposure for recanalization of peripheral arteries: early results. *Radiology* 168:359–364

6. Spears J R, Reyes V P, Wynne J, et al (1990) Percutaneous coronary laser balloon angioplasty: initial results of a multicenter experience. *J Am Coll Cardiol* 16:293–303

7. Litvack F, Grundfest W, Eigler N, et al (1989) Percutaneous excimer laser coronary angioplasty. *Lancet* ii:102–103

8. Sanborn T A, Hershman R A, Torre S R, Sherman W, Cohen M, Ambrose J A (1989) Percutaneous excimer laser coronary angioplasty. *Lancet* ii:616

9. Karsch K R, Haase K K, Mauser M, Ickrath O, Voelker W, Duda S (1989) Percutaneous coronary excimer laser angioplasty: initial clinical results. *Lancet* ii:647–650

10. Litvack F, Grundfest W S, Goldenberg T, Laudenslager J, Forrester J S (1989) Percutaneous excimer laser angioplasty of aortocoronary saphenous vein grafts. *J Am Coll Cardiol* 14:803–8

11. Karsch K R, Haase K K, Mauser M, Voelker W (1989) Initial angiographic results in ablation of atherosclerotic plaque by percutaneous coronary excimer laser angioplasty without subsequent balloon dilatation. *Am J Cardiol* 64:1253–1257

12. Karsch K R, Haase K K, Voelker W, Baumbach A, Mauser M, Seipel L (1990) Percutaneous coronary excimer laser angioplasty in patients with stable and unstable angina pectoris: acute results and incidence of restenosis during 6–month follow-up. *Circulation* 81:1849–1859

13. Sanborn T A, Torre S R, Sharma S K, Hershman R A, Cohen M, Sherman W, Ambrose J A (1991) Percutaneous coronary excimer laser-assisted angioplasty: initial clinical and quantitative angiographic results in 50 patients. *J Am Coll Cardiol* 17:94–9

14. Sanborn T A, Bittl J A, Hershman R A, Siegel R M (1991) Percutaneous coronary excimer laser-assisted angioplasty: initial multicenter experience in 141 patients. *J Am Coll Cardiol* 17:169B–173B

15. Sanborn T A, Alexopoulos D, Marmur J D, Kahn H, Badimon J J, Badimon L, Fuster V (1990) Coronary excimer laser angioplasty: reduced complications and indium-111 platelet accumulation compared with thermal laser angioplasty. *J Am Coll Cardiol* 16:502–6

16. White R A, Grundfest W S (1989) Lasers in cardiovascular disease: clinical applications, alternative angioplasty devices, and guidance systems. *Year Book Medical Publishers*, Inc., Chicago, 2nd Edition, 1–234

17. Abela G S (1990) *Lasers in cardiovascular medicine and surgery: fundamentals and techniques.* Kluwer Academic Publishers, Boston 1990, 1–480

18. Sanborn T A (1989) *Laser angioplasty.* Alan R. Liss Inc., New York, 1–121

19. Pilger E, Lammer J, Bertuch H, Stark G, Decrinis M, Pfeiffer K P, Krejs G J (1991) Nd:YAG laser with sapphire tip combined with balloon angioplasty in peripheral arterial occlusions: long-term results. *Circulation* 83:141–147

20. Parker J D, Ganz P, Selwyn A P, Bittl J A (1991) Successful treatment of an excimer laser-associated coronary artery perforation with the stack perfusion catheter. *Cath Cardiovasc Diagn* 22:118–123

21. Holmes Dr Jr., Holubkov M S, Vilietstra R E, Kelsey S F, Reeder G S, Dorros G, William Do, Cowley M J, Faxon D P, Kent K M, Bentivoglio L G, Detre K and the Co-Investigators of The National Heart, Lung and Blood Institute Percutaneous Transluminal Coronary Angioplasty Registry (1988) Comparison of complications during percutaneous transluminal coronary angioplasty from 1977 to 1981 and from 1985 to 1986: The National Heart, Lung

and Blood Institute Percutaneous Transluminal Coronary Angioplasty Registry. *J Am Coll Cardiol* 12:1149–1155

22. Torre S R, Sanborn T A, Sharma S K, Cohen M, Ambrose J A (1990) Percutaneous coronary excimer laser angioplasty: quantitative angiographic analysis demonstrates improved angioplasty results with larger laser catheters. *Circulation* 82(suppl III):III–671

23. Sanborn T A, Bittl J A, Torre S R (1991) Procedural success, in-hospital events, and follow-up clinical and angiographic results of percutaneous coronary excimer laser-assisted angioplasty. *J Am Coll Cardiol* 17:206A

19. Restenosis Following Laser Angioplasty

J. MICHAEL KOCH, STEPHAN FRIEDL, JAMES M. SEEGER,
GÉRALD BARBEAU and GEORGE S. ABELA

Symbols

cm	centimeter
CO_2	carbon dioxide
Hz	Hertz (cycle per second)
J	joule
mJ	millijoule
mm	millimeter
Nd:YAG	neodymium:yttrium aluminum garnet
nm	nanometer
W	watt
°C	degree centigrade
μs	microsecond

Introduction

Approximately ten years ago, our laboratory initiated work evaluating the use of the laser as a tool for altering vascular tissue biology to reduce the restenosis rate [1]. The attention of laser technology, however, was directed at a device to obtain immediate lumen enlargement by removing plaque [2–5]. Early limitations of laser applications in the cardiovascular system were primarily related to arterial perforation due to optical fiber stiffness and uncontrolled energy delivery [6–9]. As with balloon angioplasty, the use of a guidewire was adapted effectively to maintain coaxiality of the optical fibers within the vessel (Fig. 1) [10]. Thus, most devices currently available are capable of removing plaque and creating a lumen equivalent to the diameter of the catheter device. In addition, numerous studies have been done to evaluate the effects of various laser wavelengths and delivery modes on arterial tissue. The primary focus was on the use of continuous wave vs. pulsed laser systems. The optimum combination of laser wave-lengths and

P.W. Serruys, B.H. Strauss and S.B. King III (eds), Restenosis after Intervention with New Mechanical Devices, 385–413.
© 1992 *Kluwer Academic Publishers. Printed in the Netherlands.*

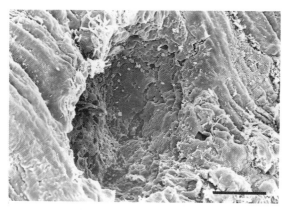

Figure 3. Scanning electron micrograph of crater immediately after lasing normal dog artery with an argon laser via a 400-μm core optical fiber. Note that the crater has a smooth border showing cut endothelial cells. Walls of the crater show exposed smooth muscle cells (Bar = 100 μm). (Fig. from Abela G S, Pepine C J *Cardiov Reviews and Reports* 6:269–278. Reproduced with permission of author and publisher.)

of acute thrombosis with no adverse long-term effect [25] (Fig. 9). Platelet deposition immediately following laser irradiation has been evaluated using both continuous wave and pulsed lasers, particularly excimer systems. Those studies have provided conflicting results due to great variability in the laser parameters used. This is not surprising since the amount of vascular trauma can be varied with any laser to result in excessive or minimal damage to the vascular wall. Thus, continuous wave lasers without temperature monitoring

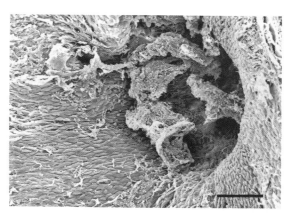

Figure 4. Scanning electron micrograph of normal dog artery 2 weeks following argon-laser irradiation (1 watt for 1 sec). Elongated neoendothelial cells are seen proliferating along the crater edges. Residual fibrin-platelet plug is seen along the upper and middle portions of crater. Bar = 100 μm. (Fig. from Chapter 9 in *Lasers in Cardiovascular Medicine and Surgery: Fundamentals and Techniques* (ed) Abela G S, Kluwer Acad. Publ. 1990. Reproduced with pesmission of author and publisher.)

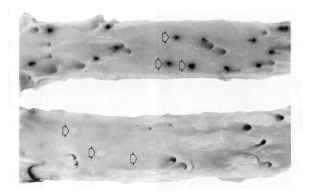

Figure 5. (Top) Gross appearance of a distal abdominal aorta from a dog at 1 week after lasing (2.5 watts for 1 sec). Numerous craters are present (arrows), but there is no thrombus present. (Bottom) Gross appearance of a distal abdominal aorta 1 month after lasing (2.5 watts for 1 sec). The number of identifiable craters (arrows) is less than at 1 week. Those that are seen have a smooth, flat, white surface. (Fig. from Abela et al (1985) *Am J Cardiol* 56: 1199–1205. Reproduced with permission from author and publisher.)

have been used to deliver energies in excess of that needed to bring about more than a sufficient amount of thermal damage required to alter biological responses [23].

Using an AV shunt model connecting the left carotid artery with the right jugular vein in dogs, arterial segments were treated with various interventional devices [26, 27]. Radioactive platelet deposition was used to evaluate the thrombogenicity of the treated surfaces [26]. These studies demonstrated that balloon angioplasty resulted in the highest amount of platelet deposition as compared to direct laser or laser thermal treatment (Figs. 10, 11). In

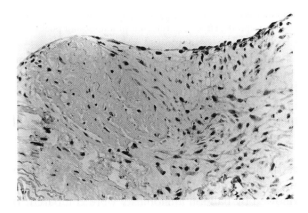

Figure 6. Light micrograph of healing artery in hypercholesterolemic monkey at 30 days following laser irradiation (1.5 watts for 1 sec). The crater is filled with organizing cellular infiltrate with little extension beyond the edges of the crater. Hematoxylin and eosin stain, magnified 55x reduced by 15%.

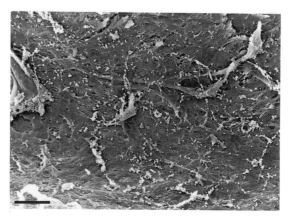

Figure 10. Scanning electron micrograph of rabbit aorta 30 min following balloon angioplasty. The endothelial layer is disrupted. Platelets and fibrin are deposited over the entire luminal surface (Bar = 100 μm).

studies using bare optical fibers were performed primarily to evaluate the feasibility of laser recanalization [8, 9, 29]. Small lumens were made using single fiber systems. All patients treated with this system alone restenosed within 6 months. Subsequent clinical trials were initiated with the intent of performing laser angioplasty with optical fiber-modified tips which would allow for larger lumen dimensions and reduced perforation rates.

These studies demonstrated improvement in lumen diameter by angiography with higher technical success in the stenotic lesions and more failures in total obstructions especially in lesions longer than 7 cm. Even with modified probes, balloon angioplasty was still needed to obtain >50% lumen dimension.

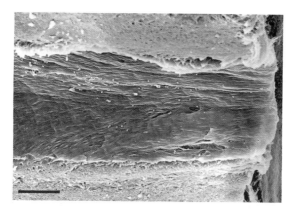

Figure 11. A low-power scanning electron micrograph from an atherosclerotic rabbit showing a vascular channel created by laser radiation in a totally occluded artery. The walls of the channel were smooth. Bar = 100 μm. (By permission of the American Heart Association. *Circulation* 1985:71–403–411. Published with authors' and publisher's permission.)

Laser Thermal Probes in the Peripheral Circulation

Sanborn and associates [30] reported outcomes and one-year follow-up in 119 patients with 129 occlusive atherosclerotic femoropopliteal lesions treated with percutaneous laser thermal angioplasty. Treatment was undertaken with a metal-capped fiber coupled to a continuous-wave argon laser which was placed in contact with the occlusive lesions under fluoroscopic guidance. Power was adjusted from 8 to 13 Watts, with exposure durations of 5 to 10 seconds. Angiographic and clinical success was defined as reduction in stenosis to <50% residual, relief of symptoms and improved pulse with an increase in the ankle-arm Doppler index of >0.15. Angiographic failure was defined as inability to cross the lesion with the thermal probe or failure to improve the stenosis to <50% residual.

The investigators reported initial overall clinical and angiographic success rates of 77%, with significantly better results in stenoses (95% success) and poorer results in occlusions (85% success), especially long (>7 cm) total occlusions (66% success). There was a 4% frequency of vessel perforation in this study, without any requirement for emergency bypass surgery. Angiographic failure occurred in 30 lesions (23%) of which 29 were total occlusions. Of these, 6 failures occurred because of inability to pass the probe due to the length of the lesion or calcium deposition. Five other failures were due to perforation. Eleven patients reportedly experienced pain during laser delivery. There were no serious complications.

At one year follow-up, 77% of the successfully treated lesions were clinically patent. Clinical patency was established by persistently improved ankle-arm Doppler indexes. Angiographic correlation was not done. Again, the clinical patency rates were significantly better for patients treated with stenosis (95% one-year clinical patency) than for long total occlusions (58% one-year clinical patency). The authors compare the one year outcome favorably to reports of one year clinical patency rates for balloon angioplasty which varied from 56 to 84%. Furthermore, one-year patency in stenoses and short (<3 cm) occlusions was reportedly 72 to 81% for balloon angioplasty. Clinical patency rates for long (>3 cm) occlusions one year after balloon angioplasty were only 50%.

The same group of patients was followed up to 21 months after treatment. At that follow-up of 42 patients with initial success, 73% continued to have clinical patency. This may suggest that clinical recurrence of disease was unlikely after the first year following treatment.

A direct comparison to balloon angioplasty is difficult to make from this data. This trial was not randomized and many of the original lesions were not approachable by balloon angioplasty, according to the investigators' opinion. Furthermore one-year clinical patency rates may differ from angiographic patency rates, due to establishment of collateral circulation. Beyond this, the results achieved with the thermal probe are at least comparable to those obtained with balloon angioplasty in treating stenoses, and potentially better than those achieved in treating occlusions. The trial does support the conclusion that the procedure was performed safely and effectively. This confirmation of feasibility would warrant further clinical trials.

In a review of 1849 peripheral thermal probe laser angioplasty procedures performed at the Arizona Heart Institute, Diethrich has observed that the primary goals of therapy have been: 1) to open a totally occluded artery to permit balloon dilatation, and 2) to ablate plaque in order to decrease the volume of material which is to be subsequently compressed by the balloon dilatation [31]. In this group of patients selection criteria were minimal. The majority of arteries treated were in the superficial femoral artery distribution, but other locations, including 45 (2% of the total procedures) occluded femoral popliteal bypass grafts, mostly synthetic, were included. In addition, 470 concomitant surgical procedures, such as patch angioplasty in other locations, endarterectomy, thrombectomy and bypass, were performed with these angioplasties. Complications in this large series included perforation in 5.0% and vasospasm in 6.5% of patients.

Successful angioplasty was defined as re-establishment of luminal continuity by angiography or restoration of pulse detectable by palpation or Doppler studies or an increase of $\geq.15$ in the ankle/brachial pressure ratio. By these criteria, laser angioplasty was initially successful in 80% of lesions. Out of the initial failures, perforation occurred in 92 (5% of attempts) and inability to cross a calcified lesion occurred in 68 (3.7% of attempts).

Following successful laser recanalization in this study, patients evaluated at 6 to 30 months had an overall patency rate of 74%. This included a 56% rate in graft occlusions. While there is no breakdown between total occlusions versus stenoses or among lesions based on length or duration, the overall patency rates seem to agree well with those in other studies reviewed. Furthermore, the distinction between 6–month and longer follow-up is not made, although other studies suggest that the majority of restenosis occurs during the first 4 to 6 months.

Of note is that all these studies were performed using laser and thermal energies of unspecified amounts. To avoid thermal build up in the vessel, the procedure was performed by a tethered to-and-fro motion resulting in a mixture of mechanical and thermal injury of unquantified amounts. Therefore, given what we know presently from the basic data, it is quite surprising how forgiving the arterial wall has been in responding to this form of injury.

Angioscopy was employed in an unspecified number of cases in this group. Observations regarding the recanalization process suggest that the effects of the probe are both thermal and mechanical. The probe may initially effect some degree of plaque ablation, but material is simply pushed aside subsequently, giving rise to dilatation, even with the laser probe as sole therapy. Furthermore, if lesions are eccentric, the probe tends to slide over them with a "roller-coaster" effect, which limits ablative potential. The author states that similar phenomena occur also with hybrid and excimer probes. Finally, as seen in angiographic and histologic studies, angioscopy documents the

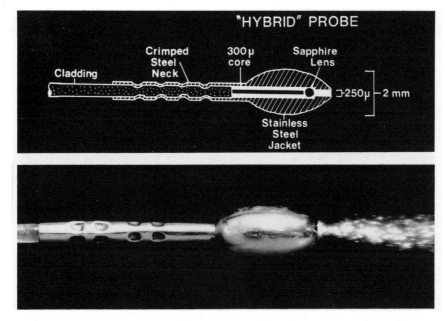

Figure 12. "Hybrid" probe (Spectraprobe-PLR™, Trimedyne Inc., Santa Anna, CA). Top panel: Schematic of a "hybrid" probe is illustrated. A metal cap 2 mm in diameter is crimped on a 300 μm core fiber. A 250-μm window allows 20% of the laser beam to exit. Behind the window, a sapphire lens is used to focus the beam as it exits. Bottom panel: Probe with exiting argon-laser beam. The beam has a waist 1 mm from the probe tip and is defocused into a diffuse light. (Fig. from Chapter 16 in: *Lasers in Cardiovascular Medicine and Surgery: Fundamentals and Techniques* (ed) Abela G S, Kluwer Acad Publ, 1990. Reproduced with permission of author and publisher.)

tendency for the probe to follow the path of least resistance, which can result in ineffective recanalization, dissection or perforation.

The Sapphire-tip Contact Probe in Peripheral Vascular Disease

In attempts to improve efficacy while maintaining the safety of the laser probe, laser fibers were fitted with a rounded sapphire tip which allowed 15 to 20% of the input laser light to escape from the contact probe [29, 32, 33]. Theoretically, the "hybrid" thermo-optical probe should permit direct laser photo-ablative, as well as thermal interactions between the laser and the occlusive atheromatous plaque.

In a series of patients using a "hybrid" laser catheter with a sapphire tip, Abela and associates treated patients with total arterial occlusions intraoperatively or by the percutaneous approach [29, 32, 33] (Figs. 12, 13, 14, and 15). The authors noted that the group was comprised of patients with a high frequency of associated conditions such as failed bypass grafts and extensive

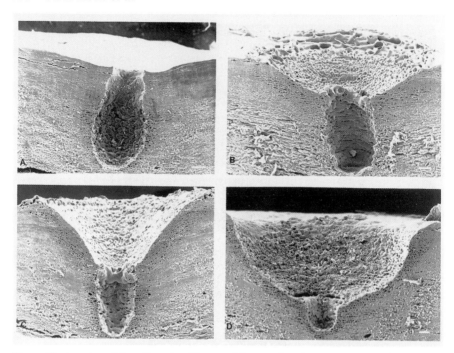

Figure 13. A series of four Scanning Electron Micrographs of craters (cross-sectional view) produced by the Spectraprobe-PLR^{TM}. Thermal compression and vaporization may be observed as well as an optically reduced central "pilot" hole. With progressive energy delivered (30–90 Joules) and fixed pressure (10 gm) layer craters are obtained with (A-D), the optical effect of the direct laser beam gradually decreasing (bars = 100 μm). (Fig. from Caravello J W et al, SPIE, Optical Fibers in Medicine V, Vol. 1201, p. 127, 1990. Reproduced with permission of author and publisher.)

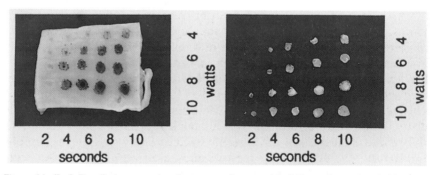

Figure 14. (Left Panel) An example of segment of aorta with diffuse atherosclerosis irradiated in air according to a dosimetry matrix. Increasing the power and exposure time resulted in larger craters. (Right panel). Paraffin casts displayed corresponding with the same dosimetry of the vaporized plaque. (Fig. from Hoffman R G et al, SPIE, *Optical Fibers in Medicine IV*, 1067:120–126, 1989. Reproduced with permission of author and publisher.)

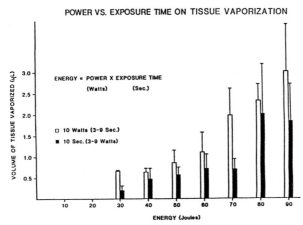

Figure 15. Tissue vaporization efficiency using "hybrid" probe. This shows that higher power (10 watts) results in a consistently greater volume of tissue ablation compared to long-time exposure (10 sec) for the equivalent amount of total energy. (Fig. courtesy of Abela G S and Barbieri E)

peripheral vascular disease. Candidates considered were only patients in whom standard balloon angioplasty attempts had failed. This was primarily those in whom a regular guidewire could not cross the lesion. Following the thermo-optical laser treatment and angiographic evaluation, balloon angioplasty was performed if the residual stenosis was >50%; otherwise laser treatment was performed as the sole therapeutic maneuver. In 32 patients treated by the percutaneous approach, the initial technical success rate was 81%. The rate of clinical improvement was only 63% (20 patients). Seven patients were treated solely with laser recanalization (no balloon angioplasty). Five cases (16%) of arterial perforation and 3 (9%) acute occlusions (thromboses) occurred. Of 20 patients with clinical and technical success, 45% had clinical evidence of restenosis at an average follow-up of 8.6 ± 4.0 months. With further modification of the "hybrid" device, temperature was monitored during laser recanalization of totally occluded peripheral arteries [34]. Temperatures were recorded with a mean of 178 ± 120 °C (range 64–503 °) at a mean time of 12.4 ± 14.1 seconds. Eleven of 16 (69%) recanalizations occurred at a probe temperature lower than 160 °C (Fig. 16). Recanalization occurred at a mean power of 7 ± 2W from an argon laser. Perforation occurred in 6 arteries at peak temperatures ranging from 73 to 502 °C. Perforations occurred in 4 of 6 densely calcific vessels requiring high probe temperature (>250 °C) during recanalization attempts (Fig. 17). No acute occlusions occurred. Initial use of lower powers and temperature with incremental rises and without a to-and-fro motion of the probe seems a more controllable method when attempting to recanalize totally occluded peripheral arteries (Figs. 18, 19).

In a variation from the sapphire-tipped probe, White and associates have

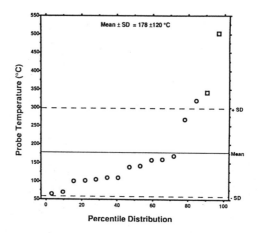

Figure 16. Percentile distribution of peak probe temperature required for recanalization of totally occluded peripheral arteries in 16 patients. Eleven of 16 recanalizations occurred at temperature below 160 °C. Peak probe temperatures in percutaneous procedures are represented as circles and peak probe temperatures in intra-operative procedures are represented as squares. Mean ± SD = 178 ± 120 °C. (Copyrighted and reprinted with the permission of Clinical Publishing Co., Inc., and/or the Foundation for Advances in Medicine and Science (FAMS), Box 832, Mahwah, New Jersey 07430, USA.) "Copyrighted and reprinted with the permission of Clinical Cardiology Publishing Co., Inc., and/or the Foundation for Advances in Medicine and Science (FAMS), Box 832, Mahwah, New Jersey 07430, USA".

modified the distal end of the laser probe with a 1.5 mm diameter spherical lens which reduces risk of perforation, while increasing the spot size of the laser beam [6]. Power is supplied by a Nd:YAG laser at 0.5 J/pulse with a pulse duration of 100μs at 10 Hz in 2- to 5-second bursts. In a series of 14 lesions, 6 total occlusions and 8 subtotal occlusions in the superficial femoral and iliac arteries, an initial success rate of 79% was obtained. No complications were reported. Restenosis occurred at 6 months in 46% of patients.

In all studies of peripheral balloon and laser angioplasty, the outcomes of failed therapeutic maneuvers have reportedly been relatively benign [33].

In a prospective, multicenter trial, Lammer and associates treated 338 patients with arteriosclerotic femoropopliteal artery occlusions with a sapphire-tip laser angioplasty catheter [35]. Only patients with total occlusions >2 cm, in whom recanalization with a guidewire was not possible were included. A Nd:YAG laser (1,064 nm), with pulse duration of 1 second at a power of 10–15 W, was coupled to a 2.2 or 3.0 mm sapphire-contact-probe catheter for recanalization. Balloon dilation was performed in all but six patients subsequent to successful laser angioplasty. Following the procedure, most patients were treated with aspirin and dipyridamole. A subset of 129 patients at one center were randomized to receive anti-platelet therapy with aspirin and dipyridamole or anticoagulation with phenprocumarol [36].

Follow-up in this study included both Doppler ultrasound at regular intervals and digital subtraction angiography at 1, 2 and 3 years. Recurrence

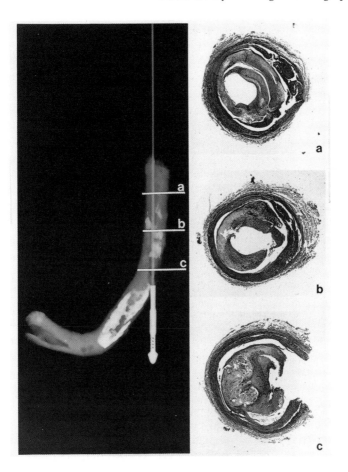

Figure 17. Left: Plain radiograph of a densely calcified artery excised during the bypass procedure done after an unsuccessful attempt that resulted in a perforation at a temperature of 250 °C. This illustrates the relation of the probe to the calcific deposit and suggests deflection of the probe by the "hard" calcific plaque resulting in perforation. Right: Histologic cross sections corresponding to three anatomic sites (a, b, c) show the increasing density and calcification of the plaque from section a to c where perforation occurred (Masson's trichrome, magnification 10×). (Copyrighted and reprinted with the permission of Clinical Publishing Co., Inc., and/or the Foundation for Advances in Medicine and Science (FAMS), Box 832, Mahwah, New Jersey 07430, USA.) "Copyrighted and reprinted with the permission of Clinical Cardiology Publishing Co., Inc., and/or the Foundation for Advances in Medicine and Science (FAMS), Box 832, Mahwah, New Jersey 07430, USA".

of stenosis was defined as angiographically documented restenosis of >50% or re-occlusion.

The initial success rate for laser recanalization was 85% (288/338), with clinical improvement in 97% of these successful cases. The recanalization rate was 89% in lesions <7 cm, and 78% in lesions >7 cm. There were 29 cases of perforation or dissection. The investigators reported 36 episodes of

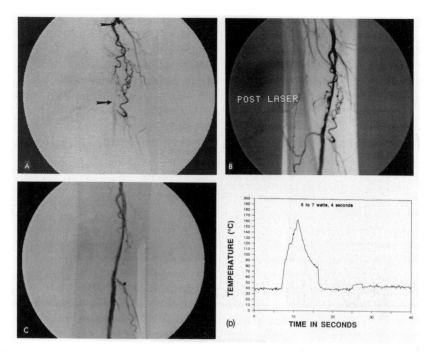

Figure 18. Sequential digital angiograms of the right superficial femoral artery (Case No. 14), (A) before laser recanalization (arrows at proximal and distal end of occlusion), (B) after laser recanalization, and (C) after balloon angioplasty. A dissection is seen in the proximal third of the balloon dilated segment. (D) Probe temperature is plotted against time during laser recanalization of the occluded segment shown in (A). Peak probe temperature of 168 °C which resulted in recanalization was reached at a power at 6 W and 4 s exposure. (Copyrighted and reprinted with the permission of Clinical Cardiology Publishing Co., Inc., and/or the Foundation for Advances in Medicine and Science (FAMS), Box 832, Mahwah, New Jersey 07430, USA.).

painful heat sensation, including all 29 cases in which there was vessel wall injury. Twenty-one patients (6.2%) had calcified plaques which could not be ablated. The patency rates for patients actually observed are shown in Table 1.

These data would suggest that the majority of recurrences would occur within the first year. Furthermore, the investigators indicate that 32 of the failures occurred due to restenosis. Six of these were asymptomatic and treated medically. Twenty-six successfully underwent repeat percutaneous angioplasty. Thirty nine more patients had a re-occlusion. Of these, 22 had bypass surgery, 5 underwent a second laser recanalization, 5 required amputation and three were managed medically. In 4 patients in whom thrombosis occurred within 2 weeks of the recanalization procedure, intra-arterial fibrinolysis was administered.

Again, it is difficult to compare the success rates and restenosis rates in this study to those of conventional balloon angioplasty. An attempt was

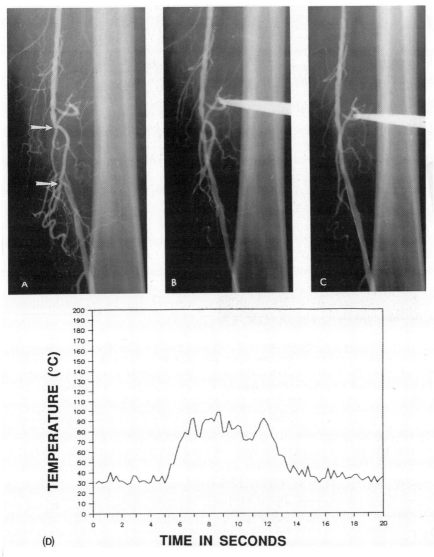

Figure 19. Sequential angiograms of a 58-year-old white male with recent onset of claudication (Case No. 7). (A) Before laser recanalization showing a 5 cm occlusion (arrows) of the superficial femoral artery with collateral filling of the distal segment and (B) Following laser recanalization, a guide wire is seen across the recanalized lumen. (C) Following balloon angioplasty. (D) Power as well as probe temperature of 95–100 °C remained constant during recanalization. (Copyrighted and reprinted with the permission of Clinical Cardiology Publishing Co., Inc., and/or the Foundation for Advances in Medicine and Science (FAMS), Box 832, Mahwah, New Jersey 07430, USA.).

Table 1.

	6 MONTHS (261 pts.)	1 YEAR (176 pts.)	2 YEARS (29 pts.)	3 YEARS (11 pts.)
Cumulative patency	80%	70%	62%	57%

Modified from Lammer et al [35].

made in each of the cases to cross the occlusions with a guidewire; however, by the authors' admission, this was not the most sophisticated approach.

In the subset analysis of patients who were randomized to anti-platelet therapy vs. anticoagulation therapy, no difference was seen in restenosis rates in the first year [36]. There were significantly more side effects in the group treated with aspirin and dipyridamole (30%) than in the group treated with phenprocumarol (6%).

Trials in peripheral angioplasty are useful in identifying areas in which the laser may offer unique outcomes and in directing focus for improvement. Lasers and thermal probes may offer selective advantages in total occlusions and long areas of disease, which have traditionally yielded poor results in trials with percutaneous devices. Calcified lesions offer a challenge which may be addressed by lasers of different wavelengths, or by application of different delivery modes or techniques.

Laser Thermal Coronary Angioplasty

Using laser activated thermal probes, studies were performed in the coronary circulation. In a preliminary study by Cumberland et al, four patients were recanalized [37]. Two of these had evidence of reocclusion within 24 hrs. In a report by Crea et al, an attempt was made to recanalize high grade stenosis intraoperatively prior to surgery [38]. One heavily calcific left anterior descending coronary artery perforated. These experiences were seen by other investigators and this program was discontinued. Unfortunately, this occurred prior to development of thermal monitoring or knowing what temperatures were needed to alter the vascular biology.

The Excimer Laser in Peripheral Vascular Disease

Excimer laser angioplasty of peripheral arteries was equally, if not more, disappointing than the thermal devices [39]. This was primarily related to small lumen sizes, difficulty in crossing heavily calcific lesions, and inability to recanalize small arteries. Thus, the use of excimer laser angioplasty for peripheral arteries is not being pursued at present.

The Excimer Laser in Percutaneous Coronary Angioplasty

The fundamental advantages of laser energy applied to atherosclerotic coronary artery disease are, as stated earlier, ablation of plaque volume and tissue structural changes which may alter short and long term re-occlusion. In addition, the excimer laser offers potential benefits of increased plaque specificity and ablation of moderately calcific plaque with minimal surrounding tissue damage.

In a clinical trial, Karsch et al operated a 308 nm XeCl excimer laser with energy fluence of $30 \pm 5 \, mJ/mm^2$ at 20 Hz via 20 concentrically-arranged quartz fibers in a 1.4 mm diameter over-the-wire catheter system [40]. Sixty patients were enrolled in the trial, including 11 patients with unstable angina and 49 who were limited by severe exertional angina. All patients were treated with aspirin prior to and following angioplasty. Following laser angioplasty, patients were treated with balloon angioplasty if adequate reduction in stenosis was not achieved. In five patients, including one with unstable symptoms, the lesion could not be engaged with the laser catheter due to severe tortuosity. Successful recanalization, defined as reduction in lesion severity of more than 50% from pre- to post-intervention was achieved in 23 of 55 patients by laser angioplasty alone. In the remaining 32 patients, balloon angioplasty was eventually performed successfully in 29, with myocardial infarction (2 patients) and death (1 patient) complicating the remaining procedures.

Of 10 patients with unstable angina treated in this study, only 2 had successful recanalization by laser alone. Four patients in this group had acute closure, requiring balloon angioplasty; all 3 significant complications were in this group. In total, 11 of the 55 patients (20%) treated with the laser catheter in this trial had acute closure, within 2 to 10 minutes following treatment, requiring subsequent balloon angioplasty.

Late follow-up angiography (6 months) was performed in 47 of these patients. Overall, 22 patients (47%) developed restenosis, defined as loss of at least 50% of the gain in the luminal diameter or a decrease in luminal diameter of ≥ 0.72 mm versus post-intervention. Of 19 patients treated by laser angioplasty alone who underwent late follow-up, only 6 (32%) had restenosis. Twenty-eight of 32 patients who underwent balloon angioplasty subsequent to laser treatment had late follow-up angiography, with 16 (57%) fulfilling criteria for restenosis.

The mechanisms for vessel closure in situations of both acute closure and restenosis are unknown. It is disturbing that acute closure occurred so frequently. The authors suggest that improvements in catheter design may help in this regard.

In an initial feasibility study of 50 patients enrolled for percutaneous coronary angioplasty, Sanborn and associates evaluated the performance of excimer laser delivered via 1.5 and 1.75 mm catheters and followed by balloon angioplasty [19]. Initial success, defined as reduction in the diameter stenosis of ≥20% was achieved by the laser in 41 (75%) of 55 lesions attempted. Subsequent balloon angioplasty was successful in all lesions in which the excimer laser failed. Limitations in the laser catheter design, including tip profile, flexibility and suboptimal energy fluence were cited as common causes for failure. Overall, mean percent stenosis was reduced from 81 ± 1% to 50 ± 3% following excimer laser angioplasty and to 20 ± 1% following balloon angioplasty. Complications were infrequent, including 2 abrupt closures (3.6%), spasm (3.6%), side branch occlusion (3.6%), and myocardial infarction (5.5%). The authors indicate that a significant proportion of complications resulted from the subsequent balloon angioplasty. Preliminary follow-up of 1 to 10 months (mean = 7) in these patients identified symptomatic recurrence in 14 patients (28%).

In an enlarging multicenter trial, Bittl et al reported treating 223 consecutive patients with improved excimer laser catheters. Initial success, defined as reduction in the diameter stenosis of ≥20%, was achieved in 192 of 245 (78%) attempted lesions. Subsequent balloon angioplasty was successfully performed in 223 of 245 (91%) lesions [41]. Complications were again reportedly infrequent. Improved catheter designs, including a larger 2.1 mm catheter, and higher energy fluence, up to 50–60 mJ/mm^2, contributed to success rates in this group which compare favorably to earlier studies in more highly selected patients.

Sharma, et al compared angiographic outcomes following excimer laser assisted coronary angioplasty versus conventional balloon angioplasty in a group of 91 patients [42]. They concluded that the arterial lumen following laser angioplasty is generally small, requiring further enlargement by balloon angioplasty. They were able to demonstrate fewer dissections and less residual stenosis in patients treated with laser prior to conventional balloon angioplasty. It is unclear how this will affect restenosis.

There is evidence that restenosis rates can be largely affected by the postprocedural luminal diameter, regardless of the type of intervention. Kuntz and co-workers reported on 191 patients, including 120 atherectomies, 72 stents, and 11 laser balloon angioplasties [43]. In this diverse group, an average loss of luminal diameter at 4 to 6 months following intervention was the same in all groups, leading to the authors' observation that the development of restenosis was principally determined by the immediate therapeutic outcome. In addition, Sanborn et al reported outcomes in 86 patients treated by percutaneous excimer laser-assisted angioplasty. At 6–month follow-up, restenosis rate was related to post-procedural residual stenosis [19]. In this group, 30 of 85 (35%) successfully treated patients had symptoms or positive treadmill tests at 6 month follow-up. Of 74 patients undergoing angiographic follow-up, 30 (41%) had restenosis, defined as ≥50% narrowing of the vessel. Importantly, patients whose post-procedural residual stenosis was ≤30% had a restenosis rate of only 25%, compared to 63 % restenosis in those whose residual stenosis was ≥30%.

In a multicenter trial of efficacy, Litvack and his associates studied 55 patients in whom a first-generation excimer laser catheter was used to treat 67 stenotic lesions and occlusions [18]. Acute success with the laser catheter, defined as >20% improvement in minimal lumen diameter with a minimum diameter of 1.0 mm was achieved in 46 of 55 (84%) patients. 36 (78%) patients underwent balloon angioplasty subsequent to laser treatment.

Clinically significant complications occurred in 3 patients. One severe dissection required CABG. One patient with dissection which was adequately treated with balloon angioplasty developed acute closure on day three following the procedure. Angiography revealed adequate collateral circulation and no further intervention was necessary. A third patient suffered marked vasospasm in response to the laser catheter, resulting in a non-Q-wave myocardial infarction. Two other patients also experienced less severe vasospasm in response to the laser.

A larger study of 958 patients, reported by Bresnehan et al reported similar initial results from excimer laser coronary angioplasty [44]. Using catheters ranging from 1.3 mm to 2.4 mm, they were able to achieve laser success rates of 85%, with overall 94% procedural success (reduction in residual stenosis to less than 50% of luminal diameter). Lesions treated included saphenous vein grafts (10%), total occlusions (10%) and stenoses >20 mm in length (22%). Forty one percent of the 1151 lesions treated were treated with laser alone. For the same cohort, Margolis et al reported 6–month follow-up in 446 patients [45]. Of these, 129 (29%) required repeat intervention or CABG. An additional 189 patients had undergone follow-up angiography, with evidence of restenosis, defined as a luminal diameter reduction to less than 50%, in 60 (32%) of them. Nineteen other patients with recurrent symptoms or positive exercise tests had not undergone catheterization. There were 7 myocardial infarctions and 6 late deaths. Overall, there were adverse outcomes in 49.6% of the 446 patients followed-up at 6 months. Within this group there was an inverse relationship between the energy delivered and restenosis, for energy fluences of 30 to 39 mJ/mm^2 versus 40 to 49 mJ/mm^2 and versus 50 to 59 mJ/mm^2.

Several reports have suggested that the laser may be useful in treating long areas of stenosis and total occlusions. Werner et al described the application of the excimer laser in 39 patients with total occlusions of 1 to 12 months of age [46]. Successful laser recanalization was performed in 25 of 27 patients in whom a standard guidewire could be advanced across the lesion. In 19 patients balloon angioplasty was required in order to reduce residual luminal narrowing to less than 50% following successful laser recanalization. There were two acute re-occlusions in the first 24 hours after angioplasty. It is notable that there was a significant difference (p = .03) between successful and unsuccessful groups in duration of occlusion (3.6 ± 3.2 versus 5.5 ± 2.9 months).

In a similar group of patients, the same authors, Buchwald et al, report in abstract format on follow-up of 104 patients with 48 stenoses and 56 occlusions [47]. These patients were treated with excimer laser at energy fluences of 37 to 64 mJ/mm^2. Initial success rates were 89% (43/48 pts.) in stenotic lesions and 70% (39/56 pts.) in occluded vessels. Subsequent PTCA was performed in 49% of stenoses and in 46% of occlusions treated successfully with the laser. Angiographic follow-up at 6 months was obtained in 68 patients, including 35 with stenoses and 33 with treated occlusions. Restenosis of ≥20% occurred in 34% of those with stenotic lesions and in 48% of those with total occlusions. These results compare favorably with balloon angioplasty.

Laser Balloon Angioplasty for Treatment of Coronary Artery Disease

Laser Balloon Angioplasty potentially delivers laser energy to "weld" arterial tissues, remodeling the vessel, reducing arterial recoil and sealing the intraluminal surface, thereby reducing thrombogenicity.

Jenkins and Spears have summarized progress to date in developing the technique and enrolling over 250 patients in a trial of conventional balloon angioplasty versus laser balloon angioplasty [48]. Their initial impression of success in treating failed angioplasty due to dissection, spasm or thrombus is borne out in other recent studies reported in abstract form. Long term outcome regarding restenosis has not been reported for this group.

Spears et al enrolled 58 patients in a multicenter trial of safety and efficacy of Coronary Laser Balloon Angioplasty [49]. Stenoses were treated with conventional balloon angioplasty using a 3.0 mm balloon dilatation catheter, followed by treatment with a 3.0 mm Laser Balloon Angioplasty catheter. Five dosing regimens, each delivering a 20 second exposure of decremental laser power, were tested. Peak exposure of 35 W × 5 seconds + 25 W × 5 seconds + 15 W × 10 seconds produced a peak in vitro temperature of 125 °C, whereas the lowest dosing regimen of 18 W × 5 seconds + 12 W × 5 seconds + 10 W × 10 seconds produced a peak in vitro temperature of only 85 °C. Technical success with Laser Balloon Angioplasty was achieved in 55 patients (95%). Three failures were due to fracture of the fiber optic within the balloon catheter.

Of 55 patients treated successfully with laser balloon angioplasty, 14 manifested unsatisfactory results following conventional balloon angioplasty. Significant dissection occurred in 8 patients (15%), including 3 who experienced acute closure of the treated vessel. Three other patients developed evidence of thrombus. All 14 of these patients underwent successful laser balloon angioplasty, with a significant increase in mean luminal diameter which persisted at angiographic follow-up at one day and one month. The mean percent diameter stenosis for 55 treated patients was 78 ± 8% before the procedure, 43 ± 18% after conventional balloon angioplasty and 26 ± 11% after laser balloon angioplasty. The mean value at one month following treatment was 23 ± 14%.

At 6 months clinical follow-up, an overall restenosis rate of 51% was found. Restenosis was defined as recurrent angina, a positive stress test, or stenosis ≥50% by coronary angiography. Restenosis rates were higher for those lesions treated by the two highest dosing regimens (67%) and in patients who had a history of restenosis prior to laser balloon angioplasty treatment (67%). Excluding these patients, the restenosis rate for other patients was only 29%, comparable to conventional balloon angioplasty.

As in the study by Spears et al, other groups have reported success in using laser balloon angioplasty as a "bail-out" technique for severe dissection or thrombus formation [49]. Reyes and associates reported on 232 patients who were enrolled in a multicenter study comparing successful PTCA + laser balloon angioplasty versus unsuccessful PTCA + laser balloon angioplasty versus PTCA alone [50]. Average minimum diameters of stenotic vessels in 102 patients at 6-month follow-up were comparable in all three groups. This led the authors to conclude that LBA is successful at improving unsuccessful PTCA acutely, with comparable results at 6 months. Mast et al reported that laser balloon angioplasty was used as a bail-out device with 100% success rate in 17 cases of conventional PTCA complicated by dissection or thrombus [51]. Safian and others, including Jenkins and Spears, reported a series of 85 patients with failed PTCA due to severe dissection or acute closure, in whom laser balloon angioplasty was used successfully in 72 patients (85%), thereby avoiding emergency CABG [49]. Despite this acute success, a re-stenosis rate of 53% was reported by Reis and associates in a series of 20 patients undergoing laser balloon angioplasty either electively (11 patients) or for acute closure after PTCA (9 patients). Pathology specimens obtained from atherectomy in 6 of these patients revealed intimal proliferation similar to that seen with restenosis following conventional balloon angioplasty [52].

The Outcome of Laser Angioplasty

Despite the anticipated benefits of less restenosis following laser angioplasty, clinical trials, particularly in the coronary circulation, have shown that re-stenosis rates are not altered when compared to PTCA. At present, it appears that feasibility of laser recanalization has shown that it can be performed safely and effectively. Long-term outcomes, however, have been adversely affected by several factors which are directly related to technique and equip-ment: 1. Patients selected are those who have failed other treatments. 2. Techniques have varied greatly making subset analysis difficult, thereby ob-scuring potential areas of benefit. 3. Mechanical and developmental problems with equipment, including optimal catheter size and flexibility result in small channels requiring balloon angioplasty. 4. Not a well defined dosimetry for both laser optical and thermal systems. 5. Lack of monitoring systems to define endpoints.

There seem to be several predictors of improved long-term outcome, reported in various studies: 1) less post-procedural residual stenosis and 2) higher energy fluence with pulsed lasers and lower thermal effects with continuous wave systems. This suggests that a therapeutic window for energy delivery seems to be present as evidenced from basic studies.

Summary

Laser recanalization appears to have some potential advantages as evidenced by the basic data in atherosclerotic models. These data suggest that there appears to be a therapeutic window for temperature effects between 75 to 100 °C. In that range there appears to be reduction in platelet deposition with the laser when compared to balloon angioplasty. This appears to be related to the coagulation of vascular collagen. At the present time, however, the clinical studies have not demonstrated any potential beneficial effects on restenosis. Unfortunately, most studies using thermal devices were conducted without any thermal monitoring. Pulsed laser systems are being used without an optimized dosimetry matrix to minimize shock wave trauma and shearing effects on the tissues. It appears that higher energy densities with pulsed lasers result in a reduction of restenosis. If this is the case, it would suggest that more efficient tissue ablation could be occuring with association of increased thermal injury. It is clear that continuous wave lasers and pulsed laser systems need to be optimized in order to influence the restenosis rate. At present clinical studies monitoring the thermal effects and shock waves with long-term follow-up are necessary to define the ideal laser parameters.

Acknowledgements

This study was supported in part by grants-in-aid from the American Heart Association, Central Florida Affiliate, Florida High Technology and Industry Council, Talahassee, Florida and the National Institutes of Health (R01-HL30320), Bethesda, Maryland. Dr. Abela is the recipient of the Research Career Development Award (K04HL01817).

References

1. Abela G S, Crea F, Seeger J M, Franzini D et al (1985) The healing process in normal canine arteries and in atherosclerotic monkey arteries after transluminal laser irradiation. *Am J Cardiol* 56:983–988.
2. Macruz R, Martins J R M, Tupinamba A, Lopes E A et al (1980) Therapeutic possibilities of laser beams in atheromas. *Arg Bras Cardiol* (Port >) 34:9–12.
3. Lee G, Ikeda R M, Kozina J, Mason D T (1981) Laser dissolution of coronary atherosclerotic obstruction. *Am Heart J* 102:1074–1075.
4. Abela G S, Normann S, Cohen D, Feldman R L et al (1982) Effects of carbon dioxide, Nd-Yag and argon laser radiation on coronary atheromatous plaques. *Am J Cardiol* 50:1199–1205.

5. Choy D S J, Stertzer Z, Rotterdam H L, Sharrock N et al (1982) Transluminal laser catheter angioplasty. *Am J Cardiol* 50:1206–1208.
6. White C J, Ramee S R, Aita M, Samson G et al (1990) Results of laser-assisted balloon angioplasty for peripheral arterial obstruction using a lensed fiber-tip delivery catheter. *Am J Cardiol* 66: 1526–1529.
7. Abela G S, Normann S, Cohen D M, Franzini D et al (1985) Laser recanalization of occluded atherosclerotic arteries: an in vivo and in vitro study. *Circulation* 71:403–411.
8. Ginsburg R, Kirr D S, Guthaner P, Tolh J et al (1984) Salvage of an ischemic limb by laser angioplasty: description of a new technique. *Clin Cardiol* 7:54–58.
9. Geschwind H, Boussignac G, Teisseire B, Vieilledent C et al (1984) Percutaneous transluminal laser angioplasty in man (letter to editor). *Lancet* II:844.
10. Anderson H V, Zaatari G S, Roubin G S, Feimgruber P P et al (1986) Steerable fiber optic catheter delivery of laser energy in atherosclerotic rabbits. *Am Heart J* 111:1065.
11. Gerrity R G, Loop F D, Golding L A R, Ehrhart A et al (1983) Arterial response to laser operation for removal of atherosclerotic plaques. *Thorac Cardiovasc Surg* 85:409–421.
12. Higginson L A, Farell E M, Walley V M, Taylor R S et al (1989) Arterial responses to excimer and argon laser irradiation in the atherosclerotic swines. *Lasers Med Sci* 4:85–92.
13. Holmes D R, Vlietstra R E, Smith H C et al (1984) Restenosis after percutaneous transluminal coronary angioplasty: initial experience (abstr). *Am J Cardiol* 53:77C–81C.
14. Chesebro J H, Lam J Y T, Fuster V (1986) The pathogenesis and prevention of aortocoronary vein bypass graft occlusion and restenosis after arterial angioplasty: role of vascular injury and platelet thrombus deposition. *J Am Coll Cardiol* 8:57B–66B.
15. Liu M W, Roubin G S, King S B III (1989) Restenosis after coronary angioplasty. Potential biologic determinants and role of intimal hyperplasia. *Circulation* 79:1374–1387.
16. Deckelbaum L I, Isner J M, Donaldson R F et al (1985) Reduction of laser-induced pathologic tissue injury using pulsed energy delivery. *Am J Cardiol* 56:662–667.
17. Fenech A, Abela G S, Crea F, Smith W et al (1985) A comparative study of laser beam characteristics in blood and saline media. *Am J Cardiol* 55:1389–1392.
18. Litvack F, Eigler N L, Margolis J R et al (1990) Percutaneous excimer laser coronary angioplasty. *Am J Cardiol* 66:1027–1032.
19. Sanborn T A, Torre S R, Sharma S K et al (1991) Percutaneous coronary excimer laser-assisted balloon angioplasty: initial clinical and quantitative angiographic results in 50 patients. *J Amer Coll Cardiol* 17:94–99.
20. Abela G S, Crea F, Smith W, Pepine C J et al (1985) In vitro effects of argon laser radiation on blood: quantitative and morphologic analysis. *J Am Coll Cardiol* 5:231–237.
21. Isner J M, Clarke R H, Donaldson R F, Aharon (1985) Identification of photoproducts liberated by in vitro irradiation of atherosclerotic plaque, calcified cardiac valves and myocardium. *Am J Cardiol* 55:1192–1196.
22. Abela G S, Franzini D, Crea F, Pepine C J, Conti C R (1984) No evidence for accelerated atherosclerosis following laser irradiation. *Circulation* 70:II–323.
23. Abela G S, Barbieri E, Friedl S E, Normann S J (1990) Direct laser and laser-thermal irradiation of normal canine coronary arteries: implications for laser delivery methods. *J Clin Laser Med Surg* 8:63–71.
24. Abela G S (1990) Immediate and chronic effects of laser angioplasty. Chapter 9 in: Abela G S (ed) *Lasers in Cardiovascular Medicine and Surgery: Fundamentals and Techniques*, Kluwer, 113–141.
25. Barbieri E, Abela G S, Khoury A, Conti C R (1987) Temperature characteristics of laser thermal probes in the coronary circulation of dogs (abstr). *Circulation* 76:409.
26. Abela G S, Tomaru T, Mansour M, Barbeau G R et al (1990) Reduced platelet deposition with laser compared to balloon angioplasty (abstr). *J Am Coll Cardiol* 15:245A.
27. Abela G S, Barbeau G, Tomaru T, Franzini D et al (1990) Thermal coagulation of vascular collagen reduces platelet adhesion following balloon angioplasty (abstr). *J Am Coll Cardiol* 15:205A.
28. Barbeau G R, Friedl S E, Saxton J M, Federman M, Abela G S (1991) Rupture of internal elastic lamina is essential for restenosis following balloon angioplasty (abstr). *Circulation* II–603.

Table 1. Properties of artificial sapphire.

Density at 25 °C	3.98	gcm-3
Moh hardness	9	
Melting point	2040	°C
Compressive strength	2.1×10^{10}	Pa

peripheral thermal damage [13]. Dispersion of the laser beam due to a different probe design can increase the volume of ablated tissue. If the transparent probe is used in combination with a Nd:YAG laser, surface coating has shown to be advantageous in order to reduce scattering of the laser photons after carbonization of the tissue surface [10]. The coating reduces the transmittance of laser light through the transparent probe so that it is between 70% and 85% [12, 14]. Thus the transparent sapphire or silica probe causes predominantly a direct laser-tissue interaction and it cannot be compared with the "hot-tip" metal probe, which completely absorbs the laser energy and causes only an indirect laser tissue interaction, or the hybrid probe (Spectraprobe, Trimedyne Inc.), which allows only 20% transmission of total laser light. Heating of the sapphire probe occurs only at the front surface, which is in contact with the plaque tissue. In air the temperature rise at the front surface was between 65 °C to 74 °C after 10 Watts for 1 second; at the lateral side it was about 10 °C after 10 Watts for 3 seconds [14].

The contact probe is attached to the end of a glass fiber 300–600 micron in diameter. This was done initially by a screw-on universal connector. Now contact probe laser angioplasty catheters have the sapphire or silica lens build into the end of the plastic catheter. To enable an over the wire technique an eccentric channel is drilled into the contact probe (Fig. 2).

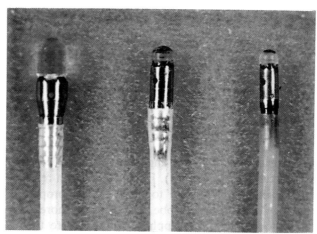

Figure 1. Transparent contact probes 1.8 mm, 2.2 mm and 3.0 mm in diameter for laser angioplasty.

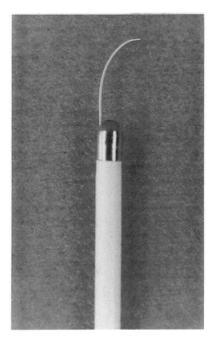

Figure 2. Laser angioplasty catheter with excentric guide wire channel.

Sapphire Probe – Tissue Reaction

Ablation of plaque tissue starts to occur at 5 Joules. A linear relationship between the laser energy and the volume of vaporized tissue can be observed. After 15 W was applied for 2 seconds, the tissue crater had a mean diameter of 2.3 mm ± 0.45 and a mean depth of 1.1 mm ± 3.35 [7, 15]. The tissue defect was surrounded by a zone of thermal necrosis with superficial carbonization followed by dehydration, cell rupture and vacuolization, plasma coagulation and perifocal edema (Fig. 3). This zone of thermal necrosis had a depth of 0.05–0.2 mm. Under scanning electron microscopy the outer crater showed a relatively smooth surface, probably due to tissue welding at lower temperatures. The tissue surface in the focal spot of the sapphire probe was highly irregular as a result of explosive tissue vaporization at very high temperatures [7].

Technique of Laser Recanalization

For laser assisted recanalization of iliac or femoropopliteal artery occlusions a neodymium-yttrium-aluminium garnet (Nd:YAG) laser (Surgical Laser Technologies, Malvern, PA) with a wavelength of 1064 nm was used with a sapphire or silica contact probe catheter 2.2 mm (7F) or 3.0 mm (9F) in

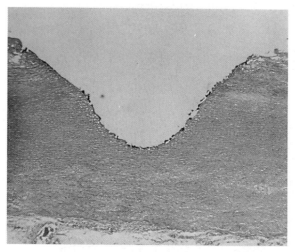

Figure 3. Histologic specimen of aortic wall. Crater after ablation with Nd:YAG laser and sapphire probe demonstrating the large volume of ablated tissue and the relative small zone of surrounding thermal necrosis.

diameter. The power setting for intravascular recanalization was 10–15 Watts in pulses of 1–second duration [15].

The recanalization procedures were done percutaneously under local anesthesia. The common femoral artery was punctured antegradely for femoropopliteal recanalizations and retrogradely for iliac recanalizations. After insertion of a 7F or 9F catheter introducer sheath the patient was anticoagulated with 5000IU of heparin intraarterially. After an unsuccessful attempt of guide-wire recanalization, the laser catheter was inserted and advanced up against the occlusion. Under minimal forward pressure of the catheter, the laser was activated. The catheter could be advanced approximately 10 mm after 20 shots of 10–15 W/second. After successful recanalization, residual stenoses within the recanalized segment were dilated by means of an angioplasty balloon. The final result was documented angiographically (Figs 4 and 5).

Adjuvant Medical Therapy/Follow-up Studies

After successful recanalization, intravenous infusion of heparin (1000/h) was continued for 1 or 2 days. Most patients subsequently underwent long-term platelet inhibition therapy (330 mg of acetyl salicylic acid and 75 mg of dipyridamole). One hundred twenty-nine patients at one hospital were included in a randomized study of platelet inhibition (n = 63) versus anticoagulation (n = 66). After 3 years of follow-up this study revealed no significant

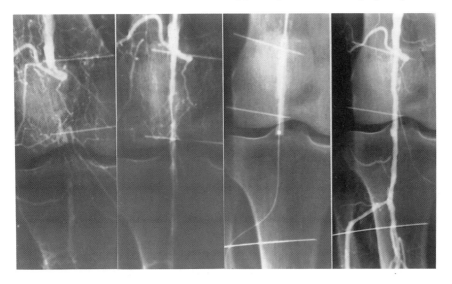

Figure 4. Laser angioplasty of popliteal artery occlusion 4 cm in length. a. Angiogram before the recanalization procedure. b. After recanalization with 2.2 mm sapphire probe. c. Balloon dilatation of the residual stenosis proximal to the joint space. d. Final angiogram of the recanalized artery.

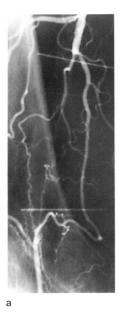 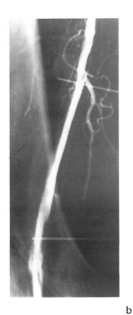

a   b

Figure 5. Laser angioplasty of a superficial femoral artery occlusion, 10 cm in length. a. Angiogram demonstrating the occlusion in the adductor channel. b. Final angiogram after laser recanalization and PTA.

Table 2. Results of Nd:YAG sapphire probe laser angioplasty of peripheral arteries.

Group	n	IRR	CR	PR 6mo	PR 12mo	PR 36mo
Lammer	341	85%	14%	80%	70%	57%
Fourrier	127	80%	74%			
Henry	104	85%	10%	77%	65%	
Horvath	122	91%	8%	72%	68%	64%
Loerelius	36	61%	59%			
Pilger	167	79%	13%	75%	67%	63%
Rees	44	76%	78%			
Rienks	123	76%	15%	87%	69%	
European-Clinical Trials total	1064	83%	12%	77%	68%	60%
US-Clinical Trial	97	72%	25%	82%	62%	

n = number of procedures, IRR = initial recanalization rate, CR = complication rate, PR = patency rate (life table analysis).

months are predominantly based on a combination of clinical examinations, Doppler measurements, and digital angiography. At 2 and 3 years only clinical examinations and Doppler ultrasound examinations were performed. At 6 months the patency rate of the successfully recanalized arteries was 59–87% (average 77%).The patency rate dropped to 65–70% (average 68%) at 1 year and 57–63% (average 60%) at 3 years. The cure rate (initial recanalization rate × patency rate) was 64%,56% and 50% at 6,12 and 36 months, respectively (Table 3). Patients with a reduced run-off had a significantly lower patency rate than patients with a normal run-off [16, 20]. In those patients with normal crural arteries, the 3 year patency rate was up to 73% [16]. The reocclusion rate after a mean observation period of 14 months was only 23% in nonsmoking and nondiabetic patients versus 44–57% in diabetic patients.

In comparison to these results the U.S.-IDE Study (#G880170) revealed an initial technical success in 70 of 97 peripheral laser assisted balloon angioplasty procedures (72%). Complications such as perforations, dissections, emboli or hematomas were observed in 25%. The cumulative patency rate of successfully angioplastied limbs was 82% at six months and 62% at one year (Medtronic Inc., personal communication), (Table 2).

Discussion

The aim of laser angioplasty was to reduce the restenosis rate.It was argued that laser ablation instead of balloon disruption of plaque tissue will leave a wider lumen and a smoother surface within the recanalized artery. This should result in a reduction of surface thrombogenicity and subsequent reduction of intima hyperplasia. However,this hypothesis has not yet been proven. Experimental work has widely concentrated on the mechanisms of plaque ablation, but has spared almost completely the influence of laser ablation on

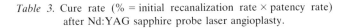

Table 3. Cure rate (% = initial recanalization rate × patency rate) after Nd:YAG sapphire probe laser angioplasty.

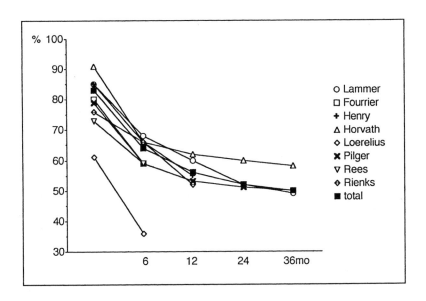

surface thrombogenicity and intimal growth rate [22, 23]. Clinical studies of laser angioplasty in coronary [24–26] or peripheral arteries [16–21] have analyzed most commonly the results of laser assisted balloon angioplasty, which is a combination of laser plaque ablation followed by additional mechanical balloon dilatation of residual stenoses. Even the so called "stand alone" procedure in the coronary arteries are associated with extensive additional mechanical trauma, such as longitudinal shear stress, due to the circumferential deadspace of multifiber laser catheters. Thus, those studies which demonstrated a 42% 6 months recurrency rate (reocclusion/restenosis) after coronary laser angioplasty (63% in stand alone procedures) and a 30% one year recurrency rate after peripheral laser angioplasty could neither prove nor disprove any advantage of laser ablation on the restenosis rate. However, these studies could demonstrate the feasibility and safety of clinical laser angioplasty and that the results were comparable with conventional angioplasty [27–31]. Due to these results further clinical work in controlled clinical trials seems to be justified. Nevertheless, experimental and clinical work has to concentrate on systems which do not need additional mechanical widening of the artery, and the influence of those systems on surface thrombogenicity, smooth muscle cell growth rate and subsequent restenosis rate.

In clinical practice laser angioplasty has turned out to be an effective

424   *J. Lammer et al*

procedure for recanalization of totally occluded peripheral arteries. Seven years ago the initial recanalization rate in total occlusions of femoropopliteal arteries using a conventional catheter/guide wire technique was reported as low as 30% [29]. This rate has improved during the last years due to the developement of high quality, surface coated, steerable guide wires [30]. However, laser plaque ablation enables recanalization even of arteries which cannot be recanalized by steerable guide wires.

The sapphire contact probe catheter system in combination with a continuous wave or long pulsed 1064 nm Nd:YAG laser has shown to be of particular advantage. The lens focuses the light to the center of the artery which reduces the thermal damage of the outer layers of the arterial wall. The continuous wave or long pulsed Nd:YAG laser effectively ablates plaque tissue with a feed-rate of about 0.5mm/second. Calcium cannot be ablated by this laser, but it has turned out that dense plaque calcifications are only present in about 10% of the cases. In comparison to the "hot-tip" laser angioplasty system, the transparent contact probe causes more tissue ablation due to the direct laser tissue interaction [7, 15]. Thus the pulse duration can be shortened which reduces heat accumulation in the arterial wall. A further fact which minimizes thermal damage to the arterial wall is that the sapphire or silica lens focuses the light whereas the "hot-tip" has a circumferential heat distribution,which sometimes caused transmural thermal necrosis of the artery. In comparison to a multifiber catheter in combination with a 308 nm excimer laser, the sapphire contact probe has no deadspace and ablation of plaque tissue is faster.

In *conclusion* laser assisted balloon angioplasty with an 1064 nm Nd:YAG laser and a sapphire/silica contact probe has demonstrated in n = 1064 cases, reported by European groups, to be an efficacious and safe procedure. The initial recanalization rate in total femoropopliteal and iliac artery occlusions was 83%. Complications such as perforations or emboli occurred in 12%. The patency rate of the successfully recanalized arteries was 77% after 6 months, 68% after 1 year and 60% after 3 years. However, it has not been demonstated for which indications laser assisted balloon angioplasty is superior to conventional balloon angioplasty. The transparent contact probe currently can not replace balloon angioplasty, although it has the potential because of its optical properties. The need for the future is to develop a probe which is able to completely clear the artery and then to prove the influence of laser angioplasty on the restenosis rate.

References

1. Lee G, Ikeda R M, Kozina J, Mason D T (1981) Laser dissolution of coronary atherosclerotic obstruction. *Am Heart J* 102:1074–1075.
2. Choy D S J, Sterzer S H, Rotterdam H Z et al (1982) Transluminal laser catheter angioplasty. *Am J Cardiol* 50:1206–1207.
3. Geschwind H, Boussignac G, Teisseire B et al (1984) Percutaneous transluminal laser angioplasty in man (letter). *Lancet* 1:844.

4. Lammer J, Ascher P W, Choy D S J (1986) Transfemorale Laser – Katheter-Thrombendarterektomie (TEA) der Arteria Carotis. *Dtsch Med Wochenschr* 11:607–610.
5. Abela G S, Norman S, Cohen D et al (1982) Effects of carbon dioxide, d:YAG, and argon laser radiation on coronary atheromarous plaques. *Am J Cardiol* 50:1199–1205.
6. Murphy-Chutorian D, Selzer P M, Kosek J et al (1986) The interaction between excimer laser energy and vascular tissue. *Am Heart J* 112:739–745.
7. Lammer J, Kleinert R, Pilger E et al (1989) Contact probes for intravascular recanalization: experimental evaluation. *Invest Radiol* 24:190–195.
8. Lee G, Ikeda R M, Chan M L (1984) Dissolution of human atherosclerotic disease by fiberoptic laser-heated metal cautery cap. *Am Heart J* 107:777–778.
9. Sanborn T A, Haudenschild C C, Faxon D P, Ryan T J (1985) Experimental angioplasty: circumferential distribution of laser thermal energy with a laser probe. *J Am Coll Cardiol* 5:934–938.
10. Daikuzono N, Joffe S N (1985) An artificial sapphire probe for contact photocoagulation and tissue vaporization. *Med Instrum* 19:173–178.
11. Lammer J, Pilger E, Kleinert R, Ascher P W (1987) Laserangioplastie peripherer arterieller Verschlüsse: experimentelle und klinische Ergebnisse. *Fortschr Roentgenstr* 147:1–5.
12. Verdaasdonk R M, Cross F W, Borst C (1987) Physical properties of sapphire fibre tips for laser angioplasty. *Lasers Med Sci* 2:183–188.
13. Bowker T J, Cross F W, Bown S G, Rickards A F (1987) Reduction of vessel wall perforation by the use of sapphire tipped optical fibres in laser angioplasty. *Br Heart J* 57:88.
14. Ashley S, Brooks S G, Gehani A A et al (1990) Thermal and optical behaviour of sapphire fibertips for laser angioplasty. *Proceedings SPIE Optical Engineering* 1201.
15. Lammer J, Karnel F (1988) Percutaneous transluminal laser angioplasty (PTLA) with contact probes. *Radiology* 168:733–737.
16. Pilger E, Lammer J, Bertuch H et al (1991) Nd:YAG laser with sapphire tip combined with balloon angioplasty in peripheral arterial occlusions. Long-term results. *Circulation* 83:141–147.
17. Fourrier J L, Marache P, Brunetaud J M et al (1987) Human percutaneous laser angioplasty with sapphire tips: results and follow up (abstr). *Circulation* 76 (suppl 4):919.
18. Horvath W, Haidinger D, Luft Ch (1989) Laserangioplastie von Extremitätenarterien – Indikationen, Ergebnisse und ergänzende interventionelle Maßnahmen. *Laser Med Surg* 5:4–8.
19. Rienks R, Berengoltz S N, Kho S N et al (1990) Laser angioplasty for peripheral arterial occlusions: results of a Dutch multicenter register. In: *Proceedings of ELA* 90. Graz, p. 14.
20. Lammer J, Pilger E, Karnel F et al (1991) Laser angioplasty: results of a prospective, multicenter study at 3-year follow-up. *Radiology* 178:335–337.
21. Rees M R, Ashley S, Gehani A A et al (1990) Comparison of the Kensey catheter and contact laser in the treatment of chronic femoropopliteal artery occlusions. *Radiology* 177P:102.
22. Abela G S, Crea S, Seeger J M et al (1985) The healing process in normal canine arteries and in atherosclerotic monkey arteries after transluminal laser irradiation. *Am J Cardiol* 56:983–988.
23. Prevosti L G, Lawrence J B, Leon M B et al (1987) Surface thrombogenicity after excimer laser and hot-tip thermal ablation of plaque: morphometric studies using an anular perfusion chamber. *Surg Forum* 38:330–333.
24. Sanborn T A, Bittl J A, Hershman R A et al (1990) Coronary excimer laser angioplasty: results in 223 patients from a multicenter registry. *Circulation* 82(suppl 3): p 670.
25. Rothbaum D A, Linnemeier T J, Landin R J et al (1991) Excimer laser coronary angioplasty: current status of investigation. In: *Proceedings of International Congress* 4: *Endovascular Therapies in Vascular Disease*. Phoenix: Arizona Heart Institute, I–2.
26. Grundfest W S, Litvak F, Eigler N et al (1991) Results of a multicenter trial of excimer laser coronary angioplasty. In: *Proceedings of International Congress* 4: *Endovascular Therapies in Vascular Disease*. Phoenix: Arizona Heart Institute, I–6.

27. Hewes R C, White R, Murray R R et al (1986) Long-term results of superficial femoral artery angioplasty. *AJR* 146:1025–1029.
28. Johnston K W, Rae M, Hogg-Johnston S A et al (1987) 5 years results of a prospective study of percutaneous transluminal angioplasty. *Ann Surg* 206:403–409.
29. Krepel V M, van Andel G J, van Erp W F M et al (1985) Percutaneous transluminal angioplasty of the femoropopliteal artery: initial and long-term results. *Radiology* 156:325–328.
30. Morgenstern B R, Getrajdman G I, Laffey K I et al (1989) Total occlusions of the femoropopliteal artery: high technical success rate of conventional balloon angioplasty. *Radiology* 172:937–940.
31. Rooke T W, Stanson A W, Johnson C M et al (1987) Percutaneous transluminal angioplasty in the lower extremities: a 5-year experience. *Mayo Clin Proc* 62:85–91.

21. Excimer Laser Assisted Angioplasty of Peripheral Vessels

G. BIAMINO, P. SKARABIS, H. BÖTTCHER,
G. KAMPMANN, J. C. RAGG, U. FLESCH and H. WITT

Introduction

Although large scale public education efforts showing the relationship between various "risk factors" and the development of arteriosclerosis may have contributed to the recent reduction in arteriosclerotic disease, it still remains the leading cause of death in industrial civilizations. It should be obvious that the main goal of treatment remains prevention; however realistic long-term therapy must be focused on the use of interventional techniques supported by pharmacological approaches.

Despite the success of arterial bypass surgery to relieve myocardial or peripheral ischemia, less invasive percutaneous techniques are appealing to relieve ischemic pain and to improve the quality of life of innumerable patients with coronary and peripheral arterial disorders. The expansion of the simple Dotter [1] concept by transcutaneous balloon angioplasty [2, 3] has dramatically changed the conception of the management of obstructive arterial disease. Technological improvements of this method during the last few years has resulted in primary success rates of 95% in attempts to recanalize stenotic peripheral or coronary arteries.

One main limitation of arterial balloon angioplasty remains, however, the inability to cross occluded vessels in more than 50% of the cases. This relevant disadvantage of the technique is magnified by the "heel of Achilles" of balloon angioplasty: the high degree of restenosis or reocclusion of about 40% [4–15] in coronary and approximately 50% in peripheral arteries [16–26].

Considering the fact that world-wide approximately 700,000 transcutaneous interventions will be performed in 1992 [27] and taking into account the approximate mean cost of each intervention, a reduction in the restenosis rate of only 15% would reduce public health expenses by at least 40 million US$ per year. At the present time due to the limitations of balloon angioplasty, more than 30 different companies are investing significant sums of money

P.W. Serruys, B.H. Strauss and S.B. King III (eds), Restenosis after Intervention with New Mechanical Devices, 427–473.

in the development of new techniques designed to remove or remodel the obstructive vessel material.

A critical analysis of the rational use of all these new crackers, breakers, stretchers, drillers, scrapers, shavers, burners, welders and melters in the treatment of obstructive atherosclerotic disease was recently considered [28]. In the early 1980s the innovative idea that laser energy might be also used to vaporize sclerotic material [29–31] convinced several groups to introduce laser angioplasty as a clinical modality very quickly [32–43]. Overly enthusiastic, maybe success-dictated reports presaged the science fiction fantasy that by aiming a laser beam through an optical fiber at the obstructive material, blood flow might be restored without spasm, embolism, dissection or perforation. The clinical debacle of the first systems using continuous wave laser irradiation was the consequence of an uncritical use of such a powerful, inadequate energy source for debulking sclerotic vessel material. Furthermore, the partial use of the acronym laser without regard to the specific tissue related properties of different laser sources led to many simplifications and misunderstandings and may explain the actual scepticism or even hostility towards laser angioplasty by a large number of interventionalists.

The main goal of our cardiovascular laser angioplasty program since November 1985 has been the development of a technology for percutaneous application of laser energy, which would remove plaque rather than mechanically reshape the obstructive material. In January 25, 1989 we successfully attempted to recanalize the occluded superficial femoral artery of a 58 year old lady with a 7 french multifiber catheter. Since then, we performed laser assisted angioplasty of peripheral vessels in more than 400 cases. In this article we will report our experiences in transcutaneous angioplasty of 306 patients with a follow-up longer than six months.

Technical Aspects

During the last few years, it has been demonstrated that the majority of laser wavelengths of the electromagnetic spectrum can debulk vessel material [41–48]. Two main parameters must be considered for laser – tissue interaction effects: the interaction time (between laser beam and tissue) and the tissue specific absorption or effective energy density [49]. Electrical fields large enough to blast chemical bonds can only be produced at very high energy densities with an extremely short interaction time. This effect, called optical breakdown or photoablation, can be obtained with the pulsed excimer laser with high energy densities [50–53].

At lower energy densities and a longer interaction time, tissue ablation is a consequence of local tissue heating with resulting desiccation and then vaporization [54]. Examples of these thermal laser effects are the continuous wave Nd:YAG or Argon laser systems. Although the laser light of the continuous wave laser sources has been transmitted via bare fibers or with metal tips [55–56], quartz windows [57] or sapphire probes [58–61] at the distal end of the optical fiber, heat can be regarded as the main cause of tissue vaporisation for all systems. Particularly when the recanalization speed is slower than 1.5 mm/sec, considerable transvasal temperature rise is observed [54] and thermal damage of adjacent tissue structures can hardly be avoided. The different transmitting systems of a continuous wave laser beam may be used with a relatively low risk of damage in non-calcified lesions when the probes are able to cross the obstruction very fast [32, 69]. Because heavily calcified material is refractory to the ablation mechanism of thermal systems [70], a recanalization stop due to a calcified obstacle will cause an unacceptably high risk of vessel wall perforation [51]. Furthermore, the increase of the vessel surrounding temperature to 60–80 °C may be deleterious with regard to the long term results of those interventions.

In contrast to the vaporisation caused by the continuous wave lasers the excimer laser is a pulsed system which induces tissue ablation during a so-called athermic process [44, 51]. This photoablation phenomenon was first described by Srinivasan in 1982 [71–73] and is only related to energy densities below 1 J/cm^2 at a wave-length of 193 nm. However, the medical systems introduced for angioplasty use a xenon chloride 308 nm excimer laser as the source of energy. At this wave-length the ablation of the irradiated tissue is no longer a consequence of a photochemical disruption of molecular chains. It is predominantly a local, very fast micro explosion provoked by an extremely high temperature rise of the irradiated volume with energy densities of about 3 to 6 J/cm^2 [74]. As a result of the excimer laser beam's small penetration depth and the extremely short pulse duration in comparison to the pulse repetition rate used, the thermal damage induced by the excimer laser is minimal even when high energy densities (7.5 J/cm^2) are used [48].

Due to contact between optical fiber and tissue during irradiation, high pressure which has developed from the ablation process can not escape. This results in high amplitude shock waves, and may partially explain the high incidence of dissections and spasms observed during coronary excimer laser angioplasties [75]. On the other hand, shock wave related complications seem to be irrelevant for peripheral revascularization interventions.

Recent studies have clearly demonstrated that the amplitude of the shock-wave becomes dramatically higher when the pulse duration is shortened [76]. A further determinant of the shock-wave's intensity seems to be the configuration of the laser pulse, indicating that a split beam profile might reduce mechanical irritations. Finally an additional factor could be the geometry of the tip of the multifiber laser catheter. For catheters with a flat tip, the amplitude of the shock waves may be higher because the volume and consequently also the pressure can not evade along the catheter during the ablation process [76]. Possible interactions between all these factors are not yet understood and may underscore the complexities in the evaluation and validation of the technique, equipment and the results obtained at the current state of the technology.

Methods and Clinical Material

Study Inclusion Criteria

Patients were included in the study if they had peripheral vascular disease for more than 6 months and were clinically symptomatic (gangrene, rest pain or claudication at a walking distance of 200 m or less). Patients who experienced claudication at a walking distance between 200–500 m were also included in the study if their quality of life was seriously affected because of their inability to walk longer distances.

All patients had single or multiple subtotal or total occlusions located in the iliac arteries or in the superficial femoral or popliteal artery with an infrapopliteal runoff of at least one vessel.

There must have been the possibility to enter the ipsilateral common femoral artery especially in case of a SFA or a popliteal lesion or the possibility to reach the lesion over the ipsilateral or contralateral side in case of an iliac or common femoral obstruction.

Follow-up

All patients underwent color Doppler flow imaging to analyze the region of interest before and 24 hours following intervention. There was a clinical follow-up including questionnaires, physical examination, treadmill exercise test, brachial-ankle index and color flow Doppler 3, 6, 12 and 24 months after the intervention. Digital subtraction angiography was performed 6 months after the intervention in all patients who wanted to have an angiographic control or earlier if patients experienced a deterioration in their clinical situation.

Patient Population

Since January 1989 we attempted recanalization with excimer laser assisted angioplasty in 306 peripheral vessels. Approximately 20% of the patients had a second laser angioplasty on the contralateral side and were included in the study twice. The age of the 250 male and 56 female patients ranged from 40 to 83 years (mean, 65). The mean ankle-brachial index before the intervention was 0.58. 20 patients (6.5%) had rest pain or gangrene, 34 patients (11%) experienced claudication at a walking distance of less than 50 m, 217 patients (71%) experienced claudication at a walking distance between 50 and 200 m, and 35 patients (11%) could walk more than 200 m.

73 patients (24%) had diabetes mellitus, 49 patients (15%) had systemic hypertension, 99 patients (32%) had additional coronary heart disease or a high-grade stenosis of the carotid arteries, and 29 patients (9.5%) had hypercholesterolemia (>250 mg / dl) at the time of intervention. Most patients had been smokers formerly, but only 31 patients (10%) admitted to heavy smoking at the time of the intervention.

35 patients (11%) had been previously treated by one, and 3 patients by two previous balloon dilatations at the site of angioplasty.

Angiographic Findings

All patients underwent diagnostic angiography before and immediately after the procedure. The severity of the lesions was visually estimated by two experienced investigators and a mean value was determined.

244 lesions were located in the superficial femoral artery, 33 in the iliac arteries and 29 lesions were in the popliteal region. Length of the lesion varied from 1 to 35 cm: 51 lesions (16.5%) were shorter than 3 cm, there were 97 lesions (31.5%) between 3–7 cm and 85 lesions (28%) between 7–12 cm; 73 lesions (24%) were longer than 12 cm (51 of them longer than 20 cm).

Laser and Laser Catheters

A 308 nm pulsed ultraviolet xenon chloride excimer laser (MAX 10, Technolas, Germany) was used as an energy source with a repetition rate of 20 Hz. Pulse duration was 60–110 ns. A 7 french multifiber catheter (containing 12 fibers with a core diameter of 260 μm, arranged around a central channel) was used in 109 cases to attempt recanalization, a 9 french multifiber catheter (containing 18 fibers in similar construction) was used in 175 cases. In 22 lesions, both catheter types were applied during the procedure. In a few cases, a 5 french catheter (42 fibers with a core diameter of 100 μm) was used in the popliteal region.

The central channel of the 9 french catheter allowed the introduction of a guide wire with a maximum size of .035 inch. Guide wires with a maximum size of .020 inch and .014 inch could be introduced into the central channel of a 7 french and 5 french catheter respectively.

Laser Angioplasty Treatment Protocol

After the non-invasive arterial evaluation, patients were taken to the laboratory in a fasting state. Patients were not pretreated with acetylsalicylic acid and were not sedated. Via antegrade puncture of the ipsilateral common femoral artery, a hemostatic introducer sheath (8 or 9 french) was introduced into the superficial femoral artery. Baseline angiography was obtained through the sheath so that the treatment site and the distal vasculature could be characterized.

When the procedure was performed in the pelvic region, the sheath was placed into the common femoral artery/external iliac artery using the standard coronary angiography technique.

Intraarterial heparin (5000 units) was administered before the laser catheter was introduced. A guide wire facilitated the navigation of the laser catheter through the non-affected proximal part of the femoral artery.

In the case of subtotal stenoses in the femoropopliteal region, the guide wire was first passed through the lesion under fluoroscopic control before the laser catheter was advanced while firing.

In the case of total occlusions, penetration of the blocking obstacle was not attempted. In fact angioscopic controls have demonstrated that when lesions were vigorously probed with guide wires, subintimal laceration or false lumina may occur and then preclude a successful laser recanalization.

Immediately prior to the laser procedure, angiography with a digital road-mapping technique was performed which permitted a better fluoroscopic control of the coaxial guidance of the laser catheter's gold marked tip. Because the 308 nm excimer laser generated only insignificant heat [77] and blood is opaque to laser light of this wavelength, the laser energy fired from fibers concentrically positioned around the central guide wire lumen will ablate only the tissue that is in direct contact with the tip of the catheter.

Taking into account the minimal penetration depth per pulse, the catheter has to be advanced very slowly to avoid mechanical or dottering effects.

After each firing period of 15–20 s we gently tried to penetrate the residual obstruction with the guide wire, controlling the coaxial position within the vessel.

Particularly in the case of long occlusions, we learned that the last few millimeters are crucial for success or failure. Avoiding subintimal dissections or other mechanical injuries of the distal patent segment of the vessel, we tried to penetrate the most distal portion of the occlusion with the guide wire. When the angiographic control through the proximal sheath clearly showed an intraluminal position of the guide wire, the laser catheter would be advanced to the conjunction. After 3 to 5 passes with firing while advancing and withdrawing the laser catheter, a control digital subtraction angiography was performed.

If the residual stenosis exceeded 50% of the lumen, the guide wire was held in position and the laser catheter was removed. An appropriate balloon dilatation catheter (4–6 mm balloon diameter) was then advanced across the lesion. This was followed by repeated overlapping balloon dilatations from distal to proximal with pressure monitoring (4–10 atm, 30s–3 min). It is our impression that by using balloons not exceeding 4 cm in length, the number of complicating dissections is significantly reduced.

At the termination of the procedure, digital subtraction angiography was performed to document the results, before the sheath was removed. Patients with successful laser assisted balloon angioplasty were treated with low dose or continuous systemic heparin for 24–36 hours after the intervention and long term acetylsalicylic acid (100–300 mg/day) in the absence of contraindications.

Prior to discharge 1–2 days after the intervention, a non-invasive evaluation of the peripheral arteries including ankle-brachial index, color-coded Doppler ultrasound and tread-mill test was performed.

Definition of Primary Success Rate

Since percutaneous angioplasty was introduced, the immediate success of the procedure has been based on the residual stenosis as estimated by angiography. It remains unknown, however, which role the so called "spoof factor" may play for such an evaluation, lulling the angioplasty operator into complacency [78]. The spoof factor should be of particular interest in evaluating the results of peripheral interventions. Estimating the degree of the obstructive lesion before and after the intervention in different projections is in fact completely unusual and in many laboratories also technically impossible. Consequently the degree of stenosis remains a subjective estimation of a static mono-plane picture with a large interobserver variability. Preangioplasty visual estimations almost uniformly rate diameter stenosis more severe than quantitative estimations do, whereas postangioplasty ones tend to underestimate the severity of the stenosis [79].

Furthermore considering the possibility of technical manipulation when using the digitally subtracted single frames, accurate visual assessment of the so called "controlled injury" regardless of the method used, remains dubious.

In an attempt to validate the semiquantitative measure of primary success, all patients underwent a color Doppler analysis of the region of interest before and after intervention. With this non-invasive technique it is possible to confirm and to substantiate the visual assessment, although the determination of a reliable "quantitative" flow level is only possible when the run-off is not obstructed. Nevertheless, this non-invasive technique seems to be helpful in the overall clinical evaluation of the primary success rate.

There is no uniform definition of the clinical primary success of angioplasty in the peripheral arteries. The following criteria have been described to validate the early clinical success of percutaneous transluminal interventions:
1) Doppler ankle / brachial index rise of at least 0.1 [93] or 0.15 [16, 83, 84] or a normalized index [83, 85] or Doppler pulsatility index increased by more than 20% [81, 83]
2) improvement of patient's symptoms by at least one clinical category [81–83, 86] or diminuition of symptoms [84]
3) doubling of the tread-mill exercise distance [81]

4) reappearance of absent relevant pulses or marked strengthening of weak pulses [16, 80, 22]
5) transformation of the monophasic Doppler waveforms to biphasic or triphasic wave forms [81, 82].

For some investigators, primary success is strictly the presence of an angiographically patent artery only (technical success). Primary success has also been defined as a combination of technical success and the presence of at least one clinical criterion; or it has been defined as a combination of technical success and all clinical criteria regarded as important.

In our study, the angiographic criterion of successful recanalization was in the case of a complete occlusion, a restoration of blood flow with a residual luminal diameter 50% of the diameter of the cranial segment of the vessel. In the case of a subtotal stenosis, the criterion was a residual stenosis 20%. The criteria for technically successful dilatation were appearance of a normal groin Doppler pulse after the iliac procedure and the appearance of an adequate flow in color-coded Doppler combined with an increase of at least 0.15 of the ankle/brachial blood pressure index within 24 hours after femoro-popliteal intervention.

The dogma that angiography should be the gold standard for the assessment of transcutaneous peripheral interventions is crumbling since new intravascular imaging techniques like angioscopy and intravascular ultrasound have been clinically introduced. Using these techniques before and after the "semi-blind" vessel recanalization, important discrepancies between the angiogram and the intravascular techniques become evident, particularly in the case of long complete occlusions of the superficial femoral artery. In contrast to the smooth angiographic picture which often gives us the impression of success, a myriad of configurations showing intimal flaps, hemorrhage, thrombotic material, cracks and crevices is directly observed with the angioscope or deduced when analyzing the IVUS frames [86].

The importance of these non-classified factors, (recently identified by non-angiographic techniques) in determining the primary success rate remains unknown. The significance of these factors in predicting restenosis will depend on comparisons between the newer techniques and well established balloon angioplasty.

Furthermore, evaluation of restenosis at the present time is complicated by at least five different angiographic definitions of restenosis for the coronary system described in literature [87] and no plausible or consistent data with regard to the definition of restenosis in peripheral arteries considering location, lesion length, risk factors and natural history of the obstructive disease.

Because of the lack of an impartial definition of restenosis after peripheral interventions, we would like to propose a more global definition including clinical, angiographic and color-coded Doppler data. Considering the pain limitation of the walking distance as a relatively objective and reproducible criterion, a patient was suspected of having developed restenosis when the

PERIPHERAL VESSELS

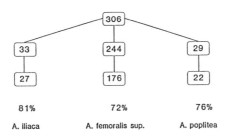

Figure 1. The recanalization of the femoral superficial artery was attempted in 244 of 306 cases (79.7%). In 33 cases (10.8%), laser assisted angioplasty of the common or external iliacal artery and in 29 cases (9.5%) of the popliteal region was performed. The overall primary success rate was 73.5%.

improvement of the exercise capability (defined on a tread-mill exercise test) after recanalization was significantly reduced. When the suspicion of restenosis was confirmed by color-coded Doppler, an angiographic control was performed.

This procedure clearly implicates an uncontrolled selection of patients because practically only patients with clinical symptoms underwent further studies. On the other hand, it is difficult to obtain consent from an asymptomatic patient for a new angiogram, particularly considering the costs, risks and laboratory's capacity.

Results

It should be stressed that in the majority of the cases, complex lesions were present in the recanalized segment. The acute and long term results of the excimer laser assisted angioplasty take into consideration only the global effects of the recanalization procedure and not the elimination or long term evolution of each single obstruction.

Recanalization of peripheral vessels was attempted in 306 cases. The overall primary success rate was 73.5% (Fig. 1).

Complications

The analysis of the procedure related serious complications indicates that the excimer laser assisted recanalization is a safe procedure. Large dissections were observed in 8 cases (2.6%), and prolonged vasospasm without clinical sequelae occurred in 6 patients (2%). The amount of serious local bleedings, not requiring surgical treatment was 1%, which is an acceptable risk. The rate of clinically symptomatic peripheral macroembolisations was low at 1%.

PRIMARY SUCCESS RATE
AFS

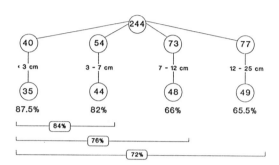

Figure 2. This diagram shows the acute results of 244 interventions in the superficial femoral
artery.

Perforation or vessel rupture occurred in 8 patients (2.6%), but in only 2
cases an elective surgical treatment was necessary. We observed 2 acute
reocclusions of the SFA a few hours after the intervention. Both patients
required acute surgical treatment because of the deterioration of the clinical
situation.

In summary, 13 complications were major (4.2%), 6 could be managed
conservatively and 7 needed a surgical intervention. There were no deaths
and no procedure related amputations.

Superficial Femoral Artery

The 244 cases of obstructed superficial femoral arteries were subdivided into
four groups: 1) subtotal stenoses and occlusions up to 3 cm, 2) total occlusions
of a length between 3 and 7 cm, 3) occlusions of a length between 7 and
12 cm, and 4) occlusions longer than 12 cm. The overall primary success
rate in these four groups was 72% (Fig. 2).
1. Irrespective of the length and multiplicity of the subtotal stenoses or
   occlusions up to 3 cm, laser recanalization was successful in 35 of 40 cases
   corresponding to a primary success rate of 87.5%. In this group of patients, a stand-alone laser procedure was performed in 12 cases with a
   satisfactory angiographic result.
   All 5 unsuccessful cases in this group were short, heavily calcified
   occlusions. Two patients were in chronic hemodialysis, two had received
   heart transplantation and one was an octogenarian with diffuse vessel
   calcification.
2. When the occlusion was located in the middle or distal part of the superficial femoral artery, and the length was between 3 and 7 cm, the primary
   success rate was high (82%). In this group of patients, 4 of 11 unsuccessful

recanalizations were due to the fact that it was not possible to reach the patent distal segment of the vessel. In these cases our inability to maintain a coaxial position of the laser catheter induced an intramural (and not an intraluminal) channel.

In three cases a perforation occurred without clinical sequelae. In two of these cases, the cause was an inadvertent cannulation of a side branch with the laser catheter, followed by a rupture of the vessel. In the remaining four cases, it was not possible to cross the occlusion either by laser or by other mechanical manipulation.

3. In the third group with occlusions of the superficial femoral artery longer than 7 cm, a lower primary success rate was achieved. This result might depend on the fact that the cases were not selected with regard to the duration of the ischemic symptoms, so that patients with clinical symptoms for more than 3–5 years were also accepted for laser angioplasty.
4. With regard to group four (12–25 cm), in contrast to previous reports [51] the relevant increase of the primary success rate from below 50% for the first 100 patients to our present overall success rate of 65%, has to be emphasized. This very encouraging result may be due to improved patient selection. In the last year each patient scheduled for laser angioplasty has undergone not only the usual blood flow analysis by color-coded Doppler ultrasound but also a careful analysis of the structure of the occluded vessel segment by ultrasound. The patient was definitively selected for laser assisted angioplasty only if the continuity of the blocked artery was detected by longitudinal ultrasound scan. Strict observance of this preselection during the last months has dramatically decreased the number of failures as well in the cases of blockage of the superficial femoral artery at the bifurcation or just below the origin of the SFA. In the future we expect an overall primary success rate of 80% or more including cases of complex and extremely long occlusions.

Inability to steer the laser catheter in the right layer of the occluded artery, despite use of a guide wire to maintain a coaxial position of the catheter, was the main reason for failure of the procedure in group three (n = 28) and in group four (n = 15).

The number of true perforations in both groups with long occlusions was insignificant and without relevant consequences. In the majority of the failed cases, the procedure had to be stopped because it was not possible to reach the distal patent part of the vessel in the correct axis.

We have observed that the procedure of excimer laser angioplasty is practically completely pain free when the catheter is advanced intraluminally. If the patient expresses discomfort or pain related to the laser firing process (presumably related to contact with the subadventional layer), the probability of a successful recanalization will decrease drastically.

Successful recanalization of totally obstructed segments with a 7 or 9 french excimer laser catheter implies the formation of an angiographically estimated channel of 2 to 3 mm in diameter. Consequently an additional

PRIMARY SUCCESS RATE
Iliac arteries

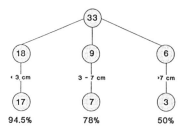

Figure 3. Primary success rate in the pelvic region. The overall recanalisation probability in this area is more than 80%.

balloon dilatation is necessary. Only in a few cases (9%) was it possible to achieve a satisfactory channel with a narrowing <50% by passing the lesion with the laser catheter forward and backward 3 to 5 times. However, it is important to stress the fact that in the majority of the cases the balloon dilatation was limited to one or two persistent stenoses, thereby avoiding dilatation along the entire length of the primarily occluded segment and thus diminishing the probability of dissection or other dilatation related complications.

Iliac Arteries

Unlike the superficial femoral artery, the iliac arteries are rarely straight, implicating a higher theoretical risk of perforation with clinical sequelae, particularly when the obstructed section includes the aortoiliac junction. Accordingly, the excimer laser multifiber catheter was only advanced after crossing the lesion with a guide wire. Only with fluoroscopic evidence of a floating guide wire in the abdominal aorta, were we convinced that a guide wire dissection in the wall of the aorta could be excluded.

With this precaution when approaching the obstruction from the ipsilateral side, we could pass 27 of 33 iliac arteries selected for angioplasty. This group included 6 successfully treated patients with an incomplete Leriche syndrome recanalized in two different sessions.

In case of an obstruction less than 3 cm, successful recanalization was achieved in 17 of 18 lesions (94.5%). The primary success rate decreased to 78% for lesions with a length between 3–7 cm. Only 3 of 6 occlusions longer than 7 cm could be successfully recanalized. In 7 of 10 cases in which the guide wire failed to cross the occlusion, clinical symptoms had been present for at least three years (Fig. 3).

Since a 9 french laser catheter can only create a channel of approximately 3 mm diameter, additional balloon dilatation was required in all cases.

In two cases a dissection of the vessel wall was suspected angiographically and confirmed by intravascular ultrasound. Implantation of a 7 mm, balloon mounted Strecker tantalum stent solved the problem.

The only serious complication in the iliac group occurred following laser dilatation of an external iliac artery in a 48 year old lady with a 6 mm balloon. An intraoperatively confirmed partial rupture occurred inducing an intensive vagal reaction and a significant hemorrhage.

Popliteal Region

Recanalization was attempted in 29 patients with obstructions of the popliteal artery and also in obstructive lesions of the trifurcational area where recanalization has always been regarded as relatively high risk.

The cases were carefully selected, and a low rate of primary failures was observed. The overall early success rate of crossing the popliteal lesions was 78%.

Our experience with lesions in the third popliteal segment and the trifurcational area seems to demonstrate that the stand-alone use of a 5–7 french multifiber catheter should be preferred instead of using it in combination with a balloon dilatation. In fact, 4 of 7 failures in this group were acute reocclusions after final balloon dilatation. Nevertheless, more experience with new types of catheters are necessary before a conclusive statement about the value of laser angioplasty in this area can be made.

Follow-up

The data collection after discharge was complicated by the fact that a large number of the patients treated in the first 18 months after the clinical introduction of the excimer laser technique lived in relatively remote parts of the country. This particularly limited our collection of repeat angiograms.

Nevertheless we could collect in 200 patients the clinical and non-invasive data 3 months after discharge and the complete data of 150 patients including angiographic studies. Figure 4 shows that evaluating the clinical and non-invasive data, the early reocclusion rate during the first 4 weeks after intervention is surprisingly low at 4%. In contrast to the results of conventional PTA, the patency rate after 3 months was maintained in 92.5% of patients.

As expected, the majority of clinical and consequently angiographic deteriorations occurred between the third and sixth month after discharge. Nevertheless, the reocclusion rate after six months was only 26%.

The non-occlusive data in 94 patients of this group one year after intervention indicates that the patency rate remains nearly constant. Despite these

6 Months Follow-up Data of 150 Patients

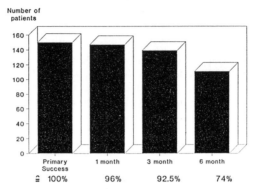

	Primary Success	1 month	3 month	6 month
	≙ 100%	96%	92.5%	74%

Figure 4. This follow-up diagram shows that restenosis or reocclusions in the FSA were predominantly observed in the first 3 to 6 months after discharge.

very encouraging results, confirmation is required in future randomized studies, including the experiences with the modern repertoire of new mechanical systems. The follow-up results of recanalisations performed in the iliac region confirm the general trend that with a satisfactory initial result, the majority of the vessels will remain patent. The patency rate in the iliac region of 95.5% six months after intervention is impressive, particularly considering the relatively large amount of initially total occluded vessels in our series (Fig. 5).

Discussion

The enthusiasm for the potential benefit of laser angioplasty has been tempered by the unsatisfactory acute and long term results using continuous wave sources [47, 32, 33, 42, 88–93].

In vitro studies showed that one of the main advantages of the excimer laser in comparison to other light sources was that even at higher energy densities ($7.5\,J/cm^2$) the damage zone around the ablated channel remains minimal within a tolerable range of 50 μm [48]. A secondary advantage of

Follow-up 6 months
Iliac arteries

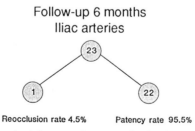

Reocclusion rate 4.5%   Patency rate 95.5%

Figure 5. 6 months follow-up after recanalisation in the pelvic area.

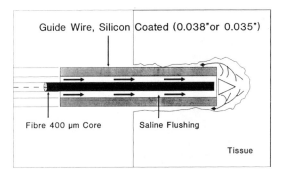

Figure 6. This picture schematically demonstrates the possible mechanism of excimer-induced recanalization using a single fiber (400mm) incorporated in an open-ended guide wire. Theoretically only the sclerotic material located just in front of the fiber should be uniformly ablated. As a result of the interaction between thermal expansion and acoustic waves generated by repetitive excimer pulses with high energy density, a 3–fold larger channel is generated.

the excimer laser may be the linear dependence of the recanalization speed to the frequency related power. Independent of the type of probe used, the average power necessary to achieve the maximum excimer recanalization speed is lower than the threshold power necessary to induce any vaporisation using a continuous wave Nd:YAG source [51]. Furthermore, the results obtained in human calcified coronary arteries demonstrate that ablation of calcified material is possible, but there will be a reduced ablation rate for heavily calcified material [51, 52, 94].

The main disadvantage associated with the excimer laser is that the size of the channel achieved is not significantly larger than the core diameter of the fiber used. However, incorporating a quartz fiber with a core diameter of 400 μm into a saline filled .038 inch open ended guide wire, channel diameters up to 1.1 mm could be achieved [51] (Fig. 6). This effect seems to be based on the absorption of short, high density light pulses leading to a local explosion of the target tissue which reacts with immediate thermal volume expansion. Using repetitive pulses with oscillating density, thermal and acoustic waves are generated applying mechanical stress and strain to the target tissue and finally causing rupture of the matter as a desired effect [49]. These mechanisms may explain why multifiber catheters incorporating 12 resp. 18 fibers with a core diameter of 260 μm can achieve a relatively smooth channel with a diameter up to 3 mm although the dead zone of the catheter's tip is extremely large compared with the sum of the fiber's ablating surfaces [76] (Fig. 7).

The results presented in this report clearly indicate that with using the described technique, a high percentage of femoropliteal stenoses and occlusions (94.5%–65%) can be recanalized, confirming our preliminary data as well as other groups [51, 94–100].

The number of stand-alone interventions without final balloon dilatation

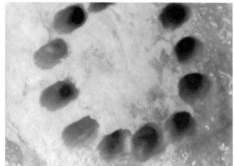

a

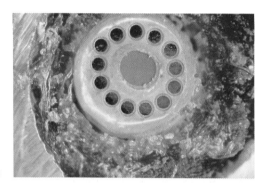

b

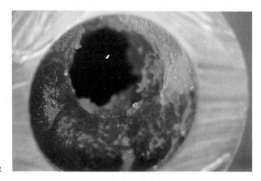

c

Figure 7.   Ablation pattern of a 7 french multifiber catheter (first generation).
a) This picture clearly indicates that a primary ablation is only achieved in front of each single fiber.
b) Using a 7 french catheter this artificial occlusion could be crossed. Note the large dead area in comparison to the relatively small ablation surface of the single fibers.
c) View of the finally achieved channel in an artificial occlusion.

remains very limited in the pelvic and femoral area, so that it seems to be more appropriate to use the term "excimer laser assisted angioplasty."

Nevertheless, this young continuously evolving technology with a primary success rate of nearly 70% in the case of total occlusions has demonstrated its superiority in comparison to the conventional balloon angioplasty, which has initial failure rates greater than 50% [3, 20–26]. Furthermore, excimer laser assisted angioplasty has succeeded in attempts to recanalize very long occlusions (exceeding 15 cm), which are normally excluded from conventional PTA. The longest femoro-popliteal segment recanalized in our series was 42 cm. With regard to long occlusions debulked by multifiber catheters, the fact that the final dilatation in many cases is limited to localized persistent narrowings should be of particular interest. The reduction of the potential injury area could have a positive influence on long term results of this technique.

The clinical appearance of the new imaging techniques angioscopy and intravascular ultrasound have raised doubts with regard to the gold standard angiography in the validation of the primary success rate. In many cases a considerable discrepancy could be observed comparing these different techniques, whereby the DSA pictures tend to overestimate the results [86]. In the mean time we are convinced that the angiographic estimation of acute early results will not be sufficient to predict the potential risk of restenosis or reocclusion of recanalized vessels, particularly in the case of long occlusions.

Nevertheless the patency rates of our patient populations, 92.5% in the femoral artery, respectively 95.5% in the pelvic region after 3 months are very high. In contrast to the femoral superficial artery where the patency rate drops to 74%, no change of patency rate of iliac arteries was observed between 3 and 6 months. Taking into account the fact that more than 60% of the recanalized vessels in the femoral region were occlusions longer than 5 cm, the follow up results confirm the clinical impression that excimer laser assisted angioplasty is superior to conventional PTA, other laser techniques and possibly other mechanical techniques.

At the present stage it is nearly impossible to compare the different techniques in a realistic and neutral way, because the patient populations treated in the different studies are too heterogenous and the number of patients in individual studies are too small. We need more experience and an intensive collaboration between the single groups outlining a generally accepted protocol that can be followed when using different equipments or techniques. The inclusion of intravascular ultrasound and angioscopy criteria in the evaluation of the restenosis process seems to be mandatory.

The evaluation of drugs for the prevention of acute and long term restenosis or reocclusion is confusing and disappointing. Nevertheless, we continue to maintain patients on heparin for at least 24 hours after intervention and to discharge them with low dose acetylsalicylic acid although there's no scientific evidence for the efficacy of the tested compounds [101].

It is our increasing feeling that the analysis of the anatomy and the semiquantitative assessment of flow in the obstructed vessel, before and 24 hours after intervention using the color-coded Doppler ultrasound [102–104] has a prognostic value with regard to the probability of restenosis or reocclusion. The integration of this and other non-invasive modalities will permit a more accurate assessment of transcutaneous interventions. In the mean time we must recognize the limitations of our current gold standard and the restriction that it imposes on the general assessment of angioplasty results [78].

Final Comment

At a meeting of the American Society of Laser in Medicine in Dallas in April 1988, we predicted the laser to be a "*l*imited *a*pplication of a *s*ophisticated and *e*xpensive *r*esearch." Although in the mean time the scientific and clinical work has transformed the sterile concept of a laser induced ablation into a realistic clinical modality, this technology remains experimental and has not yet been able to find satisfactory acceptance.

It should already be obvious at this moment that laser technology in the near future will not solve the problems related to restenosis or to other complications after transcutaneous interventions substantially. The continuing evolution of this new technology will be mandatory when the stage of "preliminary" or "encouraging" results should be surmounted.

Laser angioplasty will not survive a second "hot tip = soldering-iron" disaster. The responsibility of the involved investigators for the destiny of laser angioplasty is considerable. By presenting future results in an impartial and objective way and avoiding new unrealistic expectations or perspectives imposed by big business cardio-angiology, it may become possible for laser angioplasty to find its place in the "bag of tools" of the interventionalist in the late 1990's.

Case-reports

Case 1

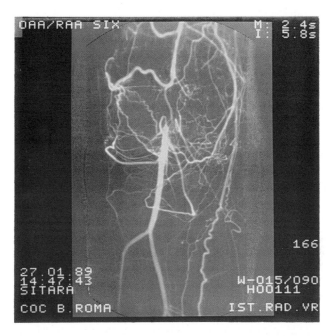

Case 1. Figure 1.

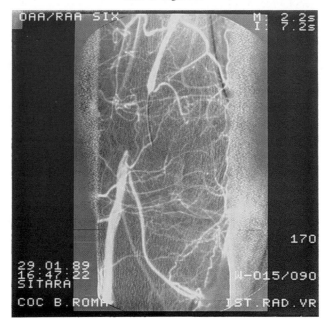

Case 1. Figure 2.

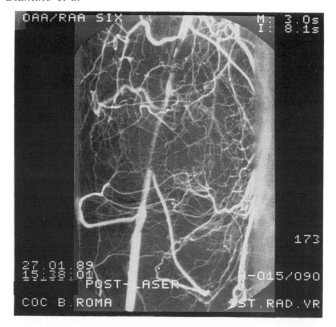

Case 1. Figure 3.

Case 1. Figure 4.

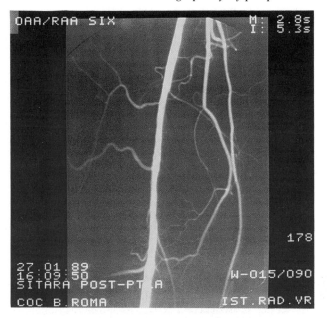

Case 1. Figure 5.

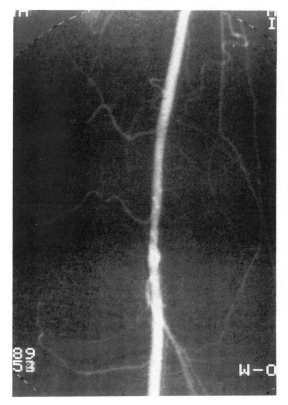

Case 1. Figure 6.

Documentation of the first case performed on January 25, 1988.
1) Total occlusion of the distal AFS up to the poplitea (5 cm). Note the intensive collateral ramification.
2) It was not possible to cross the lesion, with a guide wire directed in the collateral system.
3) After the first passage a small channel was achieved.
4) Several forward and backward lasering passes induced a sufficient channel in the proximal part of the occluded segment.
5) The remaining 75% distal stenosis was finally dilated with a 5 mm balloon. Note the disappearance of collateral vessels after successful intervention.
6) Two years after recanalisation the segment is still patent and the patient completely free of symptoms.

Case 2

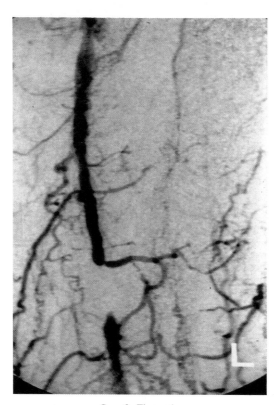

Case 2. Figure 1.

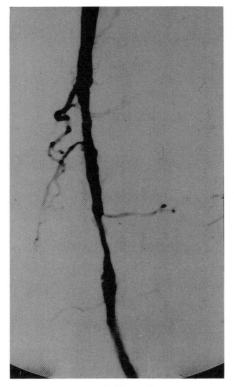

Case 2. Figure 2.

This case with claudication symptoms for three years showed a calcified 4 cm long occlusion in the mid part of the AFS (1). After recanalization with a 9 french multifiber catheter, sufficient flow with a residual stenosis of 30% was observed (2). A final PTA was not necessary.

Case 3

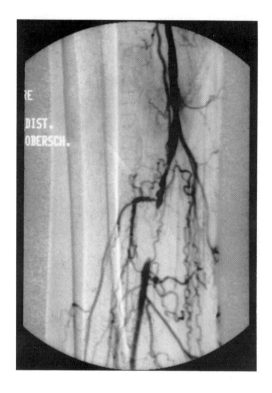

Case 3. Figure 1.

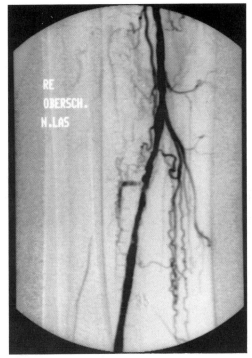

Case 3. Figure 2.

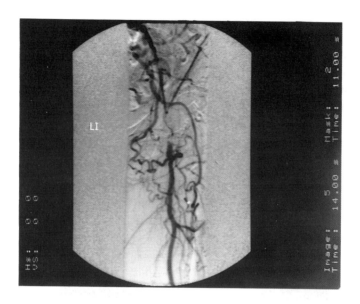

Case 4. Figure 2.

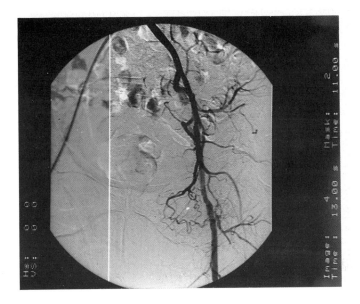

Case 4. Figure 3.

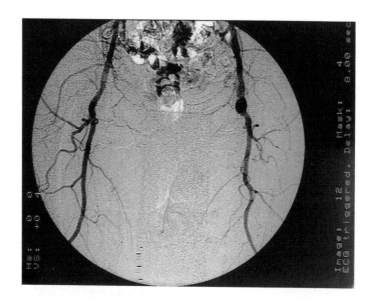

Case 4. Figure 4.

In this case (54 years, female) a total occlusion of both AFS and of the bilateral femoropopliteal bypasses three years after surgical intervention was present. During the last few months, continuous increase of the claudication (<50 m) was noted.

1) The pre-lasering angiogram shows a complete occlusion of the left common femoral artery.
2) in cross-over technique the 7F-multifiber laser catheter has reached the occlusion.
3) after lasering and final dilatation (6 mm balloon, 4 cm long) complete recanalisation.
4) 6 month follow-up shows a perfect result. The patient was at this time pain free with unlimited walking capacity.

Case 5

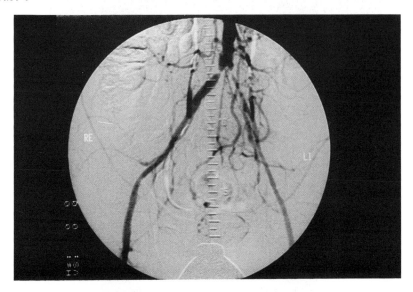

Case 5. Figure 1.

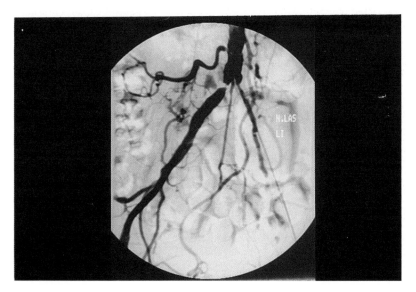

Case 5. Figure 2.

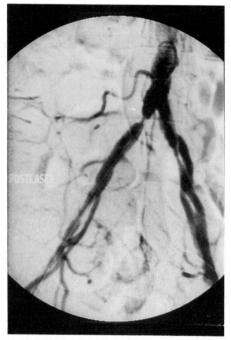

Case 5. Figure 3.

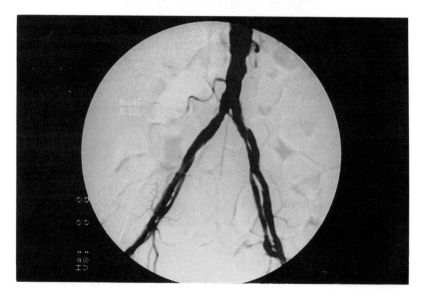

Case 5. Figure 4.

48 year old man, heavy smoker with continuously increasing claudication (<30 m) for 18 months.

1) The angiogram shows a complete occlusion of the left common iliac artery and contralateral short subtotal stenosis at the bifurcation.
2) In the first session we attempted to recanalize the left common iliac artery. The picture shows the result of the first passage. with the laser catheter.
3) Optimal angiographic result after final balloon dilatation (6 mm in diameter).
4) 2 weeks later the contralateral stenosis was likewise successfully recanalized. One year later the patient is free of symptoms, bike riding and playing tennis.

Case 6

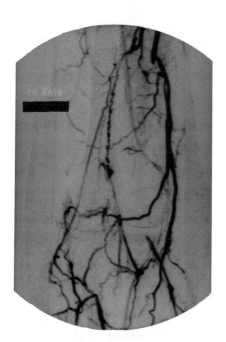

Case 6. Figure 1.

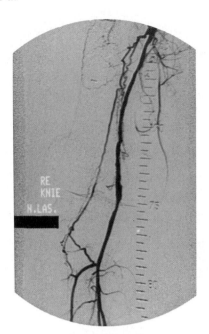

Case 6. Figure 2.

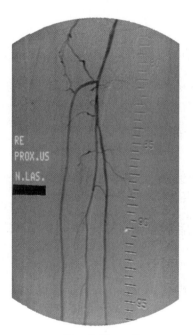

Case 6. Figure 3.

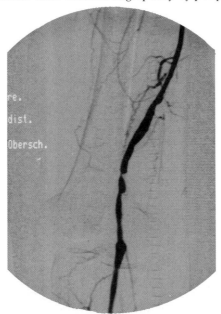

Case 6. Figure 4.

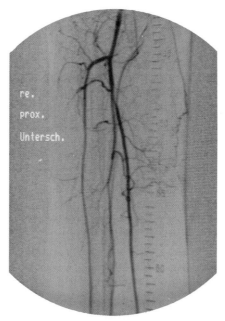

Case 6. Figure 5.

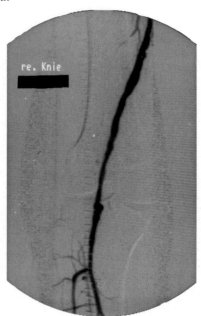

Case 6. Figure 6.

42 year old man (obesity, hypercholesterinaemia, smoker) with a walking distance less than 100 m.
1) Complete occlusion of the distal femoral- and of the popliteal artery.
2) After recanalization (June 14, 1990) with a 9 french multifiber catheter and dilatation of the mid part of the popliteal artery an angiographic perfect run-off could be shown. After recanalization the patient remained free of symptoms.
3) At the routine control 11 months later (May 2, 1991) an unexpected angiographic relevant stenosis in the first popliteal segment is detected. Is this a restenosis or an intervention-independent progression of the disease?
4) The run-off was unchanged.
5) The angioscopic and IVUS examination clearly confirmed the stenosis.
6) After dilatation with a 6 mm balloon the narrowing is gone.

Case 7

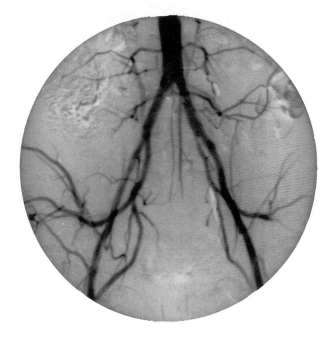

Case 7. Figure 1.

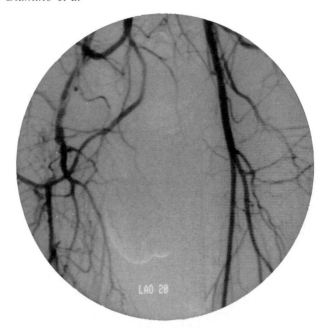

Case 7. Figure 2.

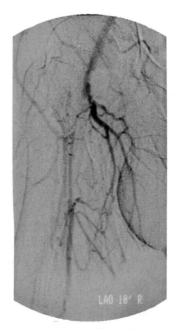

Case 7. Figure 3.

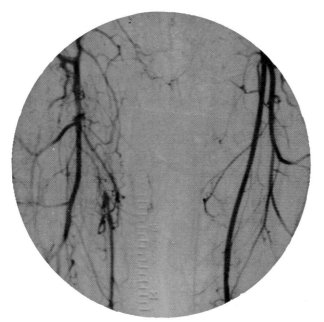

Case 7. Figure 4.

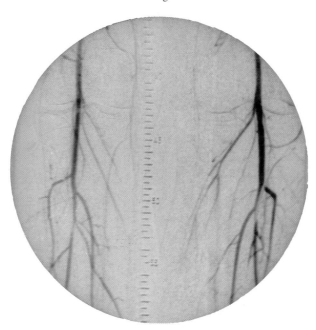

Case 7. Figure 5.

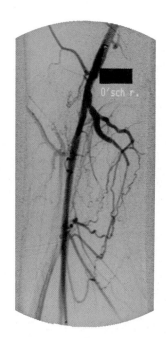

Case 7. Figure 6.

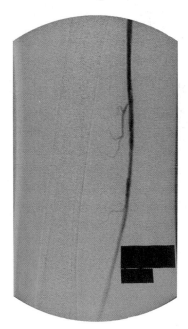

Case 7. Figure 7.

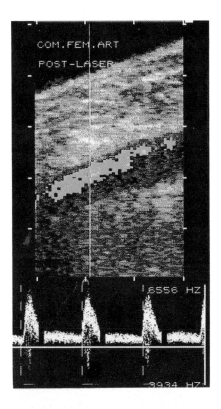

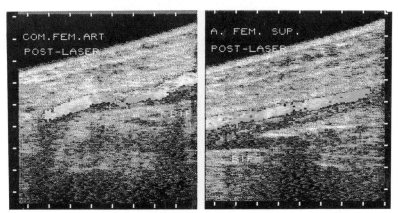

Case 7. Figure 8.

51 year old man, 6 months after AMI and following double PTCA, he developed crescendo claudication (less than 100 m).

(1) The angiogram shows a normal pelvic area, but a complete occlusion is present in the right common femoral artery (2).

The origin and the first third of the AFS is also occluded (3, 4).
(5) normal run-off.

Using a new flexible 7 french AIS-multifiber catheter connected to a
Dymer 200 it was possible in cross-over technique to reach the occlusion and
to recanalize the AFS completely (6,7).

A final dilatation with a 6 mm balloon was only necessary at the junction
of common femoral artery and AFS.

(8) The post-procedure angiodynogram shows a completely normal color-
coded flow in the initially occluded common femoral artery and proximal
AFS. The flow in the common femoral artery was above 100 ml/min.

References

1. Dotter C T, Judkins M P (1964) Transluminal treatment of atherosclerotic obstructions: description of a new technique and a preliminary report of its application. *Circulation* 30:654–670
2. Gruentzig A R, Senning A, Siegenthaler W E (1979) Nonoperative dilatation of coronary-artery stenosis: percutaneous transluminal coronary angioplasty. *N Engl J Med* 301:61–68
3. Zeitler E, Richter E I, Roth F L, Schoop W (1983) Results of percutaneous transluminal angioplasty. *Radiology* 146:57–60
4. Detre K, Holubkov R, Kelsey S et al, the Co-investigators of the National Heart, Lung, and Blood Institute's Percutaneous Transluminal Coronary Angioplasty Registry (1988) Percutaneous transluminal coronary angioplasty in 1985–1986 and 1977–1981. *N Engl J Med* 318:265–270
5. Holmes D R, Vlietstra R E, Smith H C et al (1984) Restenosis after percutaneous transluminal coronary angioplasty (PTCA): a report from the PTCA registry of the National Heart, Lung, and Blood Institute. *Am J Cardiol* 53:77C–81C
6. Mata L A, Bosch X, David P R, Rapold K J, Corcos T, Bourassa M G (1985) Clinical and angiographic assessment 6 months after double vessel percutaneous coronary angioplasty. *J Am Coll Cardiol* 6:1239–44
7. Levine S, Ewels C J, Rosing D R, Kent K M (1985) Coronary angioplasty: clinical and angiographic follow-up. *Am J Cardiol* 55:673–6
8. Leimgruber P P, Roubin G S, Hollman J et al (1986) Restenosis after successful coronary angioplasty in patients with single-vessel disease. *Circulation* 73:710–7
9. Roubin G S, King S B, Douglas J S (1987) Restenosis after percutaneous transluminal coronary angioplasty: the Emory University Hospital experience. *Am J Cardiol* 60:39B–43B
10. Vandormael M G, Deligonul U, Kern M J, Kennedy H, Galan K, Chaitman B (1987) Restenosis after multilesion percutaneous transluminal coronary angioplasty. *Am J Cardiol* 60:44B–7B
11. Val P G, Bourassa M G, David P R et al (1987) Restenosis after successful percutaneous transluminal coronary angioplasty: the Montreal Heart Institute experience. *Am J Cardiol* 60:50B–5B
12. Ernst S M P G, van der Feltz T A, Bal E T et al (1987) Long-term angiographic follow-up, cardiac events, and survival in patients undergoing percutaneous transluminal coronary angioplasty. *Br Heart J* 57:220–5
13. Bussman W, Kaltenbach M, Kober G, Vallbracht C (1987) The Frankfurt experience in restenosis after coronary angioplasty. *Am J Cardiol* 60:48B–9B
14. McBride W, Lange R A, Hillis L A (1988) Restenosis after successful coronary angioplasty. *N Engl J Med* 318:1734–7

15. King S B (1988) Percutaneous transluminal coronary angioplasty: the second decade. *Am J Cardiol* 62:2K–6K
16. Hewes R C, White R I, Murray R R, Kaufman S L, Chang R, Kadir S, Kinnison M L, Mitchell S E, Auster M (1986) Long-term results of superficial femoral artery angioplasty. *AJR* 146:1025–1029
17. Colapinto R F, Harries-Jones E P, Johnston K W (1980) Percutaneous transluminal angioplasty of peripheral vascular disease: a two year experience. *Cardiovasc Intervent Radiol* 3:213–218
18. Greenfield A (1980) Femoral, popliteal, and tibial arteries: percutaneous transluminal angioplasty. *AJR* 135:927–935
19. Johnston K W, Colapinto R F, Baird R J (1982) Transluminal dilation: an alternative? *Arch Surg* 117:1604–1610
20. Probst P, Cerny P, Owens A, Mahler F (1983) Patency after femoral angioplasty: correlation of angiographic appearance with clinical findings. *AJR* 140:1227–1232
21. Spence R K, Freiman D B, Gatenby R et al (1981) Long-term results of transluminal angioplasty of the iliac and femoral arteries. *Arch Surg* 116:1377–1386
22. Krepel V M, van Andel G J, van Erp W F M, Breslau P J (1985) Percutaneous transluminal angioplasty of the femoropopliteal artery: initial and long-term results. *Radiology* 156:325–328
23. Kumpe D A, Jones D N (1982) Percutaneous transluminal angioplasty. Radiologic viewpoint. *Appl Radiol* 11:29–40
24. Lu C T, Zairns C K, Yang C F, Cottiurai V (1982) Long-segment arterial occlusion. Percutaneous transluminal angioplasty. *Am J Roentgen* 138:119–122
25. Jorgensen B, Henriksen O, Karle A, Sager P, Holstein P, Tonnesen K H (1988) Percutaneous transluminal angioplasty of iliac and femoral arteries in severe lower-limb ischaemia. *Acta Chir Scand* 154:647–652
26. Bergentz S V, Jonsson K (1983) Percutaneous transluminal angioplasty. *Acta Chir Scand* 149:641–649
27. Brown P W (1986) *The Outlook for the Coronary Angioplasty Industry.* Report from Hambrecht and Quist Inc.
28. Waller B F (1989) Crackers, Breakers, Stretchers, Drillers, Scrapers, Shavers, Burners, Welders and Melters. The future treatment of atherosclerotic coronary artery disease? A clinical-morphologic assessment. *JACC* 13:969–987
29. Choy D S J (1988) History of lasers in medicine. *Thorac Cardiovasc Surg* 36:114–117
30. Choy D S J, Stertzer S H, Myler R K, Marco J, Fournial G (1984) Human coronary laser recanalization. *Clin Cardiol* 7:377–381
31. Forrester J S, Litvack F, Grundfest W S (1986) Laser angioplasty and cardiovascular disease. *Am J Cardiol* 57:990–992
32. Cumberland D C, Tayler D I, Welsh C L et al (1986) Percutaneous laser thermal angioplasty: initial clinical results with a laser probe in total peripheral artery occlusions. *Lancet* 1:1457–1459
33. Sanborn T A, Cumberland D C, Greenfield A J, Welsh C L, Guben J K (1988) Percutaneous laser thermal angioplasty: initial results and 1-year follow-up in 129 femoropopliteal lesions. *Radiology* 168:121–125
34. Nordstrom L A, Castaneda-Zuniga W R, Lindeke C C, Rasmussen T M, Burnside D K (1988) Laser angioplasty: controlled delivery of argon laser energy. *Radiology* 167:463–465
35. Ginsburg R, Wexler L, Mitchell R S, Profitt D (1985) Percutaneous transluminal laser angioplasty for treatment of peripheral vascular disease: clinical experience with 16 patients. *Radiology* 156:619–624
36. Sanborn T A, Faxon D P, Haudenschild C C, Ryan T J (1985) Experimental angioplasty circumferential distribution of laser thermal injury with a laser probe. *J Am Coll Cardiol* 5:934–938
37. Welch A J, Bradley A B, Torres J H et al (1987) Laser probe ablation of normal and atherosclerotic human aorta in vitro: a first thermographic and histologic analysis. *Circulation* 76:1353–1363

38. Abela G S (1988) Laser arterial recanalization: A current perspective. *J Am Coll Cardiol* 12:103–105
39. Crea F, Davies G, McKenna W, Pashazade M, Tayler K, Maseri A (1986) Percutaneous laser recanalisation of coronary arteries. *Lancet* 1:214–215
40. Ginsburg R (1988) Percutaneous laser angioplasty in the treatment of peripheral vascular disease. *Thorac Cardiovasc Surg* 36:142–145
41. Abela G S, Normann S, Feldman R L, Geiser E A, Cohen D, Conti C R (1982) Effects of carbon dioxide, Nd:YAG and argon laser radiation on coronary atheromatous plaques. *Am J Cardiol* 50:1199–1205
42. Geschwind H J, Boussignac G, Teisseire B, Benhaiem N, Bittoun R, Laurent D (1984) Conditions for effective Nd:YAG laser angioplasty. *Br Heart J* 52:484–489
43. Ginsburg R, Kirr D S, Guthaner P, Tolh J, Mitchell R S (1984) Salvage of an ischemic limb by laser angioplasty: description of a new technique. *Clin Cardio* 7:54–58
44. Pacala T J, McDermid I S, Laudenslager J B (1984) Ultranarrow linewidth, magnetically switched, long pulse, xenon chloride laser. *Appl Phys Lett* 44:658–660
45. Deckelbaum L I, Isner J M, Donaldson R F, Clarke R H, Laliberte S, Aharon A S, Bernstein J S (1985) Reduction of laser-induced pathologic tissue injury using pulsed energy delivery. *Am J Cardiol* 56:662–667
46. Grundfest W S, Litvack F, Forrester J S, Goldenberg T, Swan H J C, Morgenstern L, Fishbein M, McDermid I S, Rider D M, Pacala T J, Laudenslager J B (1985) Laser ablation of human atherosclerotic plaque without adjacent tissue injury. *JACC* 5:929–933
47. Abela G S, Norman S J, Cohen D M, Franzini D, Feldman R L, Crea F, Fenech A, Pepine C J, Conti C R (1985) Laser recanalization of occluded atherosclerotic arteries: an in vivo and in vitro study. *Circulation* 71:403–411
48. Biamino G, Dörschel K, Harnoss B M, Kar H, Müller G (1988) Experience in excimer laser photoablation of arteriosclerotic plaques. In: Biamino G, Müller G J (eds) *Advances in Laser Medicine I*. First German Symposium on Laser Angioplasty. Berlin: Ecomed Verlagsgesellschaft, 147–156
49. Berlien H P G, Müller G J (1988) Laser in medicine. In: Biamino G, Müller G J (eds) *Advances in Laser Medicine I*. First German Symposium on Laser Angioplasty. Berlin: Ecomed Verlagsgesellschaft, 45–55
50. Srinivasan R, Braren B, Dreyfus R W, Hadel L, Seeger D E (1986) Mechanism of the ultraviolet laser ablation of polymethyl methacrylate at 193 and 248 nm: laser-induced fluorescence analysis, chemical analysis, and doping studies. *J Opt Soc Am* (B) 3:785–791
51. Biamino G (1990) Coronary and peripheral laser angioplasty. In: Hogrefe & Huber (eds) *Interventional Cardiology*. Göttingen; 243–260
52. Linsker R, Srinivasan R, Wynne J J, Alonso D R (1984) Far ultraviolet laser ablation of atherosclerotic lesions. *Lasers Surg Med* 4:201–206
53. Isner J M, Donaldson R F, Decklebaum L I, Clarke R H, Laliberte M, Ucci A A, Salem D N (1985) The excimer laser: Gross, light microscopic and ultrastructural analylsis of potential for use in laser therapy of cardiovascular disease. *J Am Coll Cardiol* 6:1102–1109
54. Dörschel K, Biamino G, Brodzinski T, Axel J, Müller G (1988) Comparison of the feasibility of laser angioplasty using heater probes, sapphire tips, and bare fibers. *Eur Heart J* 9 (Suppl 1) 331
55. Abela G S, Fenech A, Crea F, Conti C R (1985) Hot tip: another method of laser recanalization. *Lasers Surg Med* 5:327–335
56. Hussein H (1986) A novel fiberoptic laser probe for treatment of occlusive vessel disease. *Optical Laser Technol Med* 605:59–66
57. Cothren R M, Hayes G B, Kramer J R, Sacks B, Kitrell C, Feld M S (1986) A multifiber catheter with an optical shield for angiosurgery. *Laser Life Sci* 1:1–12
58. Fourrier J L, Brunetaud J M, Prat A, Marache P, Lablanche J M, Bertrand M E (1987) Percutaneous laser angioplasty with a sapphire tip. *Lancet* 1:105
59. Fourrier J L, Marache P, Brunetaud J M, Mordon S, Lablanche J M, Bertrand M E (1986)

Laser recanalization of peripheral arteries by contact sapphire in man (abstract). *Circulation* 74:11–204

60. Geschwind H J, Blair J D, Mongolsmai D, Kern M J, Stern J, Delinogul U, Kennedy H L (1987) Development and experimental application of contact probe catheter for laser angioplasty. *J Am Coll Cardiol* 9:101–107

61. Borst C, Verdaasdonk R M, Boulanger L H M A, Oomen A, Berengoltz S N, Mali W P T W, Westerhof P W, Robles de Medina E O (1988) Comparison of hot tip and sapphire tip recanalization. In: Biamino G, Müller G (eds) *Advances in Laser Medicine I*. First German Symposium on Laser Angioplasty. Berlin: Ecomed Verlagsgesellschaft, 70–80

62. Sanborn T A (1988) Experimental and clinical angioplasty with a laser probe fiberoptic catheter system. *Thorac Cardiovasc Surg* 36:133–136

63. Sanborn T A, Faxon D P, Kellett M Y, Tyan T J (1986) Percutaneous coronary laser thermal angioplasty. *JACC* 8:1437–1440

64. Cumberland D C, Sanbom T A, Tayler D I, Ryan T J (1986) Percutaneous laser thermal angioplasty: clinical experience in peripheral artery occlusions (abstract). *JACC* 7:211A

65. Sanborn T A, Cumberland D C, Guben J K, Greenfield A J, Tayler D I (1986) Human peripheral percutaneous laser-assisted balloon angioplasty (abstract). *Lasers Surg Med* 6:40A

66. Abela G S, Seeger J M, Barbieri E, Franzini D, Fenech A, Pepine C J, Conti C R (1986) Laser angioplasty with angioscopic guidance in humans. *JACC* 8:184–192

67. Fourrier J L, Brunetaud J M, Lablanche J M, Bertrand M E (1986) Angioplasty by contact sapphire: in vitro study (abstract). *Lasers Surg Med* 6:177A

68. Cross F W, Bowker T J, Michaels J A, Shaw P, Brown S G (1988) Pulsed Nd:YAG laser-assisted balloon angioplasty: an early clinical assessment. In: Biamino G, Müller G J (eds) *Advances in Laser Medicine I*. First German Symposium on Laser Angioplasty. Berlin: Ecomed Verlagsgesellschaft, 124–133

69. Geschwind H, Boussignac G, Dubois-Rande J L, Leon M, Murphy-Chutorian D (1988) Sapphire touch probes for angioplasty. In: Biamino G, Müller G J (eds) *Advances in Laser Medicine I*. First German Symposium on Laser Angioplasty. Berlin: Ecomed Verlagsgesellschaft, 191–195

70. Biamino G, Kar H, Harnoss BM, Dörschel K, Müller G (1988) Feasibility of Nd:YAG laser angioplasty. In: Biamino G, Müller G J (eds) *Advances in Laser Medicine I*. First German Symposium on Laser Angioplasty. Berlin: Ecomed Verlagsgesellschaft, 134–140

71. Srinivasan R, Mayne-Bauton (1982) Self-developing photoetching of poly films by far ultraviolet laser radiation. *Appl Phys Lett* 4 (6):576–578

72. Srinivasan R, Leigh W (1982) Ablative photodecompensation: action of far ultraviolet (193 nm) laser radiation on poly films. *J Am Chem Soc* 104:6784–6785

73. Garrison B J, Srinivasan R (1984) Microscopic model for the ablative photodecompensation of polymers by far ultraviolet radiation (193 nm). *Appl Phys Lett* 44:849–851

74. Kar H (1991) Anwendungen der Photoablation in der biomedizinischen Technik. *Advances in Laser Medicine IV*, Ecomed Verlag 1991 (in press)

75. Karsch K, Haase K, Voelker W, Baumbach A, Mauser M, Seipel L (1990) Percutaneous coronary excimer laser angioplasty in patients with stable and unstable angina pectoris. *Circulation* 8:1849–1859

76. Biamino G, Kar H, Fleck E, Müller G (1991) Comparison of different excimer laser systems for coronary and peripheral angioplasty (in press)

77. Grundfest W S, Litvack I F, Goldenberg T et al (1985) Pulsed ultraviolet lasers and the potential for safe laser angioplasty. *Am J Surg* 150:220–226

78. Dietrich E B (1989) The Spoof Factor. *JACC* 14:1125

79. Califf R M, Ohman M G, Frid D J, Fortin D F, Mark D M, Hlatky M A, Herndon J E, Bengtson J R (1990) Restenosis: The clinical issues. In: Topol E J (ed) *Textbook of Interventional Cardiology*, 363–394

80. Walden R, Siegel Y, Rubinstein Z J, Morag B, Bass A, Adar R (1986) Percutaneous

transluminal angioplasty: A suggested method for analysis of clinical, arteriographic, and hemodynamic factors affecting the results of treatment. *J Vasc Surg* 3:583–90

81. Morin J F, Johnston W, Wasserman L, Andrews D (1986) Factors that determine the long-term results of percutaneous transluminal dilatation for peripheral arterial occlusion disease. *J Vasc Surg* 4:68–72

82. Johnston K W, Rae M, Hogg-Johnston S A, Math B, Math M, Colapinto R F, Walker P M, Baird R J, Sniderman K W, Kalman P (1987) 5–year of a prospective study of percutaneous transluminal angioplasty. *Ann Surg* 10:403–413

83. Borozan P G, Schulter J J, Spigos D G, Flanigan D P (1985) Long-term hemodynamic evaluation of lower extremity percutaneous transluminal angioplasty. *J Vasc Surg* 2:785–93

84. Murray R R, Hewes R C, White R I, Mitchell S E, Auster M, Chang R, Kadir S, Kinnison M L, Kaufman S L (1987) Long-segment femoropopliteal stenoses: Is angioplasty a boon or a bust? *Radiology* 162:473–476

85. Colapinto R F, Stronell R D, Johnston W K (1986) Transluminal Angioplasty of Complete Iliac Obstructions. *AJR* 146:859–862

86. Biamino G, Gross M (1991) Intravaskuläre Ultraschalldiagnostik im Vergleich zu angioskopischen Befunden. *Z für Kard* 80 (Suppl 3):208

87. Kaltenbach M, Kober C, Scherer D, Vallbracht C (1985) Recurrence rate after successful coronary angioplasty. *Eur Heart J* 6:276–281

88. Heintzen M P, Neubaur T, Klepzig M, Richter E I, Zeitler E, Strauer B E (1988) Clinical experiences with Nd:YAG laser angioplasty in the periphery. In: Biamino G, Müller G J (eds) *Advances in Laser Medicine I.* First German Symposium on Laser Angioplasty. Berlin: Ecomed Verlagsgesellschaft, 103–113

89. Sanborn T A, Greenfield A J, Guben J K, Menzoian J O, LoGerfo F W (1987) Human percutaneous and intraoperative laser thermal angioplasty: initial clinical results as an adjunct to balloon angioplasty. *J Vasc Surg* 5:83–90

90. Fourrier J L, Mordon S, Brunetaud J M, Marache P, Lablanche J M, Bertrand M E (1988) Laser angioplasty of peripheral arteries with a sapphire tip catheter. In: Biamino G, Müller G J (eds) *Advances in Laser Medicine I.* First German Symposium on Laser Angioplasty. Berlin: Ecomed Verlagsgesellschaft, 117–123

91. Geschwind H J, Kern M J, Vandormael M, Blair J D, Deligonul V, Kennedy H (1987) Efficiency and safety of optically modified fiber tips for laser angioplasty. *JACC* 10:655–661

92. Lammer J, Pilger E, Ascher P W (1988) Experimental and clinical results with Nd:YAG laser angioplasty. In: Biamino G, Müller G J (eds) *Advances in Laser Medicine I.* First German Symposium on Laser Angioplasty. Berlin: Ecomed Verlagsgesellschaft, 96–102

93. Nordstrom L A, Castaneda-Zuniga W R, Young E G, von Seggern K B (1988) Direct argon laser exposure for recanalization of peripheral arteries: early results. *Radiology* 168:359–364

94. Litvack F, Grundfest W, Adler L, Hickey A, Segalowitz J, Hestrin L, Mohr F W, Goldenberg T, Laudenslager J, Forrester J (1989) Percutaneous excimer- laser and excimer- laser-assisted angioplasty of the lower extremities: Results of initial clinical trial. *Radiology* 172:331–335

95. Litvack F, Grundfest W, Segalowitz J, Papaioanniou T, Goldenberg T, Laudenslager J, Hestrin L, Forrester J, Eigler N A, Cook S (1990) Interventional cardiovascular therapy by laser and thermal angioplasty. *Circulation* 81 (suppl IV): IV–109–IV–116

96. Huppert P E, Duda S H, Seboldt H, Karsch K R, Claussen C D (1991) Periphere Excimer-Laserangioplastie. *Dtsch med Wschr* 116:161–167

97. Katzen B, Schwarten D, Kaplan J, Cutcliff W (1988) Initial experience with an Excimer laser in peripheral lesions (A). *Circulation* 78 (Suppl II) II–47

98. Litvack F, Grundfest W, Adler L, Hickey A, Segalowitz J, Hestrin L, Goldenberg T, Laudenslager J, Forrester J (1988) Percutaneous excimer laser angioplasty in humans. *Circulation* (Suppl II);78:II–417

99. Pokrovsky A V, Volynsky J D, Konov V I, Sargin M E, Silenok A S, Goloma V V,

Puretsky M V, Belojartsev D (1990) Recanalisation of occluded peripheral arteries by excimer laser. *Eur J Vasc Surg* 4:575–581

100. McCarthy W J, Vogelzang R L, Nemcek A A, Joseph A, Pearce W H, Flinn W R, Yoa J S T (1991) Excimer laser-assisted femoral angioplasty: early results. *J Vasc Surg* 13:607–614

101. Meier B (1989) Prevention of restenosis after coronary angioplasty: a pharmacological approach. *Eur Heart J* 10:64–68

102. Klews P M (1987) The Philips Quantum Angiodynography: an ultrasound system for vascular diagnostics. *Medicamundi* Vol 32, No 2, 77–79

103. Merrit C R B (1986) Doppler blood flow imaging: integrating flow with tissue data. *Diagnostic Imaging* 8:146–155

104. Powis R L (1986) Angiodynography – a new-real-time look at the vascular system. *Applied Radiology* 1:55–59

22. Clinical Results of Percutaneous Coronary Excimer Laser Angioplasty Trials

WARREN S. GRUNDFEST, FRANK LITVACK,
JAMES MARGOLIS, JAMES LAUDENSLAGER
and TSVI GOLDENBERG

Initial experience with the excimer laser angioplasty system in the treatment of peripheral vascular disease confirmed the need for specific design criteria [1, 2]. First, the system needed to be designed in an over-the-wire fashion to facilitate use and prevent perforations. Second, the use of multiple small fibers to produce large ablation areas within a given catheter size was feasible and provided greater flexibility. Third, catheter "dead space", the area of the catheter tip which does not deliver ablative fluences, must be kept to a minimum. Fourth, most calcified lesions could be crossed. Fifth, the channels created were the size of the catheter and were generally smooth, with minimal damage to adjacent tissue [3–5].

Given the findings of the peripheral vascular trials, the FDA granted approval for trials of percutaneous coronary excimer laser angioplasty in August 1988 [6, 7]. The first patient was an 85 year old female who had 2 previous coronary artery bypass surgeries and 3 acutely successful PTCA procedures to the vein graft to her right coronary artery. After each balloon angioplasty the vein graft restenosed. After the third restenosis she presented with an episode of aborted sudden death. Given her inoperability and re-stenosis problems, excimer laser angioplasty was chosen to remove the recurrent subtotal stenosis at the site of the previous angioplasty. The procedure was accomplished without difficulty at an energy level of 35 mJ/mm^2. The procedure was acutely successful and the patient has been asymptomatic. Follow-up angiography at 1 year revealed a widely patent vein graft at the site of the laser angioplasty.

After our initial successes, approval was granted for a more extensive clinical trial at 14 centers around the United States. The following centers and principle investigators have participated in the excimer laser coronary angioplasty study.
- Cedars-Sinai Medical Center, Los Angeles, CA
    PI's: F. Litvack, N. Eigler
- South Miami Hospital, South Miami, FL
    PI's: J. Margolis, D. Krauthamer

P.W. Serruys, B.H. Strauss and S.B. King III (eds), Restenosis after Intervention with New Mechanical Devices, 475–483.

- St. Vincent's Hospital, Indianapolis, IN
  PI's: D. Rothbaum, T. Linnemeier
- Emory University Hospital, Atlanta, GA
  PI's: S. King, J. Douglas
- Mayo Clinic, Rochester, MN
  PI's: J. Bresnahan, G. Reeder
- George Washington University Hospital and The Washington Hospital
  Center, Washington, DC
  PI's: K. Kent, S. Satler, M. Leon
- Methodist Hospital, Houston, TX
  PI's: W. Spencer, A. Raizner
- Goleta Valley Community Hospital, Santa Barbara, CA
  PI: J. Vogel
- Hoag Hospital, Newport Beach, CA
  PI's: R. Haskell, P. McNalley
- Philadelphia Heart Insitute, Philadelphia, PA
  PI: W. Unterreker
- St. Luke's Hospital, Phoenix, AZ
  PI: M. Vater
- St. Luke's Hospital, Milwaukee, WI
  PI: F. Cummins
- Mercy Hospital, Pittsburgh, PA
  PI: V. Krishnaswami
- Mid-America Heart Institute, Kansas City, MO
  PI's: G Hartzler, W. Johnson

The first goal of this trial is to evaluate the safety, acute and long-term efficacy, and indications for excimer laser angioplasty. The second goal of the trial is to assess the technology and through data analysis develop patient selection criteria. The third goal of the trial is to pursue technological improvements to the system based on clinical experience. The laser and catheters used for this trial were designed, and constructed at Advanced Interventional Systems (AIS) in Irvine, CA. The laser is a 308 nm xenon chloride excimer laser operating at a laser output of 200–300 mJ/mm^2 at a pulse duration of 200 nanoseconds. This energy is delivered to the catheter by a specially designed fiber optic coupler. A family of catheters 1.3 mm, 1.6 mm and 2.0 mm diameter deliver 35–70 mJ/mm^2 to the tissue. All catheters are designed to operate in an over-the-wire fashion and ablate only on contact with tissue.

As of November 1990 1284 patients (77% male, 23% female) had been enrolled in the study [8]. All patients enrolled in the study signed an Informed Consent which was approved by the individual institutional IRB committees after FDA approval for the overall trial. The mean age of these patients was 62 years with a range from 30–87 years. Twenty-six percent of the patients had prior coronary artery bypass graft surgery and 36% of the patients had at least one prior balloon angioplasty. Symptom analysis based on Canadian Cardiovascular Society Functional Class criteria revealed that 33% of the patients were Class IV and 33% were Class III. An additional 20% of the patients were Class II, and the remaining 14% were evenly divided between Class I and Class 0. These demographics suggest a sicker than average patient population with extensive cardiovascular disease. In many cases patients were chosen for excimer laser angioplasty when all other therapeutic options had been exhausted.

1519 vessels were treated in 1284 patients. The distribution of arteries treated was as follows: left anterior descending coronary artery 41%; the right coronary artery 28%; the circumflex 16%; saphenous vein grafts 13%; and the left main (only when protected) 2%. Interestingly, 21% of the lesions were more than 20 mm in length; 31% ranged in length from 10–19 mm; and 43% were less than 10 mm in length. Mean lesion length was 14.6 mm. Ninety-one percent of the lesions were stenoses and 9% were occlusions.

Specific criteria were developed to determine if the procedure was successful [9]. Given the large potential discrepancy between the laser channel size and the arterial lumen, these criteria were designed to gauge success based upon the ability of the laser catheter to cross the lesion and the channel size created. The first 600 cases were performed only with the 1.6 mm catheter. By early 1990, larger diameter catheters were available and were used in this study. As the study progressed, improvements also occurred in catheter flexibility and trackability. Acute laser success is defined as a greater than 20% reduction in diameter stenosis with a channel diameter by laser alone of at least 0.8 mm with the 1.3 mm catheter, 1.0 mm with the 1.6 mm catheter, and 1.5 mm with the 2.0 mm catheter. Procedure success is defined as a less than 50% residual diameter stenosis at the termination of the procedure without complication, with or without adjunctive balloon angioplasty. The 1.6 mm catheter was used in 64% of the procedures; the 2.0 mm catheter was used in 24%; and although introduced late into this study, the 1.3 mm catheter was used in 11% of the procedures. Figure 1a shows a discrete calcified 11 mm long 95% stenosis in the proximal right coronary artery prior to attempted excimer laser angioplasty. This patient had 3 prior unsuccessful attempts at PTCA at 3 separate settings. Initial attempts to pass the laser catheter at 40 mJ/mm^2 were unsuccessful, however, the energy was increased to 50 mJ/mm^2 and the lesion provided little resistance as the catheter was moved across at the usual rate of 1 mm/second (Fig. 1b). The channel created by the laser permitted easy passage and completion of the procedure by balloon angioplasty. Figure 1c shows the angiogram after laser and balloon angioplasty. In this case, the laser permitted dilatation of a hard calcified lesion where previous attempts at balloon angioplasty had failed.

Laser success was achieved in 81% of the lesions and procedural success was achieved in 92% by the criteria listed above. Adjunctive balloon angioplasty was used in 56% of the lesions. Diameter stenosis at baseline was 86 ± 12%. Post-laser the stenosis decreased to 47 ± 23%, and with the ad-

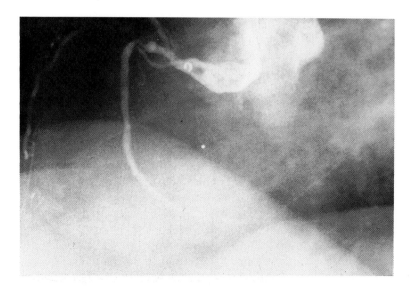

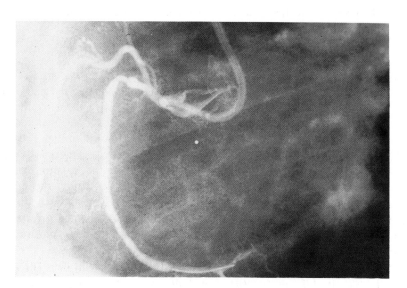

Figure 1. (A) and (B).

dition of adjunctive balloon angioplasty the residual stenosis was $25 \pm 18\%$. Success rates were dramatically uniform as assessed by both lesion location, vessel and lesion length. Procedural success was achieved in 95% of the saphenous vein grafts, 92% of both LAD and RCA lesions, 91% of circumflex lesions, and 95% of left main lesions. More dramatically, success by lesion length did not vary and was 92% in lesions longer than 20 mm, 93% in lesions less than 10 mm, and 96% in lesions of 10–19 mm length.

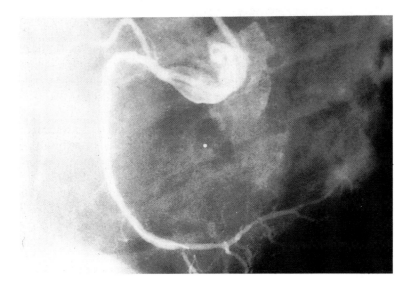

Figure 1. Excimer laser angioplasty in an undilatable lesion. These angiographic images show the right coronary artery of a 63 year old male after 3 unsuccessful attempts at PTCA. Although a wire would cross the lesion, balloon inflations to 18 atmospheres were unsuccessful (Fig. 1A). A 1.6 mm laser catheter did not pass at 40 mJ/mm², however, increasing the energy to 50 mJ/mm² resulted in easy passage of the laser catheter at 1 mm/second. This generated a 1.6 mm channel by quantitative coronary angiography (Fig. 1B). Figure 1C shows the final result after laser and balloon angioplasty produced a 3 mm diameter channel at the site of the lesion. Note the right angle bend in the coronary artery. Six month follow-up of this patient revealed no angiographic change.

Clinically significant complications occurred in 5.6% of patients including 3.1% CABG (includes emergent and in-hospital procedures), 2.1% non-Q-wave and Q-wave MI, and 0.4% death. Dissection was observed in 12.1% of the 1284 patients. However, of the patients with dissection, only half suffered any additional sequelae including acute occlusion, spasm, or perforation. Overall the acute occlusion rate was 6.5%. Most of these were readily treated with adjunctive balloon angioplasty. Embolism occurred in 0.8%, spasm in 1.6%, and aneurysm formation in 0.5%. Perforation occurred in 1.6% of patients. Of these, more than half occurred in patients with prior bypass surgery and no sequelae was reported. In 8 cases the perforation appeared to result from multiple passes in eccentric lesions at bend points. Six perforations occurred when attempts were made to enlarge the lumen without the benefit of wire guidance.

In terms of success, excimer laser angioplasty compares favorably to balloon angioplasty for treatment of long lesions [10]. Comparison of the recent study by Cook et al [11, 12] to that of Ellis et al [3] suggests that long complex lesions are ill-suited for balloon angioplasty, ACC/AHA type C lesions were successfully treated in 61% of cases by balloon angioplasty. In contrast, excimer laser angioplasty in the same type lesions showed a success rate of 84%. In B2 lesions the balloon angioplasty study revealed a 76% success rate while excimer laser angioplasty appeared successful in 95%. In type B1 lesions 96% of the lesions treated by excimer laser angioplasty were successfully opened while balloon angioplasty was successful in only 84%. However, in type A lesions balloon angioplasty was successful in 94% compared to 92% for excimer laser angioplasty. In the Cedars-Sinai experience, lesions classified by the BARI morphology suggested that laser angioplasty would be very effective in treatment of discrete, tubular, or diffusely diseased lesions, with success rates in excess of 93% [14, 15].

Comparison of complication rates between balloon angioplasty studies and excimer laser angioplasty studies is at best in its initial stages, since the patient populations may not be similar. Thus, comparisons made from this data must be interpreted with great caution. However, a review of the Cook and Ellis data clearly shows that balloon angioplasty in Type C lesions tends to produce a high rate of complications of approximately 20%, while the complication rate for excimer laser angioplasty for Type C lesions was only 7.5%. While these databases are not directly comparable, such large differences in both acute success and complication rates suggest that excimer laser angioplasty may be at least equal to if not superior to balloon angioplasty in the treatment of specific type B and C lesions.

Unlike balloon angioplasty, excimer laser angioplasty actually removes material during the process of vessel recanalization. However, the efficacy of this ablation process is dependent on many factors including the repetition rate, the force applied, the energy density at the site of ablation, the cutting area and dead space of the laser angioplasty catheter, and the biology of the lesion. Thus, it is difficult to control all of the factors which might affect the ablation process. Our research has demonstrated that the excimer laser removes tissue from the arterial lumen with minimal damage to adjacent structures. When properly performed, excimer laser recanalization of the artery leaves a smooth lumen for restoration of blood flow. The removal of tissue, coupled with the creation of a smooth recanalized artery, may produce an optimal result. By removing tissue and thus decreasing elastic recoil there may be a potential to decrease restenosis rates. However, since elastic recoil is only one component of the restenosis problem it may be difficult to prove this hypothesis.

The initial AIS protocols permitted use of energies from 30–60 mJ/mm^2 with the laser operating at 20 Hz. In this initial group 812 lesions were treated successfully with or without balloon angioplasty and were available for 6-month follow-up. Of these, 715 (88%) had clinical follow-up and 468 (58%) had angiographic follow-up at 6 months. In the follow-up period 10 patients (1.4%) died, 11 patients (1.5%) suffered myocardial infarction, 52 patients (7.3%) went on to coronary bypass grafting, and 108 patients (15%) required repeat intervention. The clinically determined restenosis rate was 29%. The angiographic restenosis rate was 51% [16–18].

Analysis of the above data showed that previous PTCA, lesion length or location, catheter size, adjunctive PTCA, gender, or presence or absence of dissection were not related to angiographic restenosis rates. The strongest predictor of restenosis after angioplasty was the per cent residual stenosis at the time of the final angiogram (laser stand-alone or laser-plus-balloon). Catheter tip energy (fluence) was statistically significant (p = .002) in predicting subsequent restenosis. The following table shows restenosis rates as a function of fluence in 445 patients [16].

Fluence (mJ/mm^2)	# Patients	# Restenosis	% Restenosis
30–34	52	36	69%
35–39	236	128	54%
40–44	89	42	47%
45–49	25	11	44%
50–54	43	11	26%

These data suggest that ablation at higher fluence rates may bring about a decrease in restenosis. The higher fluence rates potentially remove all types of tissue more effectively per pulse and may therefore produce a smooth, uniform surface during laser angioplasty. Additionally, the higher fluences prevent "Dotter" effects since complete ablation of the lesion occurs before the catheter is pushed through it.

Data collection and development of patient selection criteria is an ongoing process. The restenosis rates reported in this trial are similar to those for balloon angioplasty in similar lesions as described by Nobuyoshi et al [19], Pepine et al [20], and Vandormael et al [21]. Clinical endpoints, such as functional class, repeat intervention, MI, or death, suggest that excimer laser angioplasty is at least as safe and effective in the long-term treatment of type B and C lesions. Further data analysis and improved patient selection criteria should serve to further identify those patients who will benefit from excimer laser angioplasty. Our experience to date suggests that excimer laser angioplasty can be performed safely with risk of major complication similar to or less than that of PTCA [14, 15]. Excimer laser angioplasty is particularly effective as an alternative or adjunct to PTCA in the treatment of diffuse, calcified, long saphenous vein graft or aorto-ostial lesions. Our restenosis rates appear comparable to those found in PTCA of similar lesions [14, 15]. As catheter technology improves and higher energy densities are used uniformly, greater initial success can be expected and thus protocol modifications will occur. Investigators are now carefully examining the effects of higher energy densities and new catheter designs in an effort to determine if these factors will reduce restenosis rates. Whether these protocol modifications will have an impact on restenosis rates will require at least two to three more years of investigation.

References

1. Grundfest W, Litvack F, Forrester J (1990) Laser angioplasty. *J Coronary Artery Disease in Advances in Coronary Angioplasty*, Ed. Spencer King, III. 1(4):434–437.
2. Tsoi D, Whiting J, Eigler N, et al (1990) Excimer laser coronary angioplasty: results of quantitative coronary angiography in the first 50 patients. *J Am Coll Cardiol* 15(suppl A):246A.
3. Grundfest W S, Litvack F, Doyle L, et al (1990) Comparison of in vitro and in vivo thermal effects of argon and excimer lasers for laser angioplasty, abstracted. *Circulaɪion* 74(suppl 2):204.
4. Litvack F, Doyle L, Grundfest W S, et al (1990) In vivo excimer laser ablation: Acute and chronic effects on canine aorta, abstracted. *Circulation* , 74(suppl 2):360.
5. Litvack F, Grundfest W S, Segalowitz J, Papaioannou T, Goldenberg T, Laudenslager J, Hestrin L, Forrester J, Eigler N A, Cook S (1990) Interventional cardiovascular therapy by laser and thermal angioplasty. *Circulation* (Supplement IV) 81:3, 109–116.
6. Litvack F, Grundfest W S, Adler L, Hickey A, Segalowitz J, Hestrin L, Mohr F. Goldenberg T, Laudenslauger J, Forrester J (1989) Percutaneous excimer laser angioplasty of the lower extremities: results of an initial clinical trial. *Radiology* 172:331–335.
7. Litvack F, Grundfest W S, Eigler N L, Tsoi D, Goldenberg T, Laudenslager J, Forrester J (1989) Percutaneous excimer laser coronary angioplasty. *Lancet* 102–103, July 8.
8. Litvack F, Margolis J, Rothbaum D, Kent K, Bresnaha J, Untereker W, Cummins F, and the ELCA Investigators (1990) Excimer laser coronary angioplasty: acute results of the first 685 consecutive cases. *Circulation* 82(4):A278.
9. Shefer A, Eigler N L, Cook S L, Segalowitz J, Goldenberg, T, Laudenslager J B, Grundfest W S, Forrester J S, Litvack F (1990) Current status of excimer laser coronary angioplasty. *J of Invasive Cardio*, Health Management Publications, Inc. Vol 2, No. 6:255–264, November/December.
10. Ghazzal Z M B, Weintraub W S, Ba'albaki H A, et al (1990) PTCA of lesions longer than 20 mm: Initial outcome and restenosis. *Circulation* 82:2020 (Abstr).
11. Cook S L, Eigler N L, Shefer A, et al (1990) Percutaneous excimer laser coronary angioplasty of lesions not ideal for balloon angioplasty. Circulation. *Circulation* 84(2):632–643.
12. Cook S L, Eigler N L, Shefer A, et al (1991) Excimer laser coronary angioplasty of lesions not favorable for balloon angioplasty. *JACC* February 17(2):218A (Abstr).
13. Ellis S G, Vandormael M G, Cowley M J, et al (1990) Coronary morphologic and clinical determinants of procedural outcome with angioplasty for multivessel coronary disease: implications for patient selection. *Circulation* 82: 1193–1202.
14. Detre K M, Holmes D R, Holubkov R, et al (1990) Incidence and consequences of periprocedural occlusion: The 1985–1986 National Heart, Lung, and Blood Institute Percutaneous Transluminal Coronary Angioplasty Registry. *Circulation* 82:739–750.
15. Detre K M, Holubov R, Kelsey S, et al (1989) One-year follow-up results of the 1985–1986 National Heart, Lung, and Blood Institute's Percutaneous Transluminal Coronary Angioplasty Registry. *Circulation* 80:421–428.
16. Margolis J, Litvack F, Cummins F, Rothbam D, Bresnahan J, Untereker W, and the ELCA Investigators (1992) Affects of energy density on restenosis after excimer laser coronary angioplasty. *JACC* (Abstr in press).
17. Hartzler G, Litvack F, Margolis J, Leon M, Cummins F, Goldenberg T, and the ELCA Investigators (1992) Adjunctive excimer laser coronary angioplasty improves primary PTCA results for lesions >20 mm in length. *JACC* (abstr in press).
18. Litvack F, Margolis J, Cummins F, Breshnahan J, Goldenberg T, Rothbaum D, et al (1992) Excimer Laser Coronary Angioplasty (ELCA) Registry: report of the first consecutive 2,080 patients. *JACC* (Abstr in press).
19. Nobuyoshi M, Kimura T, Nosaka H, et al (1988) Restenosis after successful percutaneous

transluminal coronary angioplasty: serial angiographic follow-up of 229 patients. *JACC* September 12(3):616–623.
20. Pepine C J, Hirscheld J W, Macdonald R G, et al (1990) A controlled trial of corticosteroids to prevent restenosis after coronary angioplasty. *Circulation* 81:1753–1761.
21. Vandormael M G, Deligonul U, Kern M J, et al (1987) Multilesion coronary angioplasty: clinical and angiographic follow-up. *JACC* August 10(2):246–252.

23. Direct Laser Ablation of Coronary Atherosclerotic Plaque in Humans – The German Experience

ANDREAS BAUMBACH, KARL K. HAASE and
KARL R. KARSCH

Introduction

Laser angioplasty offers a new approach in the treatment of obstructive peripheral and coronary artery disease. Although the standard method balloon angioplasty has reached a high level in regard of safety and acute success [1–4], the treatment of complex lesions is still associated with increased rates of failure and complications [4]. Furthermore, despite rapid improvement throughout the past decade, we face persisting recurrence rates of 30 to 40% [5–8].

Balloon inflation results in plaque fracture, subintimal dissection and overdistension of the vessel wall [9]. This trauma is thought to be responsible for acute complications as well as the induction of a proliferative response leading to restenosis. Removal of the plaque instead of remodelling it, and the creation of a smooth channel as a result of effective laser ablation was sought as an alternative with the potential to optimize primary angioplasty success and furthermore to reduce the rate of restenosis [10].

Pulsed excimer laser irradiation results in ablation of atherosclerotic plaque with only minimal thermal side effects [11, 12]. In contrast to thermal laser angioplasty the ablation of calcified lesions is possible [13]. Laser energy has to be transmitted from the light source to the target; therefore the development of special transmission devices was the basic step towards the treatment of obstructive arterial lesions with laser energy. Experimental studies in postmortem specimens demonstrated the ablative efficacy of laser energy transmitted through a prototype catheter system consisting of quartz fibres [14]. Pulsed excimer laser angioplasty was subsequently performed to reduce coronary artery stenoses in humans [15, 16].

The first clinical experience was encouraging [15, 16], but acute success and long term results were beyond the results achieved with balloon angioplasty [16]. However, analysis of failure and procedural complications indicated, that major limitations of the procedure were linked to the current problems of the catheter system. Limited energy transmission and fibre

P.W. Serruys, B.H. Strauss and S.B. King III (eds), Restenosis after Intervention with New Mechanical Devices, 485–495.
© 1992 *Kluwer Academic Publishers. Printed in the Netherlands.*

Table 1. Procedural parameters of coronary excimer laser angioplasty in the three consecutive treatment groups.

	Series 1	Series 2	Series 3
	Xenon-chloride excimer laser Wavelength 308 nm Repetition rate 20 Hz		
Pulse width	60 ns	60 ns	115 ns
Catheters	Prototype 1.4 mm	1.3/1.5/1.8 mm	1.3/1.5/1.8 mm
No of fibres (100 μm)	20	20/30/35	20/30/35
Energy fluence	30 ± 5 mJ/mm^2	43 ± 14 mJ/mm^2	67 ± 19 mJ/mm^2
Time of laser energy delivery	123 ± 65 s	117 ± 72 s	51 ± 27 s

destruction were frequently observed. The unfavourable combination of low ablative effect and undesired mechanical effects was a reasonable cause for reduced primary success, frequent complications and a restenosis rate of 40% [16]. A new catheter system was developed and laser angioplasty with improved energy transmission was performed. With growing experience and advancing technology procedural and system parameters as well as the patient selection were modified.

In this chapter we compare the acute and long term results for three seperate treatment groups in respect of the stepwise improved clinical application of coronary excimer laser angioplasty.

Laser System

Excimer laser angioplasty was performed using a commercially available xenon-chloride excimer laser (Max 10, Technolas Inc., Munich Germany) that emitted light at a wavelength of 308 nm at a repetition rate of 20 Hz. The differences in regard of catheter devices and energy transmission in the three treatment groups are shown in Table 1.

The first series of patients (N = 60) was treated with a prototype laser catheter. This catheter had a diameter of 1.4mm, consisting of 20 quartz fibres with a core diameter of 100 μm around a central lumen for the 0.014 inch guide wire. The pulse duration was 60 ns. The time intervals for laser energy delivery and intermission were operator dependent. The energy density, measured at the catheter tip pre procedural was 30 ± 5 mJ/mm^2. The total time of laser energy delivery was 123 ± 65s. Mean loss of transmission from before to after the laser procedure was 45% in this series. Fibre destruction and total loss of energy transmission was frequently observed.

In a second series of patients (N = 40) we employed a catheter system with variable diameters of 1.3, 1.5 and 1.8 mm consisting of 20, 30 and 35 quartz fibres with a core diameter of 100 μm each. The fibre quality had been improved, resulting in a longer lifetime of the fibres and trusted energy transmission. The flexibility of the catheter devices was increased. Laser energy delivery was performed in trains of 3s with an intermission of at least 2s. Pulse duration was kept to 60 ns in this series. The mean energy density pre procedure was $43 \pm 14 \, \text{mJ/mm}^2$ with a mean loss of transmission of 30%. The total time of energy delivery was 117 ± 72 seconds. In the third and current series of patients the identical catheter system with further increased flexibility and improved coupling of the light into the fibres was used. The pulse duration was increased to 115 ns. Mean energy density before the procedure was $67 \pm 19 \, \text{mJ/mm}^2$ and mean loss of transmission was 13%. The total time of energy delivery was significantly reduced to 51 ± 27 seconds.

Laser Angioplasty

Angioplasty was performed via the transfemoral approach. 10000 U of heparin were infused intra-arterially. A 9F guiding catheter was placed in the ostium of the target vessel and the lesion was visualized after intracoronary application of 0.1 mg of nitroglycerin. The laser catheter was advanced over a 0.014 inch flexible guide wire which had been placed in the distal vessel. After reaching the proximal edge of the stenosis, laser energy application was started and the catheter was advanced, applying only moderate pressure on the device. Laser energy application was also performed during slow withdrawal of the catheter. The size of the improved catheters was selected according to the prestenotic vessel diameter and stenosis severity that was analysed in the previous diagnostic coronary angiogram. After each passage of the laser catheter, control angiography was performed to examine the result of ablation. If the control angiography after laser passage revealed a residual stenosis of more than 50% and the employment of a larger sized laser catheter was expected to be technically possible, the laser catheters were changed.

Criteria to stop laser angioplasty were: 1) a reduction of percent luminal diameter stenosis to less than 50%; 2) no further improvement of the result after the last laser irradiation cycle; 3) severe vasospasm (reduction in luminal diameter with vessel occlusion or reduced antegrade flow of contrast medium) or vessel occlusion due to dissection or thrombus formation. Additional balloon angioplasty was performed to improve an unsatisfactory result or to resolve vessel occlusion. After the final irradiation period or the last balloon inflation, vessel patency was assessed by repeat angiograms for 20 minutes. The patients were monitored in the coronary care unit for 24 hours. An early follow-up angiogram of the target vessel was routinely performed within 24 hours after the intervention.

Table 2. Patients baseline characteristics.

	Series 1	Series 2	Series 3
Number of patients	60	40	47
Male/Female	49/11	31/9	43/4
Mean age (yr)	59 ± 11	57 ± 9	56 ± 8
Extent of CAD			
1-vessel disease	41	24	27
2-vessel disease	13	12	12
3-vessel disease	6	4	8
Symptoms			
CCS 1	2	2	4
CCS 2	26	18	25
CCS 3	21	17	15
CCS 4	11	3	3
Target Vessel			
LAD	43	28	31
CX	7	3	3
RCA	10	9	14

CAD: Coronary artery disease.
CCS: Canadian Cardiovascular Society Classification.
LAD: Left anterior descending coronary artery.
CX: Left circumflex coronary artery.
RCA: Right coronary artery.

Clinical Experience

The patients baseline characteristics are presented in Table 2. Failure of the laser angioplasty attempt occurred in 5 patients in the first, 5 patients in the second and 7 patients in the third series. In 8 patients it was not possible to place the guide wire in the periphery of the target vessel, in 6 patients the target lesion could not be reached with the catheter and in three procedures the catheter failed to pass the lesion. Successful stand alone laser angioplasty with a patent vessel at the 24 hour control was performed in 23/55 patients of the first, 21/35 patients of the second and 24/41 procedures of the third group. Additional balloon dilatation was performed because of an insufficient result in 16 (29%), 6 (17%) and 5 (12%) patients of groups 1, 2 and 3 respectively. Balloon angioplasty was neccessary due to complications in 16, 5 and 12 patients. The acute results of coronary excimer laser angioplasty in the three patient series are presented in Table 3. Minor complications occurred in a high frequency in all three series. The onset of reversible vasospasm during and following laser energy delivery was consistently observed in 20 to 26% of the interventions. Membranes, indicating small dissection without reduction of antegrade flow, were also frequently angiographically documented. Additional contrast reduction, suspicious of thrombus formation, often affected the correct assessment of the angioplasty result immediately after the intervention, but in most of the cases this was not present at the routinely performed early follow-up angiography. Vessel occlusion, probably as a result of dissections, thrombus formation and vasospasm was

Table 3. Procedural outcome.

	Series 1	Series 2	Series 3
Number of procedures	60	40	48
Failure	5	5	7
% stenosis pre-intervention	81 ± 17%	72 ± 12%	70 ± 8%
Stand alone laser	23	24	24
Success	23	21	24
% stenosis post laser	27 ± 17%	31 ± 14%	35 ± 12%
MI and death	–	1	–
Early occlusion	2	–	–
Laser and balloon	32	11	17
% stenosis post laser	44 ± 14%	37 ± 15%	42 ± 15%
% stenosis post balloon	24 ± 15%	20 ± 15%	29 ± 14%
MI	2	–	–
Death	1	–	–
Early occlusion	2	–	–
Procedural complications following laser angioplasty			
Occlusion	11	7	12
Perforation	–	1	1
Dissection	10	9	6
Reversible spasm	19	7	11

MI: Myocardial infarction; % stenosis: percent luminal narrowing; Early occlusion: vessel occlusion documented at 24 hours control angiography

observed in 20 to 29% and is currently the main reason for additional balloon angioplasty. Vessel perforation with consecutive vessel closure was observed in two patients, both complications were resolved with balloon angioplasty and had no further clinical sequelae [17]. Acute myocardial infarction occurred in 3 patients. One additional patient with unstable angina pectoris developed cardiogenic shock and ventricular tachycardia and died three hours after laser and balloon angioplasty. Since the major complications in the first series occurred in patients with unstable angina pectoris, in the following series only patients with stable angina pectoris were included in the coronary excimer laser angioplasty treatment. In the second series one patient had abrupt vessel closure after laser treatment of an eccentric stenosis of the LAD, which could not be reopened by balloon dilatation. This patient developed a Q-wave infarction with an initially uncomplicated clinical course. 48 hours after discharge from the coronary care unit, this patient died suddenly. An autopsy was not performed. No fatal complication during the in-hospital period occurred in the third treatment series.

Restenosis

Angiographic control was performed within 6 months after the intervention in the majority of all patients. The endpoints of the study were follow-up angiography at 6 months, prior follow-up angiography in patients with recur-

Table 4. Follow-up data.

	Series 1	Series 2	Series 3
No. of patients for follow-up	52	32	41
Death	–	1	1
Refused CA/Lost to FU	5	5	5
Control angiography	47	26	34
Restenosis (1) or (2)	22	12	11
Restenosis (1)	22	12	10
Restenosis (2)	22	11	8
Re-PTCA	12	10	9
CABG	3	2	–

CA: Control angiography; FU: Follow-up; PTCA: Percutaneous transluminal coronary angioplasty; CABG: Coronary artery bypass grafting.
Restenosis is defined as a diameter stenosis $\geq 50\%$ and one or both of the following criteria: (1) loss of gain in luminal diameter $\geq 50\%$; (2) reduction in luminal diameter ≥ 0.72 mm.

rent symptoms of angina pectoris, re-PTCA, CABG, myocardial infarction and death. No late follow-up angiography was performed in patients with failure of laser angioplasty, persistent vessel occlusion after the treatment, in-hospital myocardial infarction and vessel occlusion at the 24-hours control. Quantitative coronary analysis was performed for the interventional and the follow-up angiography using identical projections and settings of the angiographic X-ray system. Angiographic restenosis was defined as a diameter stenosis severity $\geq 50\%$ and one or both of the following criteria:
(1) loss of gain in luminal diameter $\geq 50\%$
(2) reduction in luminal diameter ≥ 0.72 mm [7].

All clinical and angiographic data were entered in a computer-based registry. The follow-up data for the three treatment series are presented in Table 4. Figure 1 provides an illustration of the restenosis rate seperately for stand-alone procedures and combined laser and balloon interventions.

First Series

No deaths and no myocardial infarction occurred during the follow-up period. One patient was lost to follow-up and four patients refused control angiography. The latter patients had no episodes of chest pain and no signs of ischemia during treadmill exercise at maximum work load. In 47 patients an angiographic restudy could be achieved. Angiographic restenosis according to the above mentioned criteria was found in 22 patients. In 6 of these 22 patients, an occlusion of the target vessel was documented at late follow-up angiography. As shown in Fig. 1, the incidence of restenosis was higher in those patients, who were initially treated with laser and balloon angioplasty than in those patients, who were treated with laser therapy alone. In 15 patients re-PTCA (N = 12) or CABG (N = 3) was performed. Restenosis

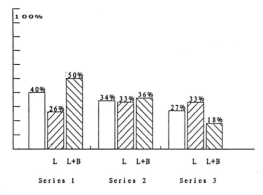

Figure 1. Incidence of restenosis in the three treatment series. Blank bar: Overall restenosis rate; L: Stand alone laser procedures; L + B: Combined laser and balloon angioplasty.

after stand alone laser angioplasty occurred more often in patients with interventions in the left circumflex and right coronary artery than in those patients, in whom the left anterior descending artery was the target vessel. (see Fig. 2).

Second Series

One patient had sudden death while participating in a tennis tournament 3 months after the intervention [18]. No myocardial infarctions were documented during the follow-up period. One patient was lost to follow-up, four patients refused control angiography, all of them being asymptomatic at rest and during exercise. Control angiography was performed in 26 patients. Restenosis was found in 12 patients and re-intervention was performed in

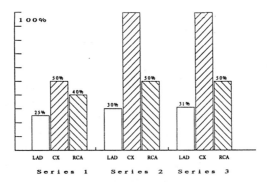

Figure 2. Restenosis after successful stand alone laser angioplasty in different target vessels. Restenosis rate = (target vessel showing restenosis/ all target vessels controlled angiographically)*100. LAD: Left anterior descending coronary artery; CX: Left circumflex coronary artery; RCA: Right coronary artery.

all of those patients (see Table 4). A difference between stand-alone laser procedures and combined treatment with additional balloon angioplasty was not found in this series (see Fig. 1). Again the incidence of restenosis after stand-alone laser angioplasty was higher in the left circumflex and right coronary artery than in the left anterior descending artery (see Fig. 2).

Third Series

During the follow-up period, one patient had sudden death while he was jogging. No patient experienced a myocardial infarction. Five patients refused control angiography, four of them having no episodes of chest pain and no signs of ischemia during treadmill exercise at maximum work load. In one patient who was asymptomatic, angiography was not performed because of a contraindication for the invasive study. In 34 patients control angiography was performed. Restenosis was observed in 11 patients, re-intervention was performed in 9 patients (see Table 4). Again we found the lowest incidence of restenosis after stand-alone procedures in the left anterior descending artery (see Fig. 2).

Discussion

The three treatment series comprise a consecutive single center patient population, therefore being good indicators for the progression in the clinical application of coronary excimer laser angioplasty. The early laser angioplasty trials [19–23], including our first series [15, 16], documented the safety and feasibility of the method. The acute results of the following series suggest, that advancement in laser and device technology resulted in improvement of the primary success rate of stand-alone laser angioplasty. The major issue in percutaneous transluminal coronary angioplasty, however, is the induction of a new local process of the disease leading to restenosis [5–8, 24, 25]. It remains to be shown, whether any method of traumatic plaque reduction provides the therapeutic capability of a persistent vessel patency [24, 25]. The long term results of our coronary excimer laser angioplasty study groups showed an improvement towards the results that are currently achieved with balloon angioplasty, but yet failed to show significant advantages.

The overall restenosis rate could be reduced from 40% in the first to 27% in the current series. Separate analysis of stand-alone procedures and combined laser and balloon interventions showed a markedly increased recurrence rate for combined interventions in the first group, suggesting that the additional trauma of balloon dilatation would lead to a higher proliferative response [16]. The comparable results of stand-alone and combined interventions in the consecutive series, suggest that other factors may have been responsible for this difference in the initial series. Balloon dilatation was frequently performed after unsuccessful laser ablation. Laser ablation was incomplete and probably ineffective in frequent cases due to limited energy transmission and fibre destruction. Therefore mechanical side effects may have been increased in this group compared to the stand-alone interventions. Additionally the combined treatment group includes 9 of 11 patients with unstable angina pectoris, who are known to have a higher risk of restenosis than patients with stable angina pectoris [5, 6]. In the second and third series higher energy transmission and longer lifetime of the fibres increased the ablation efficacy, reduced the frequency tip of fibre destruction and fluence-decrease below the ablative threshold. In combination with improved catheter flexibility, it is conceivable that the mechanical trauma was reduced. Additional balloon dilatation, either for improvement of the result or to resolve vessel occlusion did not show a negative influence on the long term result compared to stand alone procedures. The benefit of routinely performed additional balloon angioplasty for maximum stenosis reduction remains open to question. The stand-alone laser treatment group, however, is of special interest for the differentiated analysis of restenosis after plaque reduction vs. plaque remodelling. The major limitation of our patient population is the small absolute number of patients. Subgroup analysis is therefore affected by reduced statistical significance. Thus, interpretation of the stand-alone interventions, including our observation of the different longterm outcome after stand-alone laser treatment of the left anterior descending artery compared to the left circumflex and right coronary arteries will have to be verified in larger study populations. Additionally the individual influence of vessel diameter and vessel bending for the long term outcome require further analysis. Previous studies addressing restenosis after PTCA found either no significant difference for the target vessels [2, 5] or even an increased risk of restenosis after treatment of the left anterior descending artery [6, 8]. The need for multicenter trials for the future assessment of the acute and long-term success and indications for the primary employment of laser angioplasty in the treatment of coronary artery disease is obvious. Final statements, however, require a further developed system technology and device technology, comparable to the current standard in conventional PTCA.

Conclusion

Coronary excimer laser angioplasty continues to progress. Much has been learned from the early trials in terms of operating parameters, system handling and patient selection. Furthermore, improvement of the acute and long-term success rates underline the benefit of optimized energy transmission devices. Increased efficacy was documented by a significant reduction of the mean total energy delivery time per procedure in our third series. Thus far however, the most striking disadvantage of the system remains the imbalance between ablative area and total catheter tip area. Since only tissue in direct contact to the fibre tip can be transferred from the solid to the plasma phase, the amount of tissue which can effectively be ablated is directly dependent on the area of the fibres at the tip of the catheter devices. Further increase of ablative efficacy can be expected for larger catheters with an enhanced ablative area and minimized "dead space" of the catheter tip. It remains to be clarified, whether the longterm success rate has reached the final stage, or whether the increase in ablative efficacy will lead to yet further improvement of the clinical success.

References

1. Kent K M, Bentivoglio L G, Block P C, Cowley M J, Dorros G, Gosselin A J, Grüntzig A, Myler R K, Simpson J, Stertzer S H, Williams D O, Fisher L, Gillespie M J, Detre K, Kelsey S, Mullin S M, Mock M B (1982) Percutaneous transluminal coronary angioplasty: report from the registry of the National Heart, Lung, and Blood Institute. *Am J Cardiol* 49:2011–2019.
2. Myler R K, Topol E J, Shaw R E, Stertzer S H, Clark D A, Fishman J, Murphy M C (1987) Multiple vessel coronary angioplasty: Classification, results, and patterns of restenosis in 494 consecutive patients. *Cathet Cardiovasc Diagn* 13:1–15.
3. Kahn J K, Hartzler G O (1990) Frequency and causes of failure with contemporary coronary angioplasty and implications for new technologies. *Am J Cardiol* 66:858–860.
4. Ellis S G, Vandormael M G, Cowley M J, DiSciascio G, Deligonul U, Topol E J, Bulle T M and the Multivessel Angioplasty Prognosis Study Group (1990) Coronary morphologic and clinical determinants of procedural outcome with angioplasty for multivessel coronary disease. *Circulation* 82:1193–1202.
5. Holmes D R, Vlietstra R E, Smith H C, Vetrovec G W, Kent K M, Cowley M J, Faxon D P, Gruentzig A R, Kelsey S F, Detre K M, VanRaden M J, Mock M B (1984) Restenosis after percutaneous transluminal angioplasty: a report from the PTCA registry of the National Heart, Lung, and Blood Institute. *Am J Cardiol* 53:77C–81C.
6. Leimgruber P P, Roubin G S, Hollman J, Cotsonis G A, Meier B, Douglas J S, King III S B, Gruentzig A R (1986) Restenoisis after successful coronary angioplasty in patients with single-vessel disease. *Circulation* 73:710–717.
7. Serruys P W, Luijten H E, Beatt K J, Geuskens P J, De Feyter P J, Van Den Brand M, Reiber J H C, Ten Katen H J, Van Es G A, Hugenholtz P G (1988) Incidence of restenosis after successful coronary angioplasty: a time-related phenomenon. *Circulation* 77:361–371.
8. Grigg L E, Kay T W H, Valentine P A, Larkins R, Flower D J, Manolas E G, O'Dea K, Sinclair A J, Hopper J L, Hunt D (1989) Determinants of restenosis and lack of effect of dietary supplementation with eicosapentaenoic acid on the incidence of coronary artery stenosis after angioplasty. *J Am Coll Cardiol* 13:665–672.
9. Waller B F (1986) Pathology of new interventions used in the treatment of coronary heart disease. *Curr Probl Cardiol* 11 (12):665–760.
10. Forrester J S (1988) Laser angioplasty. *Circulation* 78:777–779.
11. Grundfest W S, Litvack F, Forrester J R, Goldenberg T S V I, Seran H J C, Morgenstern L, Fishbein M, Mc Dermid S, Rider D M, Pacala T J, Laudenslager J B (1985) Laser ablation of human atherosclerotic plaque without adjacent tissue injury. *J Am Coll Cardiol* 5:929–33.
12. Isner J M, Donaldson R F, Deckelbaum L I, Clarke R H, Laliberte S M, Ucci A A, Salem D N, Konstam M A (1985) The excimer laser: gross, light microscopic and ultrastructural analysis of potential disadvantages for use in laser therapy of cardiovascular disease. *J Am Coll Cardiol* 6:1102–1109.

13. Litvack F, Grundfest W S, Goldenberg T S V I, Laudenslager J, Pacala T, Segalowitz J, Forrester J S (1988) Pulsed laser angioplasty: wavelength, power and energy dependencies relevant to clinical application. *Lasers Surg Med* 8:60–65.
14. Haase K K, Wehrmann M, Duda S, Karsch K R (1990) Experimentelle intrakoronare Excimer- Laserangioplastie. *Z Kardiol* 79:183–188.
15. Karsch K R, Haase K K, Mauser M, Ickrath O, Voelker W, Duda S (1989) Percutaneous excimer laser angioplasty: initial clinical results. *Lancet* 2:647–650.
16. Karsch K R, Haase K K, Voelker W, Baumbach A, Mauser M, Seipel L (1990) Percutaneous coronary excimer laser angioplasty in patients with stable and unstable angina pectoris. Acute results and incidence of restenosis during 6–month follow-up. *Circulation* 81:1849–1859.
17. Haase K K, Baumbach A, Voelker W, Kühlkamp V, Karsch K R (1991) Gefäßwandperforation nach koronarer Excimer Laser Angioplastie. *Z Kardiol* 80:230–233.
18. Karsch K R, Haase K K, Wehrmann M, Hassenstein S, Hanke H (1991) Smooth muscle cell proliferation and restenosis after stand-alone coronary excimer laser angioplasty. *J Am Coll Cardiol* 17:991–4.
19. Litvack F, Grundfest W, Eigler N, Tsoi D, Goldenberg T, Laudenslager J, Forrester J (1989) Percutaneous excimer laser coronary angioplasty (letter). *Lancet* 2:102–103.
20. Sanborn T A, Hershman R A, Torre S R, Sherman W, Cohen M, Ambrose J A (1989) Percutaneous excimer laser coronary angioplasty. *Lancet* 2:616.
21. Litvack F, Eigler N, Margolis J R, Grundfest W S, Rothbaum D, Linnemeier T, Hestrin L, Tsoi D, Cook S L, Krauthamer D, Goldenberg T, Laudenslager J R, Segalowitz J, Forrester J S (1990) Percutaneous excimer laser coronary angioplasty. *Am J Cardiol* 66:1027–1032.
22. Werner G, Buchwald A, Unterberg C, Voth E, Kreuzer H, Wiegand V (1991) Excimer laser angioplasty in coronary artery disease. *Eur Heart J* 12:24–29.
23. Sanborn T A, Torre S R, Sharma S K, Hershman R A, Cohen M, Sherman W, Ambrose J (1991) Percutaneous coronary excimer laser-assisted balloon angioplasty: initial clinical and quantitative angiographic results in 50 patients. *J Am Coll Cardiol* 17:94–99.
24. Liu M W, Roubin G S, King III S B (1989) Restenosis after coronary angioplasty. *Circulation* 79:1374–1387.
25. Waller B F (1989) "Crackers, breakers, stretchers, drillers, scrapers, shavers, burners, welders and melters" – the future treatment of atherosclerotic coronary artery disease? A clinical-morphologic assessment. *J Am Coll Cardiol* 13:969–987.

24. Summary

SPENCER B. KING III

Introduction

The preceding chapters have been collected to review the potential for new mechanical devices to assist in producing a better long-term result than balloon angioplasty. Data as available and opinion, liberally provided, are presented in a state of the art format. Before concluding that some of these devices are leading us in the correct path toward solving restenosis, we should review the problem as we now face it with balloon angioplasty.

The first demonstration of coronary angioplasty was performed on a dog coronary artery and the obstruction was produced by an external ligature. Gruentzig's experiment demonstrated that the artery could be opened and the impressive hemodynamic result was undeniable. However, translation from this model to the atherosclerotic human plaque seemed far away. Even if the artery opened, would there not be a violent response to this injury leading if not to immediate thrombosis, then surely to later scarring and renarrowing? Gruentzig of course knew that intimal proliferation would occur during healing. He learned that from Dotter [1] and from his own early work with Dotter's technique [2] in peripheral arteries, but perhaps the healing would be self-limited leaving an adequate permanent lumen.

It was learned very early that restenosis was a frequent consequence of angioplasty but it was not inevitable. In fact in the early days of PTCA, 70% of the patients maintained open arteries without hemodynamically significant narrowing [3]. This rate of restenosis was obtained in relatively ideal candidates for PTCA. They were young with proximal discrete lesions in relatively large arteries. As PTCA has been expanded to more complex lesions, the rate of restenosis has actually increased.

Mechanism of Angioplasty and Restenosis

What is the mechanism of this renarrowing? First it is important to briefly review what is happening during PTCA. The endothelium in the area of

P.W. Serruys, B.H. Strauss and S.B. King III (eds), Restenosis after Intervention with New Mechanical Devices, 497–504.
© 1992 *Kluwer Academic Publishers. Printed in the Netherlands.*

dilatation is surely denuded but very importantly the artery is also stretched and the plaque is often split and disrupted from the vessel wall. Normal wall segments opposite large eccentric plaques are stretched and the media and internal elastic membrane are often ruptured [4]. Following the injury, since the endothelium has been denuded, platelets are deposited on the surface and begin to adhere and accumulate. Chesebro and Fuster have shown that deep injury causes much more platelet accumulation than superficial injury [5]. The altered blood flow pattern and the loss of laminar flow also promote platelet accumulation and thrombus formation. The platelets release growth factors for smooth muscle cells and fibrocytes which go on to migrate and divide. An important question which is still unanswered is how critical is the platelet thrombus formation in sending this proliferative signal. Other mediators of the restenosis process exist [6]. Endothelial denudation eliminates the elaboration of protective substances from endothelial cells like heparins and endothelial derived relaxant factor. The acutely damaged artery wall responds with an inflammatory response as well as an autocrine stimulus to smooth muscle cell migration and proliferation. Continued cell division and subsequent elaboration of extracellular matrix results in formation of a neointima of varying thickness until the process runs its course.

Even though this process occurs in all dilated arteries, the result on the final lumen opening after healing is quite variable and depends not only on the degree of proliferative response, but also on the degree of narrowing which remains following angioplasty. Two processes begin the decrement in arterial dimensions, thrombus formation and elastic recoil. Either can result in an early decrease in the area dilated when compared to the inflated balloon. Serruys showed that elastic recoil post PTCA results in a 50% loss in the lesion cross-sectional area compared to the inflated balloon [7]. Inspection of arteries post PTCA, at surgery, or post mortem examination and also by angioscopy show that the plaque is often disrupted from the wall but occupies a significant part of the lumen. Deep fissures in the plaque and between the plaque and the more normal wall segment open with balloon pressure but partially recoil after balloon deflation, thereby compromising the lumen. These geometric defects combine with the deep fissuring into highly thrombogenic material, creating a fertile field for platelet deposition, accumulation and thrombosis. Examination of post PTCA results leads one to dream of other ways to open the artery. This, in fact, is what has happened in the development of the new technologies described in this volume.

How can new technologies improve this early angioplasty result and how can such an improvement contribute to the ultimate patency of the vessel?

New Technologies for Angioplasty

New technologies have attempted to solve four failings of balloon angioplasty: to create a smoother lumen free of clefts and ridges, to remove plaque material from the lumen, to leave a larger post therapy lumen than can be obtained with balloon angioplasty, and to avoid the severe arterial stretch which disrupts the media and elastica. In the preceding chapters, we have seen that new techniques have imperfectly met these requirements. Nonetheless, they continue to be refined and the mechanisms by which each might contribute to the sustained patency is worth reviewing.

Atherectomy

Directional atherectomy by design and intent should remove plaque material while leaving undisturbed the normal portion of the vessel. In practice, however, it is impossible with current devices to avoid the stretch from the Dotter effect of passing a large 6 French or 7 French device through a tight coronary stenosis. Some goals are met, however. Plaque is removed even though it is less than one half the calculated volume and the residual lumen is usually larger than one obtains with balloon angioplasty alone. The fact that overall restenosis has not been reduced is disappointing but the apparent reduction in restenosis rates in the proximal anterior descending coronary artery is encouraging [8]. This segment just distal to the left main is difficult to dilate completely with balloons and therefore directional atherectomy holds a significant advantage in gaining a larger initial lumen. Likewise, very eccentric plaques in large vessels which do not dilate well with the balloon can be opened more completely with atherectomy. As has been pointed out, initial results with atherectomy have shown better restenosis rates when applied to primary lesions than restenotic lesions and in fact the restenosis rate in vein grafts with restenotic lesions has been prohibitive. As pointed out by Hinohara [9] and Yock [10], the amount of tissue removed may not be as important as the final artery size following atherectomy whether measured by angiography or endovascular ultrasound.

Extraction atherectomy has, by its design, not attempted to open the artery as completely as directional atherectomy. The mechanism here is forward cutting ahead of the device, thereby avoiding the stretch injury common to the balloon [11]. Ideally the surface cut should be smooth and cylindrical, however the size of the final lumen is limited by the size of the catheter which can be passed through the guide catheter and proximal coronary artery. Therefore, even though tissue is removed, the final lumen is not usually larger than that obtained with the balloon alone. The restenosis results are early returns and the effect on restenosis must be measured in subgroups to see if some exhibit better long-term results than others. Much of the investigation has concentrated on older vein grafts because of the device's unique ability to aspirate material from the vessel lumen.

Rotablator likewise produces a lumen by abrading ahead of the device and to the side. Some stretching may occur but there seems to be a preferential tissue removal from firm and even calcified tissue with relative spearing

of more normal elastic tissue [12]. Endothelial denudation is likely circumferential but less medial disruption is likely. The device must work within the
dimensions of the artery and therefore the resultant lumen is not usually as
large as one obtains with the balloon and sometimes balloon stretch is added
to achieve a larger opening. Restenosis data is still sketchy and as Bertrand
suggests, may be improved by the addition of balloon angioplasty [13].
Subgroup analysis is not yet possible.

Laser

Laser therapy in two forms has been advocated as an alternative or adjunct
to balloon angioplasty. The over-the-wire laser systems using a pulsed laser
source, usually excimer, has now been tested clinically in a large cohort of
patients [14]. The strategy regarding restenosis prevention is to avoid balloon
stretch injury by vaporizing tissue ahead of the device leaving a cleanly cut
lumen. Since the device must be contained inside the artery, device sizing is
usually limited to approximately two thirds the size of the unobstructed
portion of the artery. This strategy means that the operator must judge that
the residual narrowing left after laser therapy is adequate or that additional
balloon angioplasty is required. As with the rotablator, if the partially dilated
result is accepted, then the amount of intimal proliferation required to reach
clinically significant restenosis is relatively small. If balloon angioplasty is
added, then the planned avoidance of stretch injury is lost. Data so far have
not suggested a reduction in restenosis using the technique although many
sites selected have been in relatively small arteries with tubular lesions that
are not discrete. Guidance systems which could enable more tissue removal
without excessive arterial stretch will be necessary to evaluate whether limited trauma leaving a large residual lumen is possible and whether it can
reduce the restenosis rate.

Laser balloon angioplasty, designed to achieve a smoother lumen by
sealing cracks and flaps, and a larger lumen by inhibiting elastic recoil, has
been used in limited clinical trials. The final diameter stenosis achieved was
measurably larger than that found in control patients treated with balloon
angioplasty alone but restenosis was not reduced [15]. In fact, higher energy
levels seemed to increase the chance of restenosis over control patients.

Stents

Stent devices have been developed for balloon delivery as well as self expanding delivery systems. The mechanism by which stents reduce restenosis
is the formation of a large relatively smooth lumen which must accumulate
a significant amount of neointimal thickening in order to produce clinically
significant restenosis. The Wallstent was tested in Europe and the early

experience was encouraging as regards restenosis [16]. Core laboratory analysis has identified two mechanisms of renarrowing: the late fibrointimal proliferation and early thrombotic occlusion. Although the late restenosis figures taken alone suggest that a stent expanded to a size greater than 3.2 mm has a good chance of sustained patency, the early thrombotic occlusions have been sobering. Trials were discontinued but have resumed in limited centers for large vein graft lesions.

The Palmaz-Schatz stent has undergone extensive clinical use and encouraging results have been reported [17, 18]. These stents, however, have been used principally in large vessels with relatively short lesions in straight segments. Thrombosis has not occurred as frequently as with the Wallstent but a vigorous anticoagulation program has led to complications and is a negative aspect of stenting. Candidates for stenting have been selected for the presence of relatively straight segments and relatively large lumens. The Wiktor stent showed a slightly higher restenosis rate but patients selected all had restenotic lesions [19]. In addition, long lesions have routinely been excluded. experience with the Gianturco-Roubin stent has been limited mainly to use for acute closure. In this setting restenosis, not surprisingly, occurs in about one half of the patients [20].

Clinical Investigation

Many questions regarding the theoretical advantages of new devices in creating large smooth lumens without stretch injury will not be answered by the clinical observational studies which have been done so far. These experiences have provided valuable information on the best use niches for obtaining improved acute results and on the other hand have identified areas in which some devices are inappropriate. However, in order to judge their value in reducing restenosis compared to balloon angioplasty, controlled randomized trials will be necessary. Some of these are already underway. The STRESS trial of the Palmaz-Schatz stent in native arteries and vein grafts randomized against balloon angioplasty is to begin soon. Another trial, CAVEAT, just concluded at over 25 sites, compares directional atherectomy to balloon angioplasty. These trials, of course, study patients judged to be suitable for new technologies and are designed to detect differences in quantitatively measured restenosis on 6 month angiograms. An important issue to be examined will be which patients are entered into the studies since selection of lesions which are not suitable for directional atherectomy or stents, such as those located in small arteries, will bias results toward the balloon and selection of a great many lesions with very eccentric morphology in large vessels might bias results towards directional atherectomy or stents. The optimal situation would be to have adequate numbers to do extensive subgroup comparison but these trials will not likely carry significant statistical power to do this. Nonetheless subgroups will inevitably be examined. Other devices will have to be measured against balloons as well.

In addition to randomized trials, careful registry assessment of the activity involving new devices is underway. The NHLBI has funded a registry called NACI (New Approaches to Coronary Interventions) with a large number of centers participating. This will give a profile of the patients selected, the success rates, and the complications in new device investigation. An important aspect of this registry will be the performance of core laboratory analysis of new device results.

Adjunctive Therapy

It is unclear whether the post instrumentation adjunctive therapy should be the same for new devices as for balloon angioplasty. Some previously tried strategies, such as anticoagulation, which had not worked in balloon angioplasty, may play a more prominent role in the new technologies. Certainly vigorous prolonged anticoagulation is an integral part of stenting. Could this strategy be playing a role in reducing restenosis? Could such a strategy also help in atherectomy procedures? These questions may stimulate further trials.

One thing is clear from new technology utilization so far. All cause arterial injury and all result in neointimal regrowth. The impact of that regrowth will be less in very large arteries since the same neointimal thickening leaves a larger residual lumen at the stenosis than is the case in small arteries. Since none of the new technologies have eliminated restenosis, it will be necessary to test additional adjunctive methods for altering regrowth. Systemic therapies under investigation include anticoagulation, anti-platelet antibodies, anti-thrombin agents, lipid lowering agents or inhibitors of the mediators of restenosis.

Experience with adjunctive therapy in stented patients has shown that occasionally the healing response can be altered. Patients undergoing post-stent therapy with steroids and colchicine in addition to a vigorous anticoagulation program have been noted to develop healing defects resulting in aneurysmal formation [21].

Local Drug Delivery

Our experience with post-procedure bleeding using the new devices, all of which require large bore guide catheters, makes the prolonged use of systemic anticoagulation less than attractive. Local anti-thrombotic therapy is needed, especially for stent placement. Future research will focus on coatings for stents and possibly total polymeric stents which are not only drug delivery systems, but may also be biodegradable. Development, approval, and implementation of these systems may take a long time. It may be helpful to apply local therapy at the site of an intervention using various delivery systems. One such system is the porous balloon through which substances can be injected into the vessel wall. Experimental compounds ranging from heparin to messenger RNA have been injected in attempts to alter the regrowth pattern. This work, utilizing porcine coronary and other animal models, may point to effective strategies for the future.

What approach should be used when restenosis occurs? The syndrome of device hopping exists. Patients and physicians are not infrequently heard to say "If the balloon didn't work, let's try the laser and if that failed, how about a stent?" This attitude is understandable even though often there is little data to suggest that a new device will be more effective in preventing restenosis than another balloon dilatation. Despite important new developments described in detail in this book, balloon angioplasty remains the appropriate interventional device for most lesions requiring such therapy. Hopefully this will not always be the case and new approaches will make restenosis a rarity.

The contribution of balloon angioplasty and its offspring, the new devices, has greatly expanded our knowledge of coronary atherosclerosis and restenosis. Some of these devices will prove helpful and will be used, and some will not and will be discarded. It is a rapidly evolving field and our hope is that this volume will contribute to further advances in managing coronary artery disease not only through improved acute results but also by decreasing restenosis.

References

1. Dotter C T, Judkins M P (1964) Transluminal treatment of arteriosclerotic obstruction. Description of a new technique and the preliminary report of its application. *Circulation* 30:654
2. Zeitler E, Gruntzig A, Schoop (1978) *Percutaneous Vascular Recanalization Technique Application. Clinical Results.* Springer-Verlag, Berlin
3. Leimgruber P P, Roubin G S, Hollman J, Cotsonis G A, Meier B, Douglas J S, King S B III, Gruentzig A R (1986) Restenosis after successful coronary angioplasty in patients with single-vessel disease. *Circulation* 73:710–717
4. Waller B F (1989) Crackers, breakers, stretchers, drillers, scrapers, shavers, burners, welders and melters – the future treatment of atherosclerotic coronary artery disease? A clinical-morphologic assessment. *J Am Coll Cardiol* 13:969–987
5. Chesebro J H, Lam J Y T, Badimon L, Fuster V (1987) Restenosis after arterial angioplasty: a hemorrheologic response to injury. *Am J Cardiol* 60:10B–16B
6. Liu M W, Roubin G S, King S B III (1989(Restenosis after coronary angioplasty. Potential biologic determinants and role of intimal hyperplasia. *Circulation* 79:1374–1387
7. Serruys P W, Luijten H E, Beatt K J et al (1988) Incidence of restenosis after successful coronary angioplasty: a time-related phenomenon. *Circulation* 77:361–371
8. Hinohara T, Selmon M R, Robertson G C, Brader L, Simpson J (1990) Directional atherectomy. New approaches for treatment of obstructive coronary and peripheral vascular disease. *Circulation* 81(Suppl IV):IV79–91

9. Hinohara T, Simpson J B, Robertson G C, Selmon M R (1992) Restenosis: Directional coronary atherectomy. In: Serruys P, Strauss B, King S III (eds) *Restenosis in the Coronary Arteries Following Intervention with New Mechanical Devices*. Kluwer Academic Publishers, Dordrecht

10. Yock P G, Fitzgerald P J, Sudhir K, Hargrave V K, Ports T A (1992) Ultrasound guidance for catheter-based plaque removal and ablation techniques: potential impact on restenosis. In: Serruys P, Strauss B, King S III (eds) *Restenosis in the Coronary Arteries Following Intervention with New Mechanical Devices*. Kluwer Academic Publishers, Dordrecht

11. O'Neill W, Meany T B, Kramer B, Knopf W B, Pichard A D, Sketch M H, Stack R S (1991) The role of atherectomy in the management of saphenous vein grafts disease. *J Am Coll Cardiol* 17(Suppl A):384A

12. Arbel R, O'Neill W, Auth D, Hande N, Nixdorf U, Rupprecht H J, Dietz U, Meyer J (1989) High-frequency rotablation of occluded coronary artery during heart catheterization. *Cathet Cardiovasc Diagn* 17:56–58

13. Bertrand M E, Lablanche J M, Leroy F et al (1992)Percutaneous transluminal coronary rotary ablation with rotablator: European experience. In: Serruys P, Strauss B, King S III (eds) *Restenosis in the Coronary Arteries Following Intervention with New Mechanical Devices*. Kluwer Academic Publishers, Dordrecht

14. Grundfest W S, Litvack F, Forrester J (1990) Laser angioplasty. *Cor Art Dis* 1:430–437

15. Spears J R, Reyes V P, Wynne J, Fromm B S, Sinofsky E L, Andrus S, Sinclair I N, Hopkins B E, Schwartz L, Aldridge H E, Plokker H W T, Mast E G, Rickards A, Knudtson M L, Sigwart L, Dear W E, Ferguson J J, Angelini P, Leatherman L L, Safian R D, Jenkins R D, Douglas J S, King III S B (1990) Percutaneous coronary laser balloon angioplasty: initial results of a multicenter experience. *J Am Coll Cardiol* 16:293–303

16. Serruys P W, Strauss B H, Beatt K J, Bertrand M E, Puel J, Rickards A F, Meier B, Goy J-J, Vogt P, Kappenberger L, Sigwart U (1991) Angiographic follow-up after placement of a self-expanding coronary artery stent. *N Engl J Med* 324:13–17

17. Shaknovich A, Teirstein P S, Stratienko A A, Walker C M, Cleman M W, Schatz R A (1991) Restenosis in single Palmaz-Schatz™ coronary stents: effects of prior PTCA and interval to prior PTCA. *J Am Coll Cardiol* 17:269A

18. Fajadet J C, Marco J, Cassagneau B G, Roberts G P, Vandormael M, Jordan C G, Flores M, Laurent J P G (1991) Restenosis following successful Palmaz-Schatz intracoronary stent implantation. *J Am Coll Cardiol* 17:346A

19. De Jaegere P, Serruys P W, van der Giessen W, de Feyter P (1992) Immediate and long-term morphologic changes in stenosis geometry after Wiktor stent implantation in native coronary arteries for recurrent stenosis following balloon angioplasty. Report on the first fifty consecutive patients. In: Serruys P, Strauss B, King S III (eds) *Restenosis in the Coronary Arteries Following Intervention with New Mechanical Devices*. Kluwer Academic Publishers, Dordrecht

20. Hearn J A, King S B III, Douglas J S Jr, Roubin G S (1992) Restenosis after Gianturco-Roubin stent placement for acute closure. In: Serruys P, Strauss B, King S III (eds) *Restenosis in the Coronary Arteries Following Intervention with New Mechanical Devices*. Kluwer Academic Publishers, Dordrecht

21. Rab S T, King S B III, Roubin G S, Carlin S, Hearn J A, Douglas J S Jr (1991) Coronary aneurysms after stent placement: a suggestion of altered vessel wall healing in the presence of anti-inflammatory agents. *J Am Coll Cardiol* 18: 1524–1528